# Clinical Animal Medicine

# Clinical Animal Medicine

Editor: Gerardo Bailey

www.callistoreference.com

**Callisto Reference,**
118-35 Queens Blvd., Suite 400,
Forest Hills, NY 11375, USA

Visit us on the World Wide Web at:
www.callistoreference.com

ISBN: 978-1-63239-973-1 (Hardback)

**Cataloging-in-Publication Data**

Clinical animal medicine / edited by Gerardo Bailey.
     p. cm.
Includes bibliographical references and index.
ISBN 978-1-63239-973-1
1. Veterinary medicine. 2. Animal health. 3. Animals--Diseases. 4. Clinical medicine. I. Bailey, Gerardo.
SF745 .C55 2018
636.089--dc23

# Table of Contents

VI Contents

**Permissions**

**List of Contributors**

**Index**

# Preface

Over the recent decade, advancements and applications have progressed exponentially. This has led to the increased interest in this field and projects are being conducted to enhance knowledge. The main objective of this book is to present some of the critical challenges and provide insights into possible solutions. This book will answer the varied questions that arise in the field and also provide an increased scope for furthering studies.

Veterinary medicine refers to the field of medicine dealing with the treatment of illnesses found in animals. It is an essential area of study as it includes curing diseases like rabies, kidney disease, fleas, bone diseases, parvovirus, heartworm, etc. which are dangerous for animals. The book is an amalgamation of concepts and case studies that will provide readers with complete information about the field. This book attempts to assist those with a goal of delving into the field of veterinary medicine. It includes detailed information about the subject and its related branches. The topics covered in this extensive book deal with the core subjects of veterinary medicine. This text is a vital tool for all researching and studying this field.

I hope that this book, with its visionary approach, will be a valuable addition and will promote interest among readers. Each of the authors has provided their extraordinary competence in their specific fields by providing different perspectives as they come from diverse nations and regions. I thank them for their contributions.

**Editor**

# Histomorphologic and Immunohistochemical Characterization of a Cardiac Purkinjeoma in a Bearded Seal (*Erignathus barbatus*)

G. Krafsur,[1,2] E. J. Ehrhart,[1] J. Ramos-Vara,[3] G. Mason,[1] F. Sarren,[2]
B. Adams,[2] C. Hanns,[2] T. Spraker,[1] and C. Duncan[1,4]

[1] CSU Veterinary Diagnostic Medicine Center, Fort Collins, CO, USA
[2] North Slope Borough Department of Wildlife Management, Barrow, AK, USA
[3] Indiana Animal Disease Diagnostic Laboratory and Department of Comparative Pathobiology, Purdue University, West Lafayette, IN, USA
[4] Colorado State University Veterinary Diagnostic Laboratory, 300 West Drake Avenue, Fort Collins, CO 80526, USA

Correspondence should be addressed to C. Duncan; colleen.duncan@colostate.edu

Academic Editor: Luciano Espino López

The most common cardiac tumors of heart muscle are rhabdomyomas, solitary or multiple benign tumors of striated muscle origin. While cardiac rhabdomyomas are well described in human medical literature, limited information depicting the occurrence of cardiac rhabdomyomas in veterinary species exists. A case of multiple firm white nonencapsulated nodules in the heart of a bearded seal is described. Microscopic findings included cytoplasmic vacuolization with formation of spider cells, glycogen vacuoles, and striated myofibrils. These cells expressed immunoreactivity for neuron-specific enolase and protein gene product 9.5, a marker for neuronal tissue and Purkinje fiber cells. Immunoreactivity for protein gene product 9.5 along with other microscopic findings substantiates Purkinje fiber cell origin of the cardiac rhabdomyoma in the bearded seal and use of the term *purkinjeoma* to describe this lesion.

## 1. Introduction

Rhabdomyomas, benign tumors of striated muscle origin, most commonly occur in the heart and are the most frequently diagnosed primary cardiac tumor of infants and children [1–3]. Multiple cardiac rhabdomyomas are frequently indicative of tuberous sclerosis, an autosomal dominant condition with an array of clinical manifestations, most notably seizures, cognitive deficits, behavioral disturbances, and adenoma sebaceum [1, 3]. Additional lesions associated with tuberous sclerosis include cortical hamartomas, giant cell astrocytomas, pulmonary lymphangiomyomatosis, and renal angiomyolipomas [3]. Cardiac rhabdomyomas may be clinically silent with spontaneous regression in utero or during early childhood being the norm [1–3]. In veterinary medicine,

cardiac rhabdomyomas are most commonly identified as incidental lesions in domesticated pigs [4–6] with rare occurrence documented in sheep [4], dogs [7, 8], and deer [9]. The occurrence of cardiac rhabdomyomas in pigs appears to be breed associated, with a higher incidence of the tumors occurring in red wattle and red wattle- crossbred piglets while similar cardiac rhabdomyomas were rare in other pig breeds submitted to the same diagnostic laboratory [9].

The typical macroscopic appearance of cardiac rhabdomyomas is white to tan, single or multiple, and nodular nonencapsulated masses most commonly occurring in the left ventricular wall and to a lesser extent in the right ventricle, right atrium, interventricular septum, and the main pulmonary artery [2]. Tumor nodules are composed of pleomorphic, vacuolated cells with or without glycogen

[4]. Postmortem glycolysis with delayed formalin fixation or routine histologic processing with subsequent removal of glycogen results in the distinctive appearance of spider cells with a central nucleus suspended in a network of cross striated myofibrils; however positive periodic acid-Schiff (PAS) staining confirms glycogen content [4].

Additional phosphotungsten acid-hematoxylin staining (PTAH) permits enhanced visualization of myofibrils with cross striations [4, 6, 9]. Large nuclei with stippled chromatin, prominent nucleoli, and binucleate cells are observed. Mitotic figures are usually not appreciated [6–9].

The nature and histogenesis of cardiac rhabdomyomas remains unclear. Cardiac rhabdomyomas exhibit immunore-activity with myoglobin, desmin, vimentin, neuron-specific enolase (NSE), human natural killer cell-1(HNK-1/Leu-7), and atrial natriuretic peptide (ANP) markers, similar to normal cardiomyocytes [5, 10]. Protein gene product 9.5 (PGP 9.5), also known as ubiquitin carboxyl-terminal hydrolase-1, is frequently expressed by neuronal cells and serves as a reliable marker for Purkinje fiber cells [10]. Immunoreactivity for PGP 9.5 has been demonstrated in porcine cardiac rhab-domyomas, supporting Purkinje fiber cell origins of cardiac rhabdomyomas [5]. This report describes multiple cardiac rhabdomyomas in a bearded seal (*Erignathus barbatus*) with gross, histopathological, and immunohistochemical (IHC) findings similar to those seen in cardiac rhabdomyomas in other species and supportive of Purkinje fiber cell origin.

## 2. Case Presentation

In July 2010, as part of a long term collaborative study between Iñupiat eskimo subsistence hunters and The North Slope Borough Department of Wildlife Management, abdominal and thoracic viscera from a one-year-old female bearded seal were submitted for gross examination and diagnostic sampling. Greater than 15 discrete nodular masses ranging in size from 0.5 to 2.0 cm were present in all four chambers of the heart (Figure 1) none of which protruded into the lumen. No gross changes related to heart failure were appreciated in the heart, lungs, liver, or spleen. The pale white, variably sized nonencapsulated masses were smooth, firm, and homogenous. The masses were well demarcated from adjacent normal cardiovascular stroma and did not bulge on cut surface. Representative tissue samples from the heart, skin, thyroid and adrenal gland, lymph node, skeletal muscle, ovary, lung, spleen, liver, pancreas, stomach, and intestine were fixed in 10% buffered formalin, routinely processed, and stained with H&E, PAS, PTAH, desmin, and vimentin. To detect neuronal and Purkinje fiber cell markers, immunohistochemistry (IHC) was performed with standard indirect technique utilizing a secondary antibody conjugated to a HRP labeled polymer (DakoEnVision+, Dakocytomation) and DAB chromogen with hematoxylin counterstain. Primary antibodies used were PGP 9.5 rabbit polyclonal antibody (Z5116, Dako, Carpinteria) at 1:50 dilution and NSE mouse monoclonal antibody (M0873 clone BBS/NC/VI-H14, Dako) at 1:200 dilution and 60 min room temperature incubation. Antigen retrieval using a decloaker chamber with

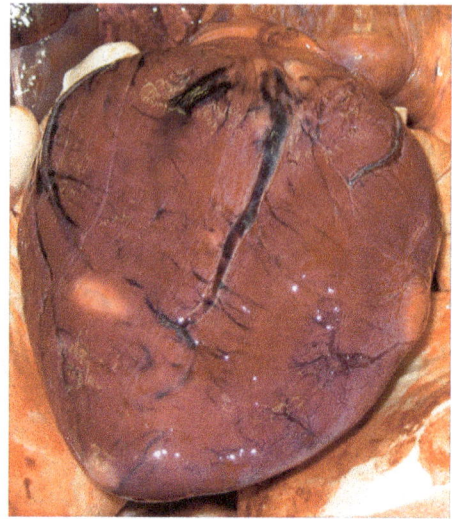

FIGURE 1: Heart; bearded seal. Multiple pale white discrete nodular masses expand the cardiac muscle (purkinjeomas).

pH 7.6 citrate buffer for NSE staining was performed prior to antibody incubation.

Histologically, the masses were nonencapsulated and variably demarcated from normal myocardium but occasionally infiltrated between cardiomyocytes as streaming bundles. Cells were polygonal with inconspicuous borders and had abundant eosinophilic cytoplasm which contained variably sized vacuoles (Figure 2). Some vacuolated cells exhibited a "spider cell" appearance characterized by a central cytoplasmic mass containing the nucleus suspended in a network of striated myofibrils (Figure 2, arrow). The nuclei were round to oval with clumped chromatin and prominent nucleoli. Anisocytosis, anisokaryosis, and occasional binucleate cells were present. Mitotic figures were not appreciated. A small focus of lymphoplasmacytic infiltration was observed in one of the masses. Neoplastic cells had PAS positive material within cytoplasmic vacuoles and within cytoplasmic projections (Figure 3); adjacent normal cardiomyocytes were PAS negative. Distinct striated myofibrils were present in PTAH stained sections of normal cardiomyocytes, but infrequent in neoplastic cells (Figure 4). Both the atypical cells and the adjacent normal myocardial cells stained similarly for desmin and vimentin. Moderate, diffuse cytoplasmic expression for PGP9.5 was present in some of the tumor cells while expression in adjacent normal cardiomyocytes was weak to absent (Figure 5). Immunoreactivity for neuron-specific enolase (NSE) was rare in the atypical cells (Figure 6).

Additional histologic lesions also present in this animal were incidental changes commonly seen in hunter harvested animals of this species (G. Krafsur, T. Spraker, unpublished personal observations) including mild exertional rhabdomyolysis with rare myositis, pulmonary nematodiasis characterized by *Parafilaroides* spp. in the alveolar spaces and airways, and occasional lymphoplasmacytic infiltrates throughout the hepatic parenchyma most likely associated with migration tracts of *Orthosplanchnus arcticus*.

Histomorphologic and Immunohistochemical Characterization of a Cardiac Purkinjeoma in a Bearded Seal...

3

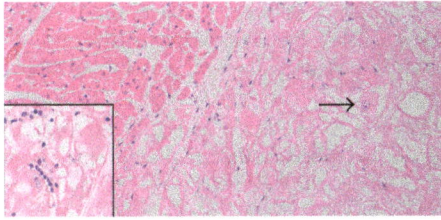

FIGURE 2: Heart; bearded seal. Neoplastic cells are large and vacuolated and occasional spider cells are also observed (arrow) and rare foci of lymphocytes are present (insert). H&E.

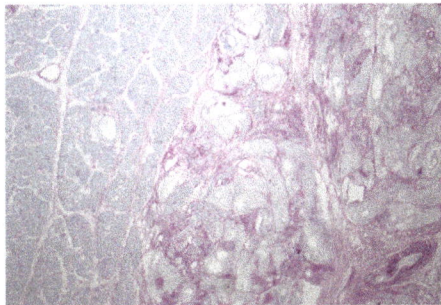

FIGURE 3: Heart; bearded seal. PAS positive granular material consistent with glycogen is present in the cytoplasm of neoplastic but not normal myocardium. PAS.

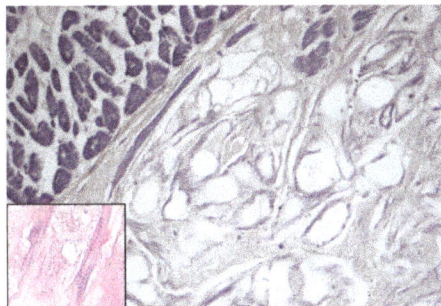

FIGURE 4: Heart; bearded seal. Normal myocardium and some rhabdomyoma cells are positive for PTAH. Striations (insert) are more common in normal cardiomyocytes but are occasionally observed in neoplastic cells. PTAH.

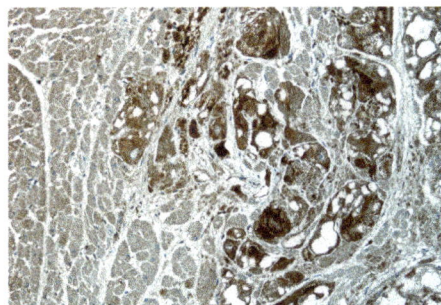

FIGURE 5: Heart; bearded seal. Neoplastic cells are moderately immunoreactive for protein gene product 9.5.

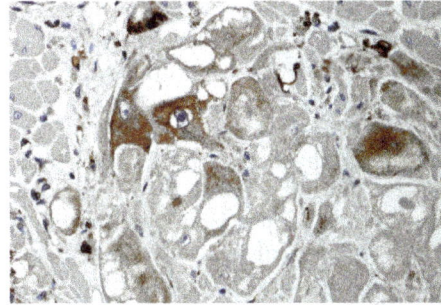

FIGURE 6: Heart; bearded seal. Neoplastic cells exhibit weak cytoplasmic staining for neuron-specific enolase.

## 3. Discussion

Limited scientific literature exists describing the incidence of cardiac rhabdomyomas in veterinary species. The veterinary literature contains only two cases describing clinical manifestations associated with cardiac rhabdomyomas including agonal convulsions with sudden death in a captive fallow deer and chylopericardium and right-sided congestive heart failure in a Staffordshire Bull Terrier that were consistent with cardiac failure likely from outflow obstruction and conduction disturbances [7, 9]. While the presence of multiple variably sized cardiac rhabdomyomas in the bearded seal heart did not appear to cause overt signs of heart failure, the numerous lesions in all four chambers of the heart may have resulted in aberrations of impulse conduction or subclinical arrhythmias.

Considerable debate exists regarding the nature and histogenesis of cardiac rhabdomyomas. Ultrastructural studies and the use of markers such as NSE and PGP 9.5 have been used to gain insight regarding the cells of origin and whether they derive from striated myocardium or Purkinje fiber cells. Purkinje fibers, located in the subendocardial and ventricular myocardium, are the conducting fibers of the heart that permit coordinated contraction of the ventricles. Purkinje fibers are neither neurons nor nerve cells but rather specialized myocytes arranged in aggregates or fibers. Larger than cardiomyocytes, Purkinje fibers are not contractile and lack a sarcoplasmic reticulum, $t$-tubules, and intercalated discs, features typical of cardiomyocytes [2]. The microscopic appearance of Purkinje fiber cells is different from cardiomyocytes; Purkinje fiber cells are larger, with scant myofibrils, and abundant glycogen resulting in less intense eosin staining than adjacent myocardium [2, 4]. The histogenesis of cardiac rhabdomyomas is complicated with ultrastructural characteristics indicative of both cardiomyocyte and Purkinje fiber cell origins reported in studies of human cardiac rhabdomyomas [2]. Intercalated discs, specialized cell-cell attachments between adjacent cardiomyocytes, were identified in one of the rhabdomyomas while desmosomal attachments, typical for Purkinje fiber cells, were visualized in the remaining two rhabdomyomas [2]. Microscopically, nodules from the bearded seal cardiac rhabdomyomas were composed of a preponderance of large, polygonal vacuolated cells with a paucity of striated myofibrils, characteristic features of

Purkinje fiber cells. PAS stains did demonstrate the presence of a granular material consistent with glycogen suggesting the rhabdomyoma cells are of a Purkinje fiber cell origin. Sparsely distributed myofibrils were appreciated within the vacuolated cells from identical sections of PTAH stained bearded seal cardiac rhabdomyoma cells. The myofibrils were microscopically indistinguishable from those in adjacent normal myocardium. The paucity of cross striations in PTAH stained sections of bearded seal cardiac rhabdomyoma cells offers further evidence that these cells derive from Purkinje-fiber cells. Studies investigating cardiac innervation and the conduction system of the fetal and adult camelid heart have shown that PGP 9.5 is a reliable marker for the identification of Purkinje fiber cells [10]. These findings along with strong PGP 9.5 immunoreactivity appreciated in swine cardiac rhabdomyomas support the use of PGP 9.5 as a reliable marker for the identification of Purkinje fiber cells [5, 10].

This report provides the first description of multiple cardiac rhabdomyomas in a bearded seal. The enlarged pleomorphic vacuolated spider cells, glycogen positive staining, limited striated myofibrils, and immunoreactivity for Purkinje fiber markers NSE and PGP 9.5 strongly characterize the Purkinje fiber origin of these cardiac rhabdomyomas and support the use of *purkinjeoma* as a descriptor for this tumor.

## Conflict of Interests

The authors declare that there is no conflict of interests regarding the publication of this paper.

## Acknowledgments

G. Krafsur wishes to thank Jill-Marie Seymour and Sara Carroll, graduate students from the University of Alaska-Fairbanks School of Fisheries and Ocean Sciences, for their assistance with the collection of tissues. Thanks are due to Lara Horstmann-Dehn, professor in the School of Fisheries and Ocean Science at the University of Alaska-Fairbanks, for her expertise in aging the bearded seal. Thanks are due to Barrow subsistence hunter Felton Sarren for allowing the lead investigator to examine and collect tissues from the subsistence harvested bearded seal. Finally, the authors are deeply indebted to Billy Adams and the rest of the scientists and staff at the North Slope Borough Department of Wildlife Management for their technical assistance and generous financial support of this work. Financial support for the costs associated with tissue processing and slide preparation was provided by the North Slope Borough Department of Wildlife Management, Barrow, Alaska.

## References

[1] A. Nir, A. J. Tajik, W. K. Freeman et al., "Tuberous sclerosis and cardiac rhabdomyoma," *The American Journal of Cardiology*, vol. 76, no. 5, pp. 419–421, 1995.

[2] J. F. Silverman, S. Kay, C. M. McCue, R. R. Lower, A. J. Brough, and C. H. Chang, "Rhabdomyoma of the heart: ultrastructural study of three cases," *Laboratory Investigation*, vol. 35, no. 6, pp. 596–606, 1976.

[3] D. M. Weiner, D. H. Ewalt, E. S. Roach, and T. W. Hensle, "The tuberous sclerosis complex: a comprehensive review," *Journal of the American College of Surgeons*, vol. 187, no. 5, pp. 548–561, 1998.

[4] R. Bradley, G. A. H. Wells, and J. B. R. Arbuckle, "Ovine and porcine so-called cardiac rhabdomyoma (Hamartoma)," *Journal of Comparative Pathology*, vol. 90, no. 4, pp. 551–558, 1980.

[5] B. Jacobsen, M. Kreutzer, D. Meemken, W. Baumgärtner, and C. Herden, "Proposing the term purkinjeoma: protein gene product 9.5 expression in 2 porcine cardiac rhabdomyomas indicates possible purkinje fiber cell origin," *Veterinary Pathology*, vol. 47, no. 4, pp. 738–740, 2010.

[6] B. J. McEwen, "Congenital cardiac rhabdomyomas in red wattle pigs," *Canadian Veterinary Journal*, vol. 35, no. 1, pp. 48–49, 1994.

[7] C. S. Mansfield, J. J. Callanan, and H. McAllister, "Intra-atrial rhabdomyoma causing chylopericardium and right-sided congestive heart failure in a dog," *Veterinary Record*, vol. 147, no. 10, pp. 264–267, 2000.

[8] Z. A. Radi and A. Metz, "Canine cardiac rhabdomyoma," *Toxicologic Pathology*, vol. 37, no. 3, pp. 348–350, 2009.

[9] C. Kolly, A. Bidaut, and N. Robert, "Cardiac rhabdomyoma in a juvenile fallow deer (Dama dama)," *Journal of Wildlife Diseases*, vol. 40, no. 3, pp. 603–606, 2004.

[10] A. A. El Sharaby, M. Egerbacher, A. K. Hammoda, and P. Böck, "Immunohistochemical demonstration of Leu-7 (HNK-1), Neurone-Specific Enolase (NSE) and Protein-Gene Peptide (PGP) 9.5 in the developing camel (*Camelus dromedarius*) heart," *Anatomia, Histologia, Embryologia*, vol. 30, no. 6, pp. 321–325, 2001.

# Unilateral Subconjunctival and Retrobulbar Hemorrhage Secondary to Brodifacoum Toxicity in a Dog

## Sonia E. Kuhn and Diane V. H. Hendrix

*Department of Small Animal Clinical Sciences, College of Veterinary Medicine, University of Tennessee, 2407 River Drive, Knoxville, TN 37996, USA*

Correspondence should be addressed to Sonia E. Kuhn; skuhn3@utk.edu

Academic Editors: A. F. Koutinas and J. S. Munday

An 8-year-old spayed female mixed-breed dog was presented for an acute onset of bleeding around the left eye. Mild exophthalmos and massive subconjunctival hemorrhage on the globe and nictitating membrane were present in the left eye. Retrobulbar hemorrhage was suspected, and pain was implied on opening of the mouth because the patient resisted and vocalized. No other abnormalities were found on ophthalmic or physical examination. Further questioning of the owner confirmed potential brodifacoum ingestion, and prothrombin time and partial thromboplastin time were both markedly elevated. Treatment with oral vitamin $K_1$ was implemented, and the subconjunctival hemorrhage was significantly improved within a few days of instituting treatment. All clinical signs of coagulopathy were completely resolved within 4 weeks of presentation. Coagulopathy secondary to brodifacoum ingestion can manifest as severe unilateral bulbar and nictitating membrane subconjunctival hemorrhage and exophthalmos due to retrobulbar hemorrhage without other clinical signs.

## 1. Introduction

Intraocular and periocular bleeding can occur with primary disease of the globe and adnexa or as manifestations of systemic disease. Clinical signs are hyphema and hemorrhage of nearly any aspect of the eye, including the uvea, vitreous, retina, subretinal space, conjunctiva, subconjunctival, and retrobulbar space. Periocular and intraocular hemorrhages are most commonly associated with uveitis or retinal detachment [1] caused by infectious diseases, including systemic fungal [2] and rickettsial diseases [3–5]; immune-mediated diseases such as uveodermatologic syndrome [6]; bleeding and vascular disorders such as hypertension [7, 8], thrombocytopenia [9, 10], anemia [11] and coagulopathy [1]; neoplasia [1, 12]; diabetes mellitus [13]; and hyperviscosity syndrome from multiple myeloma [8, 14] and polycythemia vera [8]. Additionally, persistent hyperplastic primary vitreous [15], retinal dysplasia, preiridal fibrovascular membrane formation [16], and blunt or penetrating trauma [1, 17] can also cause intraocular hemorrhage. Retrobulbar hemorrhage occurs because of trauma or coagulopathy and can cause exophthalmos [18–21].

Conjunctival or scleral hemorrhage in dogs usually occurs focally as petechiae from a primary hemostatic disorder, which is typically due to thrombocytopenia. Although subconjunctival hemorrhage is uncommon, it can occur secondary to coagulopathy, trauma, and vasculitis [21]. It has also been reported to occur with Rocky Mountain spotted fever [3] and scleral rupture [17]. The aim of this report is to describe an atypical presentation of brodifacoum rodenticide toxicity where the only clinical signs were unilateral subconjunctival and retrobulbar hemorrhages.

## 2. Case Presentation

An 8-year-old spayed female mixed-breed dog was presented for an acute onset of bleeding around the left eye. The bleeding began 6 hours prior to presentation and was progressively worsening. The dog had been alone in a fenced yard for most of the day. Her activity level was appropriate, and thirst and appetite were normal. No known trauma had occurred. Prior medical history was unremarkable. The dog had been sprayed by a skunk (*Mephitis mephitis*) 2 weeks prior to presentation but did not seem to suffer any ill effects from that incident. Appropriate vaccinations were current, and she was not receiving any medication aside from heartworm and flea prophylaxis.

On ophthalmic examination, direct and consensual pupillary light responses were normal in both eyes (OU). A menace response was present OU, and the dog exhibited behavior consistent with vision bilaterally. The Schirmer tear test 1 (Schirmer tear test strips, Merck Animal Health) showed normal tear production in the right eye (OD) at 19 mm/min and was not evaluated in the left eye (OS) due to the bleeding (reference range > 15 mm/min). A drop of 0.5% proparacaine hydrochloride ophthalmic solution (Alcaine, Alcon Laboratories) was applied topically OU, and applanation tonometry (Tono-Pen Vet, Reichert, Inc.) was performed. Intraocular pressure was 15 mmHg OU (reference range 6–24 mmHg) [22]. Massive hemorrhage was present beneath the bulbar conjunctiva for 360° around the left globe as well as beneath the palpebral and bulbar conjunctiva of the nictitating membrane OS (Figure 1(a)). Mild serosanguinous discharge was also present OS. The left globe was mildly exophthalmic (Figure 1(b)), and retropulsion seemed to cause moderate pain. The left eyelids were mildly swollen, and palpation of the left bony orbit was unremarkable. Slit-lamp biomicroscopy (Kowa SL-15, Kowa) and indirect ophthalmoscopy (20 D handheld lens, Volk Optical Inc.; Vantage Plus Wireless Headset, Keeler Instruments Inc.) were performed OU. Examination of the left and right anterior and posterior segments were unremarkable aside from prominent suture tip opacities in the lens OD. Nuclear sclerosis was noted OU. No evidence of bleeding was detected in or around the right eye.

The only abnormality found on physical examination was pain on opening of the mouth, as the patient resisted and vocalized during this maneuver. Temperature, pulse, and respiratory rate were within normal limits. The patient was bright, alert, and responsive. The mucous membranes were pink with a capillary refill time of <2 seconds. Thoracic auscultation and abdominal palpation were unremarkable. Neither petechiae nor ecchymoses were found, and no evidence of trauma was present.

Initial differential diagnoses for the subconjunctival hemorrhage OS were coagulopathy and trauma. Upon further questioning of the owner, it was confirmed that brodifacoum rodenticide (d-CON rat and mice bait pellets, Reckitt Benckiser) had been placed in the yard occupied by the dog 10 days prior to presentation. Prothrombin time (PT) and partial thromboplastin time (PTT) were tested. The PT was prolonged beyond quantification (reference range 6.8–8.7 seconds), and PTT was markedly prolonged at 146.5 seconds (reference range 14.5–25.6 seconds). A complete blood count, including platelet estimation, was within normal limits. Total protein and hematocrit were both normal at 7.0 g/dL (reference range 5.7–7.9 g/dL) and 55.7% (reference range 41–60%), respectively. Pleural fluid was not seen on thoracic ultrasound, and a small amount of free abdominal fluid was seen around the bladder on abdominal ultrasound. This fluid was presumed to be blood, but abdominocentesis for confirmation was not performed due to the coagulopathy.

The patient was admitted to the hospital for overnight monitoring and treatment. A subcutaneous injection of 93 mg (5 mg/kg) vitamin K$_1$ was given at admission and was repeated 12 hours later. Oral treatment with 25 mg (1.3 mg/kg) of vitamin K$_1$ twice daily was then instituted for 4 weeks. The left eye was lubricated with artificial tears ophthalmic ointment (15% mineral oil with 83% white petrolatum, Rugby Laboratories) four times daily to prevent exposure keratitis secondary to exophthalmos and lagophthalmos from nictitating membrane and eyelid swelling. Exercise restriction to prevent additional bleeding was also instituted.

Two days later, PT and PTT were within normal limits at 7.7 seconds and 17.8 seconds, respectively. The subconjunctival hemorrhage and eyelid swelling OS were markedly improved (Figure 2(a)). Artificial tears ointment was discontinued since the globe was no longer exophthalmic. The Schirmer tear test 1 was within normal limits OU at 15 mm/min OD and 21 mm/min OS. Applanation tonometry showed normal intraocular pressures OU of 8 mmHg OD and 10 mmHg OS. Examination of the anterior segment and fundus was unchanged OU.

The patient was reevaluated 1 month after initial presentation. Oral vitamin K$_1$ had been discontinued 2 days prior to examination. The PT was within normal limits at 7.4 seconds, and PTT was slightly prolonged at 26.4 seconds. The subconjunctival and periocular hemorrhage OS was fully resolved (Figure 2(b)). Examination of the anterior and posterior segments was unchanged OU from the initial presentation. Oral vitamin K$_1$ therapy was not reinstituted since the coagulopathy had resolved. Communication with the owner 3 months later revealed the dog to be completely asymptomatic and free of any remaining detectable abnormalities.

## 3. Discussion

Ocular lesions have been documented with anticoagulant rodenticide exposure but are rarely mentioned in texts that discuss clinical signs of this toxicity. This may be because ocular lesions are uncommon relative to other signs, or because they are usually mild in comparison to the more life-threatening hemorrhage that typically occurs, such as hemothorax. Hyphema as well as scleral and subconjunctival hemorrhage has been previously reported with anticoagulant rodenticides [1, 21, 23–25]. The previously reported scleral hemorrhage may have been referring to subconjunctival hemorrhage, though photographs of the lesions were not provided [23, 26]. Concurrent exophthalmos or suspected retrobulbar hemorrhage was not mentioned in those cases where scleral hemorrhage was noted, and one of the cases had other obvious concurrent clinical signs of coagulopathy [26]. In one retrospective study evaluating clinical signs of coagulopathy due to anticoagulant rodenticide, scleral hemorrhage was an uncommon finding that was seen in only 3 of 52 cases [23]. Whether this hemorrhage occurred with or without other clinical signs of coagulopathy was not discussed.

Massive subconjunctival hemorrhage of the nictitating membrane has not been previously documented as a clinical

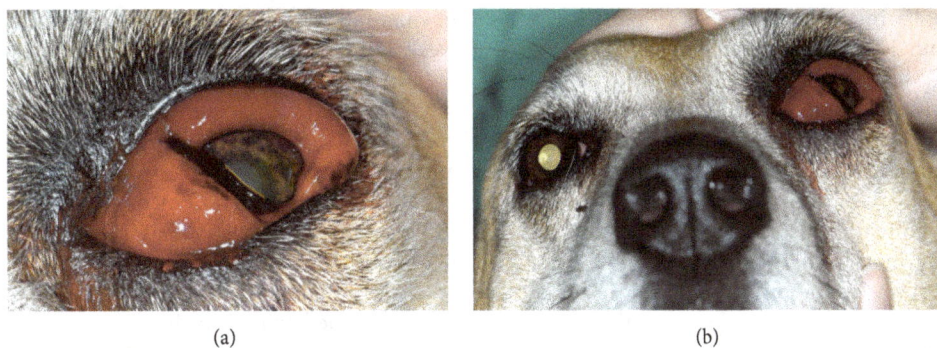

FIGURE 1: At initial presentation, severe subconjunctival hemorrhage of the globe, and nictitating membrane were present around the left eye. Mild exophthalmos, frank bleeding, and serosanguinous discharge were also seen. These were the only clinical signs of coagulopathy secondary to brodifacoum ingestion.

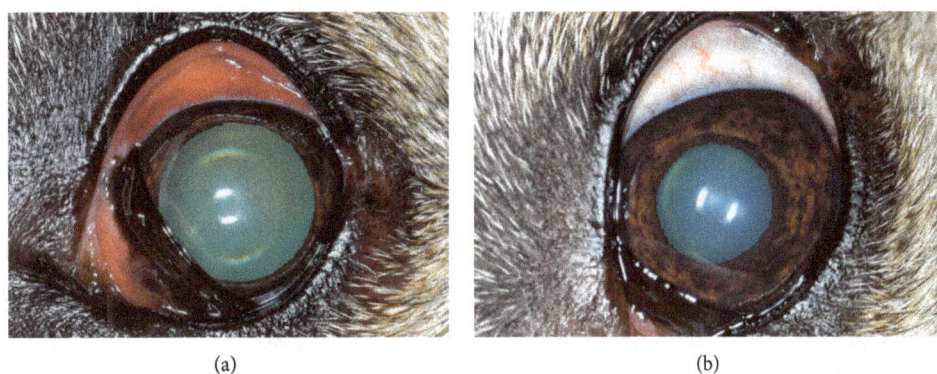

FIGURE 2: (a) Two days after therapy with oral vitamin $K_1$, the exophthalmos was resolved and the subconjunctival hemorrhage greatly improved. (b) The subconjunctival hemorrhage was resolved after treatment with oral vitamin $K_1$ for 4 weeks.

sign of anticoagulant rodenticide toxicity, though exophthalmos secondary to retrobulbar hemorrhage is known to occur [19–21]. Retrobulbar hematoma secondary to warfarin toxicity has also been reported to cause exophthalmos in humans [27]. Other causes of acquired coagulopathy that could cause subconjunctival or retrobulbar hemorrhage in dogs are severe liver disease; vasculitis; autoimmune disease directed against a coagulation factor; disseminated intravascular coagulation (DIC); anticoagulant therapy; or low levels of vitamin K secondary to obstructive hepatopathy, malabsorption, or low dietary vitamin K [21, 28, 29].

Bleeding disorders can be classified as diseases that affect fibrinolysis, primary hemostasis, and secondary hemostasis. Fibrinolysis is responsible for fibrin clot dissolution and depends on the conversion of plasminogen to plasmin [29]. Clot dissolution forms fibrin degradation products, which subsequently are removed from circulation by the liver. Accumulation of these products causes bleeding tendencies by interfering with platelet function and thrombin inhibition [29]. Primary hemostasis seals injured blood vessels with the creation of the primary hemostatic plug via the interactions of platelets and endothelium. Platelet or endothelial diseases, such as thrombocytopenia, thrombocytopathia, and vasculopathies, cause primary hemostatic disorders [29].

Secondary hemostasis has traditionally been defined using a cascade model where the intrinsic and extrinsic enzymatic pathways converge into a common pathway that results in the conversion of fibrinogen to fibrin [29]. The fibrin produced by secondary hemostasis solidifies the primary hemostatic plug. Factors VIII, IX, XI, and XII are involved in the intrinsic pathway, while tissue factor and factor VII constitute the extrinsic pathway. The common pathway involves factor X and the conversion of prothrombin to thrombin (factor II), which ultimately leads to the cleavage of fibrin from fibrinogen. While PT evaluates the extrinsic and common pathways, PTT evaluates the intrinsic and common pathways. More recently, coagulation has been described with a cell-based model, which explains *in vivo* deficiencies seen with the cascade model [30]. The cell-based model views coagulation as occurring in distinct yet overlapping phases rather than separate enzymatic pathways [30]. It also accounts for the role of cell surfaces in fibrin formation as well as the additional functions of coagulation proteins beyond the coagulation cascade [30]. The liver produces most of the coagulation factors necessary for secondary hemostasis [29]. Factors II, VII, IX, and X are known as vitamin K-dependent coagulation factors since they contain glutamyl residues that must be activated with carboxylation, which requires reduced vitamin $K_1$ as a cofactor [28, 31]. These glutamyl residues allow for binding of the coagulation protein to a cell membrane surface via calcium binding, and calcium binding cannot occur unless carboxylation occurs [30].

Carboxylation results in the oxidation of vitamin $K_1$, and the enzyme vitamin $K_1$ epoxide reductase is necessary to reduce vitamin $K_1$ back to its active form so that it can be recycled to activate additional coagulation factors [28]. Disorders of secondary hemostasis are due to decreased concentrations of or ineffective coagulation factors and result in coagulopathies.

Anticoagulant rodenticides, as described in this case, cause coagulopathy by depletion of vitamin K-dependent coagulation factors via inhibition of vitamin $K_1$ epoxide reductase [20, 31]. Warfarin and pindone are first-generation anticoagulants, while brodifacoum, bromadiolone, and diphacinone are second-generation anticoagulants [31]. The second-generation anticoagulants have longer half-lives, less drug-acquired resistance, and increased potency [20, 31, 32]. Clinical signs of coagulopathy secondary to brodifacoum manifest 2 to 5 days after ingestion and vary based on the location and severity of the hemorrhage [20, 29, 31]. The most common are dyspnea, lethargy, coughing, hemoptysis, pale mucous membranes, and tachycardia [23, 24]. Bleeding typically occurs into body cavities causing hemothorax, hemoabdomen, and retroperitoneal hemorrhage [20, 23]. Less frequent signs are melena, hematochezia, prolonged bleeding at injection sites, epistaxis, gingival bleeding, and neurologic signs [23, 24]. Case reports of atypical presentations of coagulopathy due to anticoagulant rodenticide include lameness from hemarthrosis [33], pericardial effusion [34], hematometra [35], hydronephrosis secondary to blood clots in the urinary bladder [36], tracheal obstruction [37], and submucosal gastric hemorrhage [38].

The earliest laboratory abnormality detected after second-generation anticoagulant rodenticide toxicity is elevation of the proteins induced by vitamin K absence or antagonism [31]. Prolongation of PT occurs within 36–72 hours of ingestion and precedes prolongation of PTT because of the short half-life of factor VII [20, 29]. Neither PTT nor activated clotting time is prolonged until greater than 72 hours after ingestion [20]. Decontamination of the patient is not indicated after signs of coagulopathy have developed since the toxin was consumed several days before examination. Patients with severe hemorrhage and subsequent anemia may require transfusions of whole blood or fresh frozen plasma to provide red bloods cells and coagulation factors to halt bleeding. Oral vitamin $K_1$ at 1.25–2.5 mg/kg twice daily for 4 weeks is needed to resolve coagulopathy caused by second-generation anticoagulants [31]. Therapy is needed for only 2 weeks for first-generation anticoagulants and for 3 weeks with bromadiolone since these agents are shorter acting [20]. Absorption of oral vitamin $K_1$ is improved if given with a fatty meal [20]. A subcutaneous loading dose of 2.5–3.3 mg/kg of vitamin $K_1$ is recommended by some clinicians and discouraged by others [19, 20, 31, 39, 40]. Injections can cause additional bleeding and hematoma formation and are not more bioavailable than the oral formulation [19]. Intravenous administration is not recommended due to the risk of anaphylaxis [39]. Treatment should be discontinued for 2 days before repeated testing of PT to ensure that the patient is able to produce active coagulation factors without supplementation. If PT is still prolonged after discontinuation

of vitamin $K_1$, then supplementation is continued for another week and the patient is then retested [20].

This case is an unusual presentation of coagulopathy secondary to brodifacoum ingestion in that unilateral subconjunctival and retrobulbar hemorrhages were the only apparent clinical signs. Subconjunctival hemorrhage can occur because of scleral or conjunctival bleeding, or anterior migration of retrobulbar blood [21, 25]. Retrobulbar hemorrhage was presumed because of the exophthalmos and severe subconjunctival hemorrhage OS, though this was not confirmed with imaging or sample collection. While fresh frozen plasma is usually indicated for patients with active bleeding, it was not administered in this case since no other significant detectable body cavity effusion had occurred at the time of diagnosis and the patient was not anemic. Anemia is present in the majority of coagulopathic dogs after rodenticide ingestion and can be seen in 83% of cases [24]. Monitoring was continued for the first 24 hours of vitamin $K_1$ therapy so that fresh frozen plasma could have been administered if necessary. This patient had complete resolution of all clinical signs with oral vitamin $K_1$ supplementation, and no permanent adverse effects occurred to the globe or periocular structures OS. The mild prolongation of PTT seen in this patient at the conclusion of vitamin $K_1$ therapy was not indicative of an unresolved coagulopathy since the PT was normal. Mild elevations of PTT are often clinically insignificant, and PT is a more sensitive indicator of coagulopathy secondary to vitamin K deficiency [29].

As with other reports of atypical presentations of coagulopathy secondary to anticoagulant rodenticide ingestion, this case further reinforces that patients with this syndrome can present with bleeding in nearly any location. Prognosis is excellent as long as a prompt diagnosis is made and proper treatment instituted. An incorrect initial diagnosis occurs in up to 25% of cases of coagulopathy due to anticoagulant rodenticide toxicity, which can be life threatening because treatment is delayed and hemorrhage continues [24]. Patient history can also be misleading, as owners denied pet exposure to anticoagulant rodenticide in over 50% of confirmed cases in one study [41]. The massive unilateral subconjunctival hemorrhage in this case allowed for rapid diagnosis of the patient's coagulopathy before more serious bleeding and anemia occurred. In summary, anticoagulant rodenticides should be strongly considered in cases of unilateral subconjunctival hemorrhage of the globe and nictitating membrane or when retrobulbar hemorrhage is suspected.

## References

[1] A. Trbolova, "Hyphema in dogs: 91 cases," *Veterinary Ophthalmology*, vol. 12, no. 1, pp. 61–70, 2009.

[2] K. N. Gelatt, L. D. McGill, and V. Perman, "Ocular and systemic cryptococcosis in a dog," *Journal of the American Veterinary Medical Association*, vol. 162, no. 5, pp. 370–375, 1973.

[3] M. G. Davidson, E. B. Breitschwerdt, M. P. Nasisse, and S. M. Roberts, "Ocular manifestations of Rocky Mountain spotted fever in dogs," *Journal of the American Veterinary Medical Association*, vol. 194, no. 6, pp. 777–781, 1989.

[4] A. A. Komnenou, M. E. Mylonakis, V. Kouti et al., "Ocular manifestations of natural canine monocytic ehrlichiosis (*Ehrlichia canis*): a retrospective study of 90 cases," *Veterinary Ophthalmology*, vol. 10, no. 3, pp. 137–142, 2007.

[5] J. F. Wilson, "*Ehrlichia platys* in a Michigan dog," *Journal of the American Animal Hospital Association*, vol. 28, pp. 381–383, 1992.

[6] J. L. Laus, M. G. Sousa, V. P. Cabral, F. V. Mamede, and M. Tinucci-Costa, "Uveodermatologic syndrome in a Brazilian Fila dog," *Veterinary Ophthalmology*, vol. 7, no. 3, pp. 193–196, 2004.

[7] N. L. LeBlanc, R. L. Stepien, and E. Bentley, "Ocular lesions associated with systemic hypertension in dogs: 65 cases (2005–2007)," *Journal of the American Veterinary Medical Association*, vol. 238, no. 7, pp. 915–921, 2011.

[8] I. F. Lane, S. M. Roberts, and M. R. Lappin, "Ocular manifestations of vascular disease: hypertension, hyperviscosity and hyperlipidemia," *Journal of the American Animal Hospital Association*, vol. 29, no. 1, pp. 28–36, 1993.

[9] S. K. O'Marra, A. M. Delaforcade, and S. P. Shaw, "Treatment and predictors of outcome in dogs with immune-mediated thrombocytopenia," *Journal of the American Veterinary Medical Association*, vol. 238, no. 3, pp. 346–352, 2011.

[10] I. Aubert, M. Carrier, M. Desnoyers, and L. Breton, "A case of bilateral hyphema secondary to an immune-mediated thrombocytopenia in a dog," *Medecin Veterinaire Du Quebec*, vol. 27, no. 3, pp. 103–108, 1997.

[11] C. L. Cullen and A. A. Webb, "Ocular manifestations of systemic diseases part 1: the dog," in *Veterinary Ophthalmology*, K. N. Gelatt, Ed., pp. 1470–1537, Blackwell, Ames, Iowa, USA, 4th edition, 2004.

[12] S. G. Krohne, N. M. Henderson, R. C. Richardson, and W. A. Vestre, "Prevalence of ocular involvement in dogs with multicentric lymphoma: prospective evaluation of 94 cases," *Veterinary and Comparative Ophthalmology*, vol. 4, pp. 127–135, 1994.

[13] M. P. Landry, I. P. Herring, and D. L. Panciera, "Funduscopic findings following cataract extraction by means of phacoemulsification in diabetic dogs: 52 cases (1993–2003)," *Journal of the American Veterinary Medical Association*, vol. 225, no. 5, pp. 709–716, 2004.

[14] D. V. H. Hendrix, K. N. Gelatt, P. J. Smith, D. E. Brooks, C. J. G. Whittaker, and N. T. Chmielewski, "Ophthalmic disease as the presenting complaint in five dogs with multiple myeloma," *Journal of the American Animal Hospital Association*, vol. 34, no. 2, pp. 121–128, 1998.

[15] A. Bayón, M. C. Tovar, M. J. Fernández Del Palacio, and A. Agut, "Ocular complications of persistent hyperplastic primary vitreous in three dogs," *Veterinary Ophthalmology*, vol. 4, no. 1, pp. 35–40, 2001.

[16] B. H. Grahn and R. L. Peiffer, "Fundamentals of veterinary ophthalmic pathology," in *Veterinary Ophthalmology*, K. N. Gelatt, Ed., pp. 355–437, Blackwell, Ames, Iowa, USA, 4th edition, 2004.

[17] A. Rampazzo, C. Eule, S. Speier, P. Grest, and B. Spiess, "Scleral rupture in dogs, cats, and horses," *Veterinary Ophthalmology*, vol. 9, no. 3, pp. 149–155, 2006.

[18] B. M. Spiess, "Diseases and surgery of the canine orbit," in *Veterinary Ophthalmology*, K. N. Gelatt, Ed., pp. 539–562, Blackwell, Ames, Iowa, USA, 4th edition, 2004.

[19] C. Means, "Anticoagulant rodenticide toxicosis," in *Clinical Veterinary Advisor Dogs and Cats*, E. Coté, Ed., pp. 76–77, Mosby, St. Louis, Mo, USA, 1st edition, 2007.

[20] C. DeClementi and B. R. Sobczak, "Common rodenticide toxicoses in small animals," *Veterinary Clinics of North America Small Animal Practice*, vol. 42, pp. 349–360, 2012.

[21] C. L. Martin, "Conjunctiva and third eyelid," in *Ophthalmic Disease in Veterinary Medicine*, C. L. Martin, Ed., pp. 183–218, Manson, London, UK, 1st edition, 2005.

[22] H. E. Klein, S. G. Krohne, G. E. Moore, A. S. Mohamed, and J. Stiles, "Effect of eyelid manipulation and manual jugular compression on intraocular pressure measurement in dogs," *Journal of the American Veterinary Medical Association*, vol. 238, no. 10, pp. 1292–1295, 2011.

[23] B. Haines, "Anticoagulant rodenticide ingestion and toxicity: a retrospective study of 252 canine cases," *Australian Veterinary Practitioner*, vol. 38, no. 2, pp. 38–50, 2008.

[24] S. E. Sheafor and C. Guillermo Couto, "Anticoagulant rodenticide toxicity in 21 dogs," *Journal of the American Animal Hospital Association*, vol. 35, no. 1, pp. 38–46, 1999.

[25] C. L. Martin, "Ocular manifestations of systemic disease part 1 the dog," in *Veterinary Ophthalmology*, K. N. Gelatt, Ed., pp. 1401–1448, Lippincott Williams & Wilkins, Philadelphia, Pa, USA, 3rd edition, 1999.

[26] M. Schaer and C. Henderson, "Suspected warfarin toxicosis in a dog," *Journal of the American Veterinary Medical Association*, vol. 176, no. 6, pp. 535–536, 1980.

[27] D. Thompson, C. Stanescu, P. Pryor, and B. Laselle, "Retrobulbar hematoma from warfarin toxicity and the limitations of bedside ocular sonography," *Western Journal of Emergency Medicine*, vol. 11, no. 2, pp. 208–210, 2010.

[28] D. C. Baker, "Dgnosis of disorders of hemostasis," in *Veterinary Hematology and Clinical Chemistry*, M. A. Thrall, Ed., pp. 179–196, Blackwell, Ames, Iowa, USA, 2nd edition, 2006.

[29] S. G. Hackner, "Bleeding disorders," in *Small Animal Critical Care Medicine*, D. C. Silverstein and K. Hopper, Eds., pp. 507–514, Elsevier Saunders, St. Louis, Mo, USA, 1st edition, 2009.

[30] S. A. Smith, "The cell-based model of coagulation," *Journal of Veterinary Emergency and Critical Care*, vol. 19, no. 1, pp. 3–10, 2009.

[31] R. M. DuFort and L. Matros, "Acquired coagulopathies," in *Textbook of Veterinary Internal Medicine*, S. J. Ettinger and E. C. Feldman, Eds., pp. 1933–1937, Elsevier Saunders, St. Louis, Mo, USA, 6th edition, 2005.

[32] M. Lund, "Comparative effect of the three rodenticides warfarin, difenacoum and brodifacoum on eight rodent species in short feeding periods," *Journal of Hygiene*, vol. 87, no. 1, pp. 101–107, 1981.

[33] J. R. Bellah and J. P. Weigel, "Hemarthrosis secondary to suspected warfarin toxicosis in a dog," *Journal of the American Veterinary Medical Association*, vol. 182, no. 10, pp. 1126–1127, 1983.

[34] D. J. Petrus and A. Rosemary, "Pericardial effusion and cardiac tamponade secondary to brodifacoum toxicosis in a dog," *Journal of the American Veterinary Medical Association*, vol. 215, no. 5, pp. 647–648, 1999.

[35] S. L. Padgett, J. E. Stokes, R. L. Tucker, and L. G. Wheaton, "Hematometra secondary to anticoagulant rodenticide toxicity," *Journal of the American Animal Hospital Association*, vol. 34, no. 5, pp. 437–439, 1998.

[36] N. Hansen and C. Beck, "Bilateral hydronephrosis secondary to anticoagulant rodenticide intoxication in a dog," *Journal of Veterinary Emergency and Critical Care*, vol. 13, no. 2, pp. 103–107, 2003.

[37] T. L. Blocker and B. K. Roberts, "Acute tracheal obstruction associated with anticoagulant rodenticide intoxication in a dog," *Journal of Small Animal Practice*, vol. 40, no. 12, pp. 577–580, 1999.

[38] S. L. Marks, T. L. Gieger, and J. Williams, "Presumptive intramural gastric hemorrhage secondary to rodenticide intoxication in a dog," *Journal of Veterinary Emergency and Critical Care*, vol. 11, no. 1, pp. 27–31, 2001.

[39] A. J. Brown and L. S. Waddell, "Rodenticides," in *Small Animal Critical Care Medicine*, D. C. Silverstein and K. Hopper, Eds., pp. 346–350, Elsevier Saunders, St. Louis, Mo, USA, 1st edition, 2009.

[40] B. J. Woody, M. J. Murphy, A. C. Ray, and R. A. Green, "Coagulopathic effects and therapy of brodifacoum toxicosis in dogs," *Journal of Veterinary Internal Medicine*, vol. 6, no. 1, pp. 23–28, 1992.

[41] L. W. Tseng, R. H. Poppenga, and D. Hughes, "Anticoagulant rodenticide toxicity and serum anticoagulant rodenticide concentrations in 43 dogs (1997–2000)," in *Proceedings of the Seventh International Veterinary Emergency and Critical Care Symposium*, p. 798, 2000.

# Surgical Correction of Patellar Luxation in a Rabbit

## J. Riggs and S. J. Langley-Hobbs

*The Queen's Veterinary School Hospital, Department of Veterinary Medicine, University of Cambridge, Madingley Road, Cambridge CB3 0ES, UK*

Correspondence should be addressed to J. Riggs; jr393@cam.ac.uk

Academic Editors: C. M. Loiacono and S. Stuen

A two-and-a-half-year-old giant lop-eared rabbit, weighing 5.1 kg, presented with a one-month history of intermittent right hind limb lameness. The limb locked in extension during hopping. On examination, a grade-2 medial patellar luxation of the right hind was diagnosed, with associated stifle joint swelling. Radiographic findings of the right stifle comprised periarticular osteophyte formation consistent with mild degenerative joint disease and joint effusion. Surgical correction involving right trochlear wedge recession sulcoplasty and lateral imbrication was carried out to stabilise the patella in the trochlear groove. The right hind limb lameness resolved, and the patella was stable at a 6-month postoperative examination. One year postoperatively, the right patella was luxating again concurrent with bilateral stifle effusions. Euthanasia was performed twenty months after surgery due to recurrent lameness in the right hind limb.

## 1. Introduction

Patellar luxation is a common disorder of the stifle, predominantly affecting small-breed dogs [1] but increasingly prevalent in larger-breed dogs [2] and cats [3, 4]. Medial luxation is reported more commonly in young, small-breed dogs with developmental disease and in cats [3, 5]. Approximately 50% of medial patellar luxation cases in dogs display bilateral involvement [6]. Clinical signs vary, according to the severity of the anatomical derangements and the degree of luxation, from intermittent, nonpainful, "skipping" lameness, reluctance to jump, and crouched gait to severe lameness and skeletal deformities.

In contrast to patellar luxation in dogs and cats, there is a lack of the literature regarding this condition, and other developmental orthopaedic abnormalities, in the rabbit species. Unilateral (left) medial patellar luxation with degenerative joint disease of the stifle has been described in a 1-year-old rabbit, concurrent with a shortened left femur, a shallow trochlear groove, a rotated proximal left tibia, and a left hip subluxation [7]. As this rabbit was ambulatory and not apparently painful, no treatment was given. Another report described bilateral medial patellar luxation in a 5-month-old rabbit [8] resulting in impaired mobility, but conservative

management was elected. To the authors' knowledge, no reports of surgically corrected patellar luxation in the rabbit currently exist. This case report describes clinically significant patellar luxation in a pet rabbit in the UK and demonstrates the role of surgery in its management.

## 2. Case Presentation

A two-and-a-half-year-old, male neutered, lop-eared rabbit weighing 5.1 kg presented to the referring veterinarian with a one-month history of right hind limb lameness, reported to be acute in onset by the owners. The lameness was characterised as intermittent locking of the right hind limb in extension during normal hopping motion. The rabbit was deemed otherwise healthy. No gait abnormalities of the contralateral hind limb were noted, and the stance of the rabbit at rest was considered normal. Initial examination revealed right medial patellar luxation as the only orthopaedic abnormality. The rabbit underwent indoor cage rest for four weeks prior to being reexamined. Over this period, there had been no improvement in the lameness, and repeat clinical examination again revealed right medial patellar luxation, this time with significant soft-tissue swelling medial to the stifle joint.

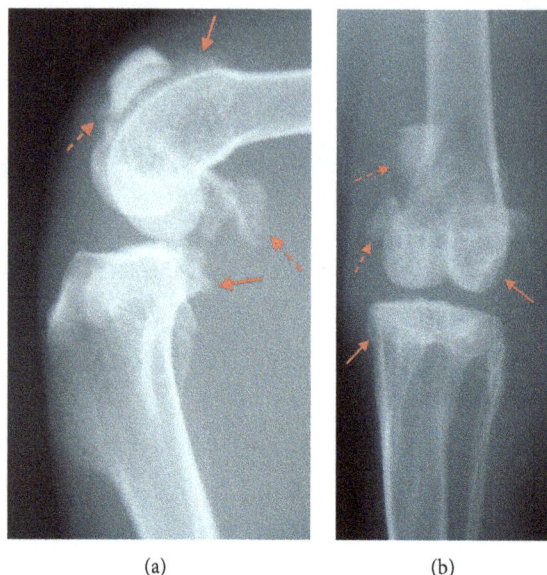

(a)                                                                      (b)

FIGURE 1: (a) Mediolateral view of the right stifle joint. Osteophytes (solid arrows) present on the trochlear ridge, femoral condyles, and tibial plateau and enthesophytes (dashed arrows) present on the fabellae and poles of the patella are likely secondary to medial patellar luxation. (b) Craniocaudal radiographic view of the right stifle, again demonstrating osteophytosis of the femoral condyles and tibial plateau (solid arrows), and enthesophytosis of the fabellae and patella (dashed arrows), along with medial patellar luxation. Reproduced from the BSAVA Manual of Rabbit Surgery, Dentistry and Imaging, edited by F. Harcourt-Brown and J. Chitty, with the permission of BSAVA Publications.

The rabbit was then referred to the Queen's Veterinary School Hospital for further investigation and treatment. On presentation, the patient was bright, alert, and in reasonable body condition, although poorly muscled around the hindquarters. Orthopaedic examination and manipulation of the stifle joint confirmed right medial patellar luxation, soft-tissue swelling particularly localised to the medial aspect of the joint, and a mild stifle joint effusion. The luxation was classified as grade-2 according to the clinical examination findings [9]. A grade-1 medial luxation of the left patella was elicited on left stifle extension; no lameness was associated with this finding.

Light preanaesthetic sedation was achieved with buprenorphine (20 μg/kg), and anaesthesia was induced with a combination of medetomidine (0.2 mg/kg) and ketamine (10 mg/kg), all injected intramuscularly. A 4 mm cuffed endotracheal tube was placed for delivery of oxygen and isoflurane to maintain anaesthesia following induction. A 22 G intravenous catheter was placed into the marginal ear vein for perioperative fluid therapy (lactated Ringer's solution at 10 mL/kg/hour), and for subsequent injections of meloxicam (0.1 mg/kg) and cefradine (15 mg/kg) each given once during surgery.

Standard radiographic views (mediolateral and craniocaudal) of both stifles were taken once the patient was anaesthetised. Radiographic findings included an increased soft-tissue opacity in the cranial compartment of the right stifle joint with loss of definition of the parapatellar fat pad, consistent with stifle joint effusion. Marked osteophytosis of the femoral trochlear ridge, femoral condyles, and tibial plateau and enthesophytosis of the fabellae and patellar poles were evident (Figures 1(a) and 1(b)). The patella was displaced medially (Figure 1(b)). The radiological diagnosis

was degenerative joint disease of the right stifle with medial patellar luxation. No radiographic abnormalities were seen in the left stifle (Figures 2(a) and 2(b)).

Manual manipulation of both stifle joints was performed in an attempt to elicit a cranial or caudal draw, indicative of concurrent cruciate ligament rupture. No craniocaudal instability was detected in either limb. Synoviocentesis of the right stifle joint with subsequent cytological examination demonstrated low cellularity of the synovial fluid; 95% of the nucleated cell population comprised mononuclear cells and 5% neutrophils. No bacteria were visualised. The sample was deemed normal synovial fluid [10].

In the absence of any other significant abnormalities, the rabbit's right hind limb lameness was considered to be due to the medial right patellar luxation. As the lameness had failed to improve with rest and conservative management, surgical therapy was initiated. A lateral parapatellar approach to the right stifle joint was made [11] with medial dislocation of the patella. Examination of the cruciate ligaments following arthrotomy confirmed these structures to be intact. Osteotomies were made using an X-acto saw (Veterinary Instrumentation) axial to each trochlear ridge to create a triangular-shaped osteochondral wedge, which was temporarily removed from the trochlea [12]. Two further osteotomies were then performed, parallel to the initial osteotomies, and a thin "V"-shaped piece of subchondral bone was removed. The osteochondral wedge was replaced, and the patella was repositioned in the groove. Lateral imbrication of the joint capsule was carried out using metric size-3 polydioxanone (PDS II, Ethicon) in an interrupted modified mayo mattress-suture pattern. The fascia lata was imbricated in a similar fashion prior to closure of the subcutaneous tissues using metric-2 poliglecaprone (Monocryl, Ethicon) in

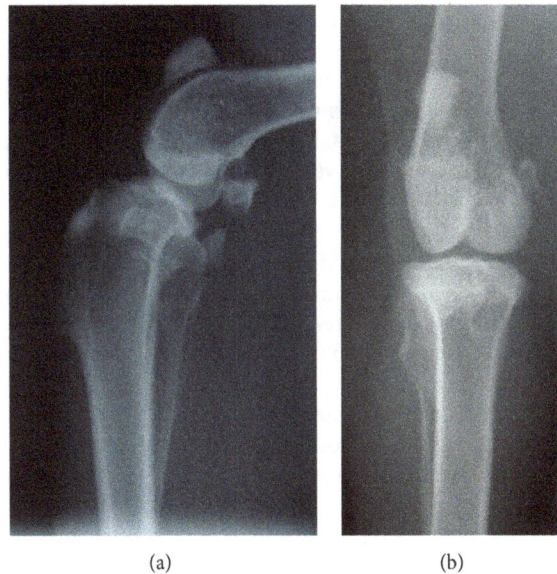

(a)          (b)

FIGURE 2: (a) Mediolateral view of the contralateral left stifle joint. (b) Craniocaudal radiographic view of the left stifle joint.

a simple continuous pattern. An intradermal suture layer, also using metric-2 poliglecaprone, was used to attain cutaneous apposition, and skin glue was applied to avoid the need for transcutaneous sutures. Postoperative radiographs were not taken because no surgical implants had been placed and due to the concern over the length of anaesthesia and associated hypothermia in this species.

The patient's blood glucose was monitored closely during the anaesthetic and in the recovery period, until the patient was eating well by himself. Whilst being hospitalised, analgesia was provided by administration of buprenorphine (20 μg/kg q8 hrs, IM) and meloxicam (0.1 mg/kg q24 hrs, PO). By twelve hours after surgery, the rabbit was starting to use the limb normally, the incision site looked good, and swelling was minimal. Whilst being hospitalised, the rabbit developed a muco-purulent left ocular discharge consistent with conjunctivitis. Ophthalmic examination also revealed bilateral cataract formation. Treatment with topical ketorolac and gentamicin was initiated at an eight-hour frequency and continued for five days. Forty-eight hours after admission, the rabbit was discharged from the hospital. Instructions were given to implement three weeks of cage rest at home and to continue with ten days of meloxicam (0.1 mg/kg q24 hrs, PO) for analgesia.

At a recheck appointment two days after surgery, the rabbit was using the limb well, and there was evidence of normal incisional healing. Three months later, the continued normal use of the limb was reported with no signs of recurrent lameness, leg locking, or reluxation. At six months following surgery the rabbit represented with right stifle swelling; examination confirmed the patella to be in place. One week later, left stifle swelling had also developed. An anti-inflammatory steroid injection was administered by the referring practice, and no further diagnostics pursued. One year following surgery, due to persistence of right stifle swelling, repeat examination of the rabbit was carried out—this time, patellar reluxation was detected. Further surgery

was declined. The patient was managed conservatively until the client elected for euthanasia twenty months after surgery due to recurrent lameness in the right hind limb.

## 3. Discussion

In this case report, wedge recession sulcoplasty for unilateral medial patellar luxation resulted in the resolution of clinical signs for six months following surgery. However, bilateral stifle swelling subsequently developed, and reluxation of the right patella was documented one year postoperatively.

Reluxation of the patella is a known complication of surgical correction in dogs, along with wound dehiscence, septic arthritis, impaired stifle extension, wedge migration, and degenerative joint disease [2, 13]. One study reported an 18% frequency of postoperative complications following surgical correction of patellar luxation in dogs, with an 8% frequency of reluxation [14]. Surgical correction was not attempted in a previous case report describing clinically significant patellar luxation in a rabbit [8] due to the authors' concerns about the possibility of recurrence. However, the frequency of reluxation following surgery was found to be lower in dogs weighing less than 20 kg compared with those of larger sizes, and when the sulcoplasty technique was employed [14], both of which suggest that this management modality may be indicated for the rabbit species. Whilst some authors [15, 16] advocate the use of soft-tissue reconstruction techniques alone in the treatment of grade-1 and -2 luxations, failing to overcome skeletal malformations through application of soft tissue reconstruction techniques in isolation is reported to be the main cause of poor surgical outcomes for patellar luxation in dogs [17]. Following application of the sulcoplasty technique in the rabbit reported herein, potential alternative reasons for ultimate failure of the surgical technique include inadequate depth of the groove created by osteotomy, the presence of an underlying congenital tibial alignment abnormality which was not overcome by sulcoplasty alone, and an underlying stifle condition causing joint capsule swelling.

The normal volume of synovial fluid in the rabbit stifle has been reported to be $100\,\mu L$ [18], and a grading system has been suggested for objective documentation of synovial fluid volume changes following the induction of degenerative joint disease in experimental rabbit models [18]. On initial presentation to the Queen's Veterinary School Hospital, the joint effusion would have been characterised as grade-1 (mild: fluid volume greater than normal but did not fill the stifle joint and did not pour out on arthrotomy). As the rabbit did not re-present to the Queen's Veterinary School Hospital following surgery, no accurate comment can be made on the subsequent joint effusion that developed, but the fact that it became apparent bilaterally and persisted over a six-month period would be suggestive of degenerative joint disease progression [19] or another stifle disease.

Whilst degenerative joint disease is not commonly reported in pet rabbits, which might be due to lack of observed clinical signs rather than lack of occurrence [20], this species has been used extensively as an experimental model for degenerative joint disease development and to assess response to different treatment options [18, 21–24]. Studies have shown that degenerative joint disease in this species is associated with synovial effusion, synovitis, capsular fibrosis, meniscal tears, medial collateral and posterior cruciate ligament damage, and osteophyte formation [18, 25]. Osteophyte formation as part of degenerative joint disease progression in experimental models of unilateral cruciate ligament transection has been shown to be rapid [25] occurring within two weeks of surgical intervention.

A significant degree of degenerative joint disease was present in the right stifle of the rabbit at the time of presentation to the Queen's Veterinary School Hospital, two months following the reported onset of clinical signs. Degenerative joint disease is a recognised sequela of patellar luxation [16, 26], and it is associated with augmented pain and lameness. The radiographic findings associated with patellar luxation-induced degenerative joint disease are usually mild [26] unless concurrent joint diseases are present. In the absence of other diagnosed orthopaedic conditions, it was therefore somewhat unusual that the rabbit in this case report had such marked radiographic changes consistent with degenerative joint disease after just two months of clinical signs.

Although surgical correction does not inhibit degenerative joint disease development [13, 26], by permitting normalisation of joint loading and range of motion it reduces lameness and improves mobility and thus should be undertaken early in the disease process. The presence of joint effusion at six months after surgery would suggest that the rate of degeneration was high in this rabbit in spite of patellar correction. Possible suggestions for this include synovial inflammation following arthrotomy, trochlear cartilage damage [13], presence of concurrent undiagnosed joint pathology prior to surgery, and subsequent injury incurred in the same joint following surgery. Patellar luxation has been suggested to be a risk factor for cranial cruciate ligament damage, through increased strain on the ligament brought about by abnormal forces acting across the stifle joint [26].

Interestingly, swelling was also noted in the left stifle joint approximately six months after presentation even though this limb was not affected by clinically significant patellar luxation. It is possible that bilateral cruciate ligament rupture could have occurred, either as a result of trauma or secondary to degenerative changes in the ligaments themselves [27, 28].

One predisposing factor for the development of patellar luxation in this rabbit may have been its giant-breed signalment. Studies have shown that large-breed dogs have an increased susceptibility to developmental skeletal deformities due to their increased growth rates and differential calcium metabolism compared with smaller-breed dogs [29]. One might postulate that a rapid growth rate, and/or inadequate nutrition during growth, may have resulted in skeletal weakness or deformity (coxa vara, genu vara, and medial rotation of the tibia, e.g.) due to abnormal loading of the limbs against open physes which may support a developmental aetiopathogenesis of patellar luxation in the rabbit, as suggested for the dog [16].

## 4. Conclusion

This case report highlights the clinical significance of medial patellar luxation as a cause of hind limb lameness in the rabbit. The exact cause of the condition is unknown. This report demonstrates the application of trochlear wedge recession sulcoplasty in the rabbit species, which was temporarily successful in alleviating clinical lameness for six months postoperatively. The reason for ultimate failure of the technique in this case is not known, but it may be related to the concurrent joint effusions. As the rabbit is now established as the UK's third most popular mammalian pet, and breeding is likely to be intensified to meet consumer demand, one can postulate that the prevalence of orthopaedic conditions, such as patellar luxation [16], is likely to increase. Consequently, further studies into the prevalence and aetiopathogenesis of patellar luxation in the rabbit are required, and surgical techniques need to be adapted and refined for use in this species.

## Conflict of Interests

The authors declare that they have no conflict of interests.

## References

[1] W. A. Priester, "Sex, size, and breed as risk factors in canine patellar dislocation," *Journal of the American Veterinary Medical Association*, vol. 160, no. 5, pp. 740–742, 1972.

[2] A. M. Remedios, A. W. Basher, C. L. Runyon, and C. L. Fries, "Medial patellar luxation in 16 large dogs. A retrospective study," *Veterinary Surgery*, vol. 21, no. 1, pp. 5–9, 1992.

[3] M. E. Johnson, "Feline patellar luxation: a retrospective case study," *Journal of the American Animal Hospital Association*, vol. 22, pp. 835–838, 1986.

[4] J. E. F. Houlton and S. E. Meynink, "Medial patellar luxation in the cat," *Journal of Small Animal Practice*, vol. 30, pp. 349–352, 1989.

[5] R. D. Horne, "Canine patellar luxation (a review)," *Veterinary Medicine, Small Animal Clinician*, vol. 66, no. 3, pp. 211–218, 1971.

[6] E. J. Trotter, "Medial patellar luxation in the dog," *Compendium on Continuing Education for the Practising Veterinarian*, vol. 2, article 58, 1980.

[7] R. Duran-Struuck, L. A. Colby, M. Rogers, K. D. Hankenson, T. R. Meier, and D. Rosenstein, "What is your diagnosis?" *Journal of the American Veterinary Medical Association*, vol. 232, no. 6, pp. 839–840, 2008.

[8] G. D. Araujo and C. Y. Kanayama, "Luxação de patela em coelho (*Oryctolagus cuniculus*)," *PubVet*, vol. 5, article 39, 2011.

[9] *Adapted from Putnam R. Patellar Luxation in the Dog*, University of Guelph, Ontario, Canada, 1968.

[10] T. W. Campbell and C. K. Ellis, "Comparative cytology," in *Avian and Exotic Animal Haematology and Cytology*, T. W. Campbell and C. K. Ellis, Eds., Blackwell, 3rd edition.

[11] D. L. Piermattei and K. A. Johnson, *An Atlas of Surgical Approaches to the Bones and Joints of the Dog and Cat*, Saunders, 4th edition, 2004.

[12] B. Slocum, D. B. Slocum, T. Devine, and E. Boone, "Wedge recession for treatment of recurrent luxation of the patella. A preliminary report," *Clinical Orthopaedics and Related Research*, vol. 164, pp. 48–53, 1982.

[13] R. G. Roy, L. J. Wallace, G. R. Johnston, and S. L. Wickstrom, "A retrospective evaluation of stifle osteoarthritis in dogs with bilateral medial patellar luxation and unilateral surgical repair," *Veterinary Surgery*, vol. 21, no. 6, pp. 475–479, 1992.

[14] G. I. Arthurs and S. J. Langley-Hobbs, "Complications associated with corrective surgery for patellar luxation in 109 dogs," *Veterinary Surgery*, vol. 35, no. 6, pp. 559–566, 2006.

[15] J. R. Campbell and M. J. Pond, "The canine stifle joint. II. Medical luxation of the patella. An assessment of lateral capsular overlap and more radical surgery," *Journal of Small Animal Practice*, vol. 13, no. 1, pp. 11–18, 1972.

[16] J. K. Roush, "Canine patellar luxation," *Veterinary Clinics of North America—Small Animal Practice*, vol. 23, no. 4, pp. 855–868, 1993.

[17] D. L. Piermattei and G. L. Flo, "The stifle joint," in *Handbook of Small Animal Orthopaedics and Fracture Repair*, W. O. Brinker, D. L. Piermattei, and G. L. Flo, Eds., pp. 516–580, WB Saunders, 3rd edition, 1997.

[18] D. Amiel, T. Toyoguchi, K. Kobayashi, K. Bowden, M. E. Amiel, and R. M. Healey, "Long-term effect of sodium hyaluronate (Hyalgan) on osteoarthritis progression in a rabbit model," *Osteoarthritis and Cartilage*, vol. 11, no. 9, pp. 636–643, 2003.

[19] S. Laverty, C. A. Girard, J. M. Williams, E. B. Hunziker, and K. P. H. Pritzker, "The OARSI histopathology initiative—recommendations for histological assessments of osteoarthritis in the rabbit," *Osteoarthritis & Cartilage*, vol. 18, supplement 3, pp. S53–S65, 2010.

[20] S. J. Langley-Hobbs and N. Harcourt-Brown, "Chapter 23: joint surgery," in *BSAVA Manual of Rabbit Imaging, Surgery and Dentistry*, F. Harcourt-Brown and J. Chitty, Eds., 2013.

[21] A. Hulth, L. Lindberg, and H. Telhag, "Experimental osteoarthritis in rabbits. Preliminary report," *Acta Orthopaedica Scandinavica*, vol. 41, no. 5, pp. 522–530, 1970.

[22] H. A. Barcelo, J. C. M. Wiemeyer, C. L. Sagasta, M. Macias, and J. C. Barreira, "Effect of S-adenosylmethionine on experimental osteoarthritis in rabbits," *American Journal of Medicine*, vol. 83, no. 5, pp. 55–59, 1987.

[23] G. Tiraloche, C. Girard, L. Chouinard et al., "Effect of oral glucosamine on cartilage degradation in a rabbit model of osteoarthritis," *Arthritis and Rheumatism*, vol. 52, no. 4, pp. 1118–1128, 2005.

[24] M. Saito, T. Sasho, S. Yamaguchi et al., "Angiogenic activity of subchondral bone during the progression of osteoarthritis in a rabbit anterior cruciate ligament transection model," *Osteoarthritis & Cartilage*, vol. 20, no. 12, pp. 1574–1582, 2012.

[25] M. Bouchgua, K. Alexander, M. d'Anjou et al., "Multimodality imaging of temporal changes in knee osteoarthritis lesions in an in vivo rabbit model," *Osteoarthritis & Cartilage*, vol. 15, p. 324, 2007.

[26] C. C. Willauer and P. B. Vasseur, "Clinical results of surgical correction of medial luxation of the patella in dogs," *Veterinary Surgery*, vol. 16, no. 1, pp. 31–36, 1987.

[27] M. A. van Zuijlen, P. W. F. Vrolijk, and M. A. G. van der Heyden, "Bilateral successive cranial cruciate ligament rupture treated by extracapsular stabilization surgery in a pet rabbit (*Oryctolagus cuniculus*)," *Journal of Exotic Pet Medicine*, vol. 19, no. 3, pp. 245–248, 2010.

[28] P. B. Vasseur, R. R. Pool, S. P. Arnoczky, and R. E. Lau, "Correlative biomechanical and histologic study of the cranial cruciate ligament in dogs," *American Journal of Veterinary Research*, vol. 46, no. 9, pp. 1842–1854, 1985.

[29] M. A. Tryfonidou, M. S. Holl, M. Vastenburg et al., "Hormonal regulation of calcium homeostasis in two breeds of dogs during growth at different rates," *Journal of Animal Science*, vol. 81, no. 6, pp. 1568–1580, 2003.

# 4

# Two Cases of Lacaziosis in Bottlenose Dolphins (*Tursiops truncatus*) in Japan

Keiichi Ueda,[1] Ayako Sano,[2] Jyoji Yamate,[3] Eiko Itano Nakagawa,[4] Mitsuru Kuwamura,[3] Takeshi Izawa,[3] Miyuu Tanaka,[3] Yuko Hasegawa,[3] Hiroji Chibana,[5] Yasuharu Izumisawa,[6] Hirokazu Miyahara,[1] and Senzo Uchida[1]

[1] *General Research Center, Okinawa Churaumi Aquarium, Aza Ishikawa 888, Motobu-Cho, Kunigami-Gun, Okinawa 905-0206, Japan*
[2] *Department of Animal Sciences, Faculty of Agriculture, University of the Ryukyus, Sembaru 1, Nishihara-Cho, Nakagusuku-Gun, Okinawa 903-0213, Japan*
[3] *Laboratory of Veterinary Pathology, Division of Veterinary Sciences, Rinku-Campus, Osaka Prefecture University, Rinku Ohrai Kita 1-58, Izumisano, Osaka 598-8531, Japan*
[4] *Department of Pathological Science, CCB, State University of Londrina, P.O. Box 6001, 86051-970 Londrina, PR, Brazil*
[5] *Medical Mycology Research Center, Chiba University, Inohana 1-8-1, Chiba 260-8673, Japan*
[6] *Department of Veterinary Medicine, Rakuno Gakuen University, Bunkyodai Midorimachi 582, Ebetu, Hokkaido 069-0836, Japan*

Correspondence should be addressed to Ayako Sano; aya_grimalkin@yahoo.co.jp

Academic Editors: J. Lakritz, F. Mutinelli, R. L. Santos, and S. Stuen

Lacaziosis, formerly called lobomycosis, caused by *Lacazia loboi*, is a zoonotic mycosis found in humans and dolphins and is endemic in the countries on the Atlantic Ocean. Although the Japanese coast is not considered an endemic area, photographic records of lacaziosis-like skin lesions were found in bottlenose dolphins (*Tursiops truncatus*) that were migrating in the Goto Islands (Nagasaki Prefecture, Japan). We diagnosed 2 cases of lacaziosis in bottlenose dolphins captured simultaneously at the same coast within Japanese territory on the basis of clinical characteristics, cytology, histopathology, immunological tests, and detection of partial sequences of a 43 kDa glycoprotein coding gene (*gp43*) with a nested-PCR system. The granulomatous skin lesions from the present cases were similar to those found in animals from endemic areas, containing multiple budding and chains of round yeast cells and positive in the immune-staining with anti-*Paracoccidioides brasiliensis* serum which is a fungal species related to *L. loboi*; however, the *gp43* gene sequences derived from the present cases showed 94.1% homology to *P. brasiliensis* and 84.1% to *L. loboi*. We confirmed that the causative agent at the present cases was different genotype of *L. loboi* from Amazon area.

## 1. Introduction

Lacaziosis is a granulomatous chronic skin infection caused by the fungus *Lacazia loboi* and is endemic in the Atlantic coastal waters of Latin American countries [1–3]. Interestingly, *L. loboi* is a sister taxon with a close phylogenetic relationship to *Paracoccidioides brasiliensis*, which is a highly pathogenic fungal species also endemic in Latin American countries [4]. The disease it causes, lacaziosis, is formerly known as Jorge Lobo's disease [5, 6] or lobomycosis until 2005 [7].

The characteristics of the disease are chronic keloidal skin lesions accompanied by pruritus, sensations of burning, and pain [2]. The hosts include humans and 3 species of dolphins: the bottlenose dolphin (*Tursiops truncatus*), the Indian Ocean bottlenose dolphin (*Tursiops aduncus*), and the estuarine dolphin, "costero" (*Sotalia guianensis*) [8]. Only one case of dolphin-to-human infection has been reported in a dolphin

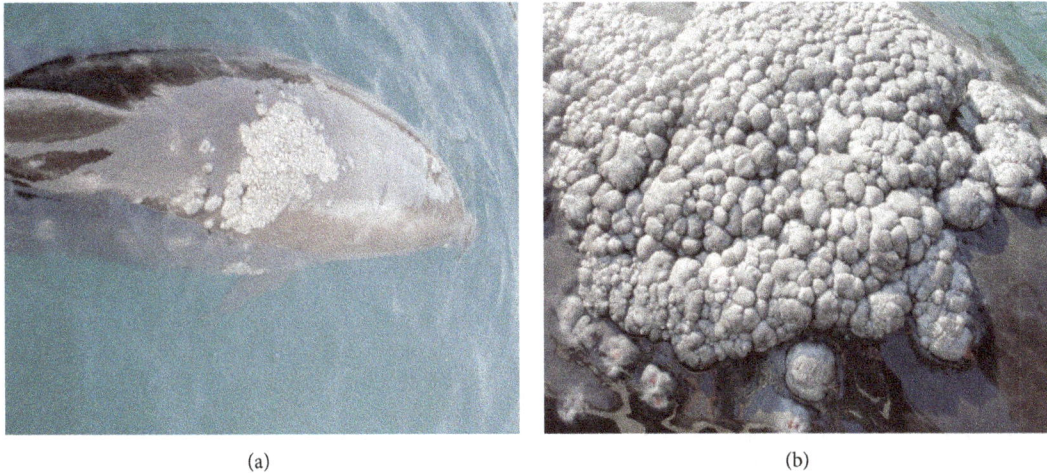

(a)                                                      (b)

FIGURE 1: The skin lesion (approximately 25 × 25 cm) in Case 1 in August 2010 (a, b).

trainer in The Netherlands who contacted the infected animal, suggesting that lacaziosis should be considered a zoonotic fungal infection [9, 10].

Lacaziosis is usually found at altitudes above 200 m in tropical, humid, or subtropical forests with an average temperature of 24°C and more than 2,000 mm of annual rainfall [1–3, 8]. The natural reservoir of *L. loboi* is unknown; however, its habitat is likely to be in rural environments on the basis of the observed distribution of the disease, and soil and vegetation seem to be probable sources of infection. Lacaziosis in dolphins suggests that some aquatic reservoir also exists [2, 3].

Human cases have been reported in Brazil, Costa Rica, Panama, Venezuela, Colombia, Guiana, Surinam, French Guiana, Ecuador, Peru, Bolivia, Honduras, and Mexico. Some cases have also been reported in the United States, but those patients thought to have been infected in Venezuela, Canada, The Netherlands, Surinam, France, South Africa [1–3, 8, 10], and Greece [11] bordering countries to the Atlantic Ocean. Interestingly, an unconfirmed case was reported from Bangladesh [12] which is not an endemic area.

On the other hand, cetacean cases have been reported in Brazil [13], Surinam [14], Florida and North Carolina (United States) [15–18], Mexico [19], the Bay of Biscay (Spain) [9], Spain in a dolphin that originated in Cuba [20], and Hawaii in a bottlenose dolphin transported from Florida [21]. Furthermore, lacaziosis-like cases have been observed in Indo-Pacific bottlenose dolphins in Mayotte waters located close to Madagascar, in the Indian Ocean [22], Venezuela, Colombia, Ecuador, Peru, Chile, Brazil [23], and in the Goto islands, Nagasaki Prefecture at the Kyushu area of the Japanese Sea [24]. Therefore, lacaziosis and lacaziosis-like diseases are endemic in the Atlantic, Pacific, and Indian Oceans [23]. According to Kiszka et al. [22], this lacaziosis-like disease is very similar to lobomycosis but lacks a histologic diagnosis [24]. Except for one case from Spain, most cases were diagnosed by photography and macroscopy without histopathologic, serologic, or molecular biological data [20].

The causative fungal species *L. loboi*, is difficult to culture except by animal passages [2, 3, 8, 10]. Therefore, the diagnosis of lacaziosis is based on clinical symptoms, histopathologic observations, and immunologic tests by cross-reaction to *Paracoccidioides brasiliensis*, a closely related fungal species of *Onygenales* [1–4, 7, 8, 10]. Furthermore, the diagnosis seems to be very difficult confirm outside of endemic areas, where no doctor or veterinarian would consider lacaziosis when they encountered chronic granulomatous keloidal skin lesions either in humans or dolphins.

The present study aims to establish a diagnosis in two cases of lacaziosis in bottlenose dolphins captured simultaneously on the same coast of Japan and cared for in individual aquariums, on the basis of clinical characteristics, cytology, histopathology, immunological testing, and detection of partial sequences of the 43 kDa glycoprotein coding gene (*gp43*) corresponding to those of *P. brasiliensis* [4, 7].

## 2. Cases

*2.1. Case 1.* A male bottlenose dolphin (*Tursiops truncatus*), estimated to be 17 years old, was captured in 2007 in a coastal area of Japan and cared for under outdoor conditions at an aquarium. The body weight and body length at the time of death were 280 kg and 303 cm, respectively.

The dolphin's testosterone level decreased to less than 1 ng/mL beginning in March 2010. The skin of the back of the dolphin became swollen in July 2010. In August 2010, the skin developed a cauliflower-like eczema approximately 20 × 25 cm in size (Figures 1(a) and 1(b)). The animal received antibiotics without effect. The blood $\beta$-glucan level was 22.4 pg/mL (>6 pg/mL is regarded as positive for fungal infection according to a commercial laboratory). The biopsied skin lesions contained yeast-like structures, as determined by a commercial pathology laboratory. The dolphin's condition was diagnosed as fungal infection, and terbinafine hydrochloride was administered orally at a dose of 2 mg/kg SID. However, no improvement was noted.

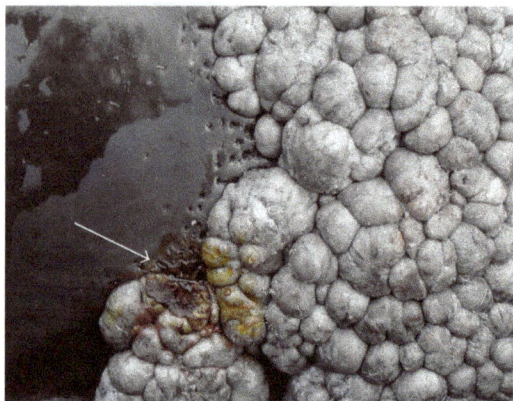

FIGURE 2: The margin of the skin lesion with abundant small fistulae appeared in November 2010. The arrow indicates the biopsy site.

In October 2010, the lesion had expanded, and pain was detected by palpation. Administration of fluconazole orally at a dose of 800 mg (2.7 mg/kg) was initiated; however, no effect was seen. The animal's body temperature was elevated slightly at 37°C or more. According to Hampton et al., the deep body temperature normally ranges from 37°C to 37.5°C during the active time; however, temperatures decrease during sleeping and after feeding times [25].

In November 2010, the body temperature decreased (35°C), and the number of blood white cells increased to 33,000 cells/$\mu$L, while the normal number varies from 5,000 to 9,000/$\mu$L in captive dolphins [26]. The size of the lesion was approximately 30 × 35 cm. There were abundant small fistulae at the margin of the lesion (Figure 2). The biopsy was also done. The lesion had a topical temperature of approximately 40°C, as detected by thermography (Figure 3(a)). The echo image of the lesion suggested that the invasion was limited to the subcutaneous connective tissue and did not extend to the muscle (Figure 3(b)). Round or multiple budding yeast cells consisting of a spherical to piriform mother cell (4~12 $\mu$m in diameter) with some small daughter cells (less than 0.5~6 $\mu$m mm in diameter) connected by a narrow base (less than 0.5 $\mu$m in width and 0.5 $\mu$m in length) were detected in the smear of the biopsied skin samples of the dermis stained with Giemsa, periodic acid-Schiff reaction (PAS), and Gomori methenamine method (GMS) (Figures 4(a)–4(c)).

On 19 December 2010, the animal showed a spontaneous increased respiratory ratio indicating lower vital signs. We speculated that the dolphin was suffering from sepsis and tried to administrate fluid replacement; however, there was no response. By the next day, the animal had died.

Purulent pneumonia and hepatic failure were detected at the autopsy. *Staphylococcus aureus* and *Morganella morganii* were isolated both from the lung and the blood. We concluded that the cause of the death was sepsis. In addition, the autopsied skin samples cultured on potato dextrose agar (Difco potato dextrose agar, Becton, Dickinson and Company Japan, Tokyo, Japan) supplemented with 100 mg/L of chloramphenicol and Mycosel agar (BBL Mycosel agar, Becton, Dickinson and Company Japan) plates at 25 and 35°C for 4 weeks produced negative results.

Abundant yeast-like cells were detected in the skin lesions stained with hematoxylin and eosin, PAS, and GMS (Figures 5(a)–5(c)). Most of the yeast cells appeared as chains, while multiple budding yeast cells connected by narrow bases to the mother cells were also detected.

For immunohistochemistry, sections from skin lesions were incubated with a rabbit polyclonal antibody against *P. brasiliensis* which is a related species to *L. loboi* for 16 hrs at 4°C. The bounded antibodies were detected with horse radish peroxidase conjugated to anti-rabbit secondary antibody (Histofine Simple Stain MAXPO; Nichirei, Tokyo, Japan) and 3,3′-diaminobenzidine tetrahydrochloride (DAB, Vector Laboratories Inc., Burlingame, CA, USA) as chromogen. The yeast cells reacted positively to immune-staining by anti-*P. brasiliensis* rabbit serum (Figure 5(d)).

The serum obtained at death showed a slight precipitation line in the immunodiffusion test against a fungal cell antigen of *P. brasiliensis* detected by macroscopical observation on a slit lighting system.

Detection of the 43 kDa glycoprotein coding gene (*gp43*) with reference to the sequences of *P. brasiliensis*, *P. lutzii*, and *L. loboi* was tried because of adequate sequence data in the GenBank database and its high homology [7].

The biopsied or paraffin-embedded specimens were examined. The fresh samples were fixed with 70% ethanol at least overnight, cut into approximately 5 × 5 × 5 cm$^3$ sized pieces, and placed into a 1.5 mL sized sterile microtube. The samples were washed 3 times with sterile water by centrifugation at 13,201 g for 5 min, 0.5 mL of DEXPAT (TaKaRa, Otsu, Japan) solution for DNA elution was added, and they were heated at 100°C for 10 min. Then the microtubes containing the tissue samples and DNA eluting solution were cooled on ice and centrifuged at 13,201 g for 10 min. The supernatant was collected and stored as a crude DNA solution. For paraffin-embedded tissue samples, 3 sections of 10 $\mu$m thick paraffin-embedded tissues were placed into micro tubes (1.5 mL), and 0.5 mL of DEXPAT solution was added. After being boiled for 10 min., the tubes were centrifuged at 13,201 g for 10 min, and the supernatants were stored as crude DNA solutions. After being purified by an ethanol precipitation method, the DNA solutions were processed to amplify *gp43* using a primer set for *gp43* of *P. brasiliensis* [27]. It is because that both *P. brasiliensis* and *L. loboi* are closely related fungal species [7] and showed higher homology in the gene sequences [4].

We placed 2.5 $\mu$L of the sample, 2.5 $\mu$L of 20 pM primers MAE (5′-TGCTGCGGCGGGGTTAAACCATGTC-3′) and ATO (5′-GTTGTGGTATGTGTCGATGTAGACG-3′) [27], and 17.5 $\mu$L of distilled water in a 0.2 mL PCR tube with one Ready-to-Go bead (Amersham Pharmacia, Tokyo, Japan). The reaction mixture was subjected to 1 cycle of denaturation at 95°C for 4 min, 40 cycles of amplification at 94°C for 1 min, 50°C for 1.5 min, 72°C for 2 min, and then a final extension step at 72°C for 10 min in a PCR Thermal Cycler MP (TaKaRa, Otsu, Japan). For amplification in the second-round PCR, the first PCR product was processed by the ethanol precipitation method, and the same PCR reaction was repeated.

The PCR products were approximately 550-base pair sized bands amplified from both fresh and paraffin-embedded tissue samples. The sequences were determined by

(a)  (b)

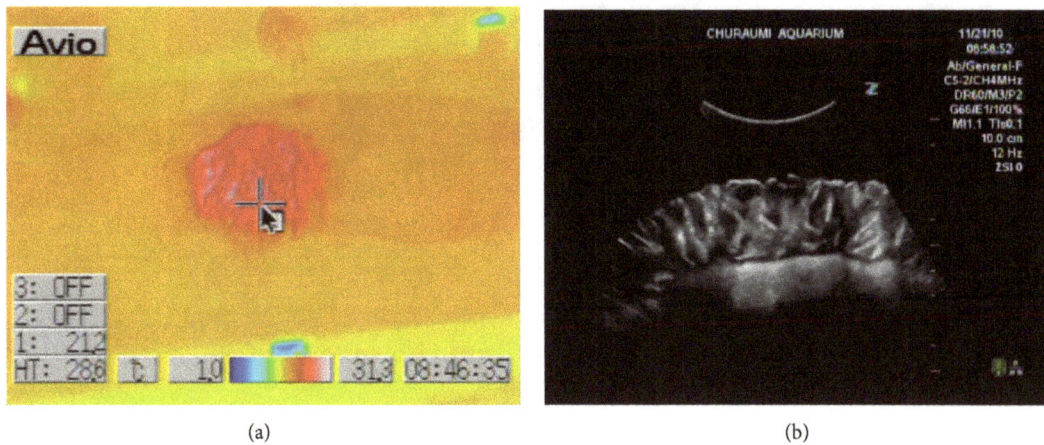

FIGURE 3: A topical temperature of approximately 40°C (arrow) was determined by a thermographic image of the lesion (a), and the depth of invasion was detected by an echo system (b).

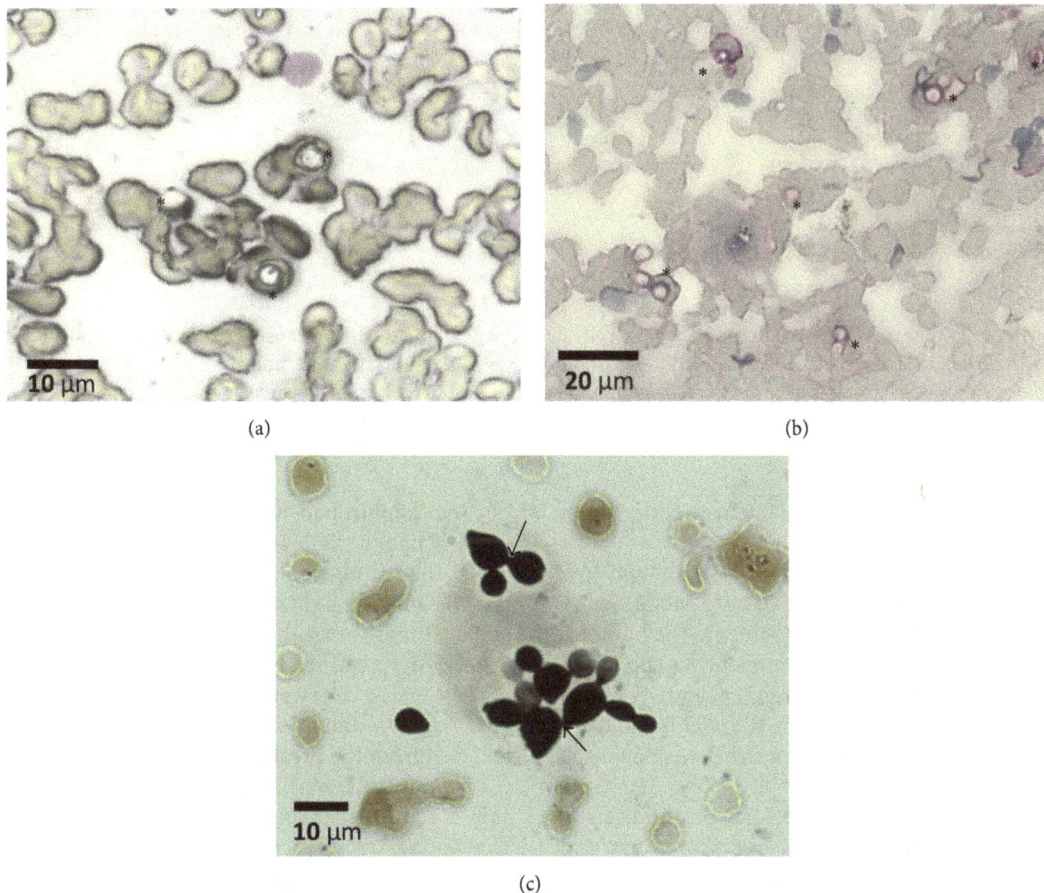

(a)  (b)

(c)

FIGURE 4: Spherical yeast cells (∗) stained with Giemsa (×200, (a)), with PAS (×200, (b)), and spherical to piriform mother cells with some small daughter cells connected by a narrow base (arrows) stained with GMS (×400, (c)).

a direct sequencing method using ABI PRISM 3100 sequencer (Applied Biosystems) labeled with the primers MAE and ATO [28]. DNA sequences were aligned with the GENETEX-MAC genetic information processing software (Software Development Co., Ltd., Tokyo, Japan). The reliable sequence comprised 471 bases obtained from the paraffin-embedded tissue sample; however, the biopsied sample failed to confirm the sequence. The accession numbers of this sequence were registered as AB811031 in the GenBank database. The sequence was localized in the cluster containing P. brasiliensis,

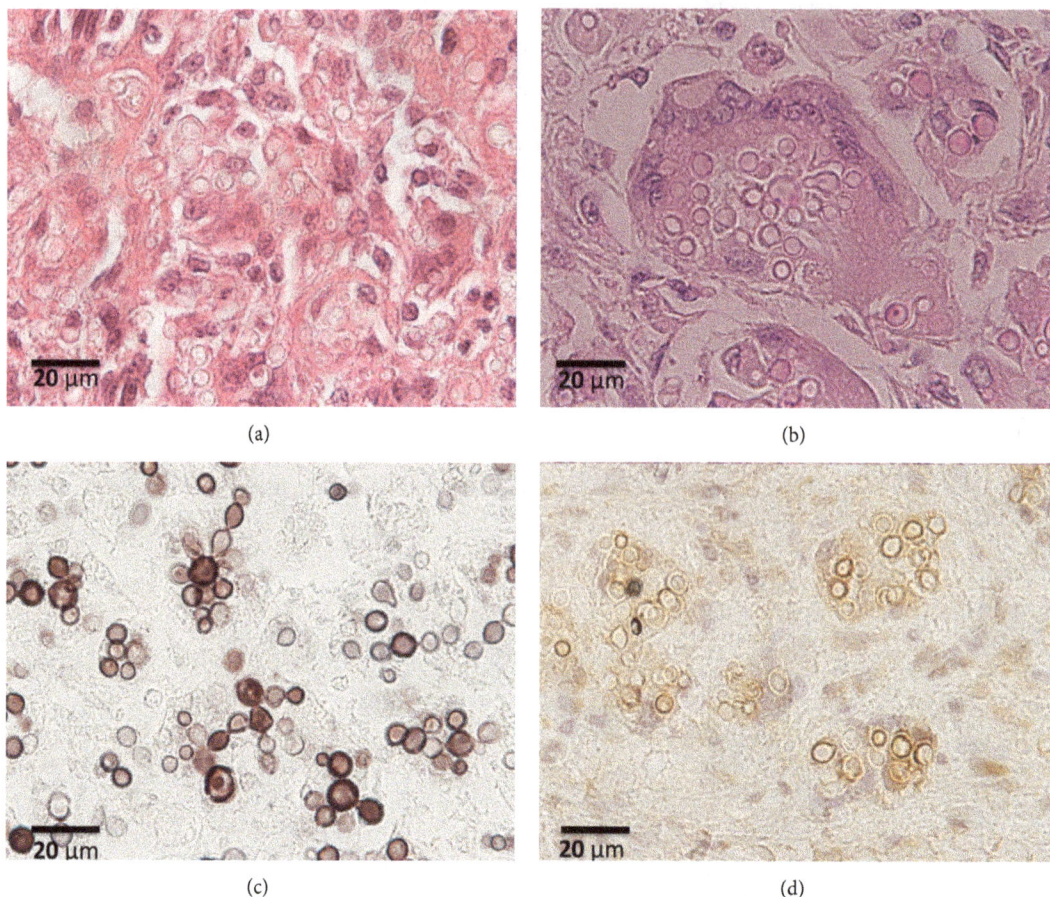

FIGURE 5: Yeast-like cells appeared as abundant round hyaline cells stained with hematoxylin and eosin (×200, (a)), PAS positive cells arranged in a multiple budding detected in a giant cell stained with PAS (×200, (b)), well-defined chains or multiple buddings stained with GMS (×200, (c)), and positive in immune-staining with anti-*P. brasiliensis* rabbit serum (×200, (d)) in the dermis.

*P. lutzii*, and *L. loboi* through a BLAST search (http://blast .ncbi.nlm.nih.gov/).

The 471 base pairs sequence showed 94.9% homology to *P. brasiliensis* (PBU26160) [29], 87.7% to *P. lutzii* (XM00279244), and 84.1% to *L. loboi* (EU109947) [4] (Table 1). The homologies to fungal species related to *Paracoccidioides* spp., such as *Ajellomyces dermatitidis* (XM_002624715) and *A. capsulatus* (XM_001540694) retrieved from the GenBank database (http://www.ncbi.nlm.nih.gov/genbank/), were 66.3 and 63.6%, respectively (Table 1).

We diagnosed the dolphin as lacaziosis on the basis of the clinical characteristics of the skin lesion, cytologic and histopathologic findings, immunostaining and immunodiffusion test, and the molecular biological study.

2.2. Case 2. A female bottlenose dolphin (*Tursiops truncatus*), estimated to be 5 years of age, was captured in 2007 in the coastal region of Japan simultaneously with the Case 1 dolphin and cared for under outdoor conditions in an aquarium at the same institution as Case 1 for 2 years. Then the animal was transported to the present aquarium where it was cared for until its death. The body weight and body length at the time of death were 175 kg and 240 cm.

The dolphin had two granulomatous lesions in the skin of both upper eye lids in February 2011 (Figures 6(a) and 6(b)). The lesions expanded by March 2011. We hypothesized that the animal might suffer from lacaziosis and performed a biopsy. There were some yeast-like components on the smears of the lesions stained by Giemsa solution (data not shown); however, yeast cells were not detected by histopathology, and *gp43* was not amplified. In addition, *Candida glabrata* was detected from the breath.

In May 2011, we biopsied and cauterized the lesions. *C. glabrata* and *Aspergillus niger* were detected on the breath. The animal received topical applications of ketoconazole cream and oral administration of itraconazole 1,000 mg/body BID followed by antibiotics and hydrocortisone. In addition, a granulomatous mass at the oral cavity appeared (Figure 7(a)).

We started to measure the blood $\beta$-glucan levels in June 2011 and found 8–41 pg/mL during July and August 2011, which indicated a fungal infection.

In September 2011, a new skin lesion appeared on the back fin (data not shown). Several scars caused by shark bites also became granulomatous (Figure 7(b)). We biopsied these lesions and detected multiple budding yeast-like cells

TABLE 1: Homologies of the partial sequence of *gp43* to *Paracoccidioides brasiliensis*, *P. lutzii*, *Lacazia loboi*, *Ajellomyces dermatitidis*, and *A. capsulatus*.

| GenBank accession no. | bps | Position (total bases) | Identity (%) | Isolate or ID [ref] |
|---|---|---|---|---|
| Present case | 471 | 1–471 (471) | — | SUM |
| *Paracoccidioides brasiliensis* | | | | |
| PBU26160 | 466 | 2603–3068 (3702) | 94.9 | B339 [29] |
| *P. lutzii* | | | | |
| XM_002792442* | 466 | 1136–1601 (2016) | 87.7 | Pb01 |
| *Lacazia loboi* | | | | |
| EU109947 | 463 | 1–463 (483) | 84.1 | 10-RMS [4] |
| *Ajellomyces dermatitidis* | | | | |
| XM_002624715* | 469 | 484–952 (1260) | 66.5 | SLH14081 |
| *A. capsulatus* | | | | |
| XM_001540694* | 469 | 475–943 (1251) | 63.3 | Nam1 |

*The sequence was retrieved from the GenBank database.

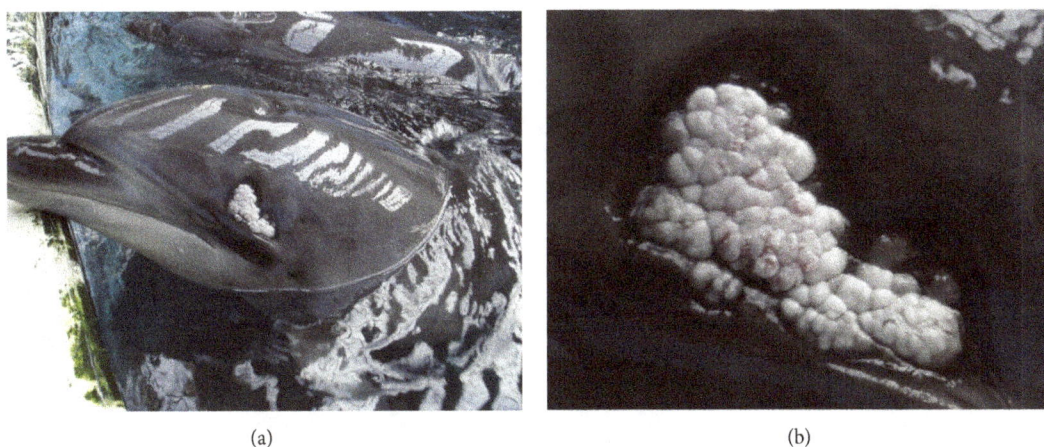

(a)

(b)

FIGURE 6: Granulomatous skin lesions of Case 2 at the left upper eye-lid in February 2011 (a, b).

by cytologic observation of samples stained by Giemsa (Figure 8(a)), mounted with 5% KOH (Figure 8(c)), and added with lactophenol cotton blue (Figure 8(c)) and GMS (Figure 8(d)). All biopsied skin samples from May, June, and September 2011 cultured on potato dextrose agar supplemented with 100 mg/L of chloramphenicol and Mycosel agar plates at 25 and 35°C for 4 weeks were negative.

The DNAs derived from Case 2 were not amplified through the PCR conditions used in Case 1. Therefore, we designed an inner primer set: SUM F1 (5′-GTCATC-GATCTCCATGGTGTTAAG-3′) and SUM R2 (5′-GGC-AGARAAGCATCCGAAA-3′) with reference to the *gp43* sequences from *P. brasiliensis* (PBU26160, AY005408, and AB304681) and *L. loboi* (AY697436 and EU109947); the sequence determined in the Case 1-derived DNA was aligned by GENETYX-MAC ver. 12.0 genetic information processing software (GENETYX CORPORATION, Tokyo, Japan). The PCR condition was as the same as the first PCR.

We detected 382 base pairs of a partial sequence of *gp43* showing 100% identity to those from Case 1 by the nested-PCR system from the biopsied sample collected at the above times.

The serum also showed a slight precipitation line in the immunodiffusion test against a fungal cell antigen of *P. brasiliensis* (data not shown).

On the basis of these clinical characteristics and cytologic and molecular biological observations, we made a diagnosis of lacaziosis.

The dolphin died suddenly in December 2012. The animal had shown a higher respiratory ratio at 7 times per min since the summer of 2012. The macroscopic findings were intestinal occlusion caused by cardiac disorder, pulmonary chronic inflammation, and one purulent cyst at the scar from cauterization of the animal's lesion without yeast-like cells.

## 3. Discussion

The present 2 dolphins showing chronic granulomatous skin lesions represent the first examples of lacaziosis from Pacific Ocean diagnosed on the basis of clinical, cytologic, histologic, serologic, and molecular biological data. Although many cases of lacaziosis-like diseases in dolphins from Ecuador, Colombia, Peru, and Chile along the coast of the Pacific Ocean have been recorded, they were diagnosed by

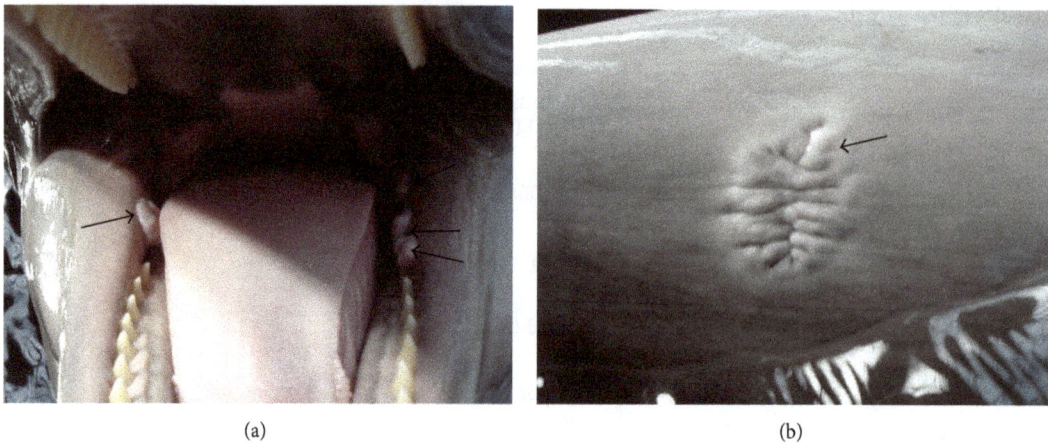

FIGURE 7: Granulomatous masses at the oral cavity appeared in May 2011 (arrows, (a)). One of the newly appeared skin lesions on the scars caused by a shark bite in September 2011 (arrow, (b)).

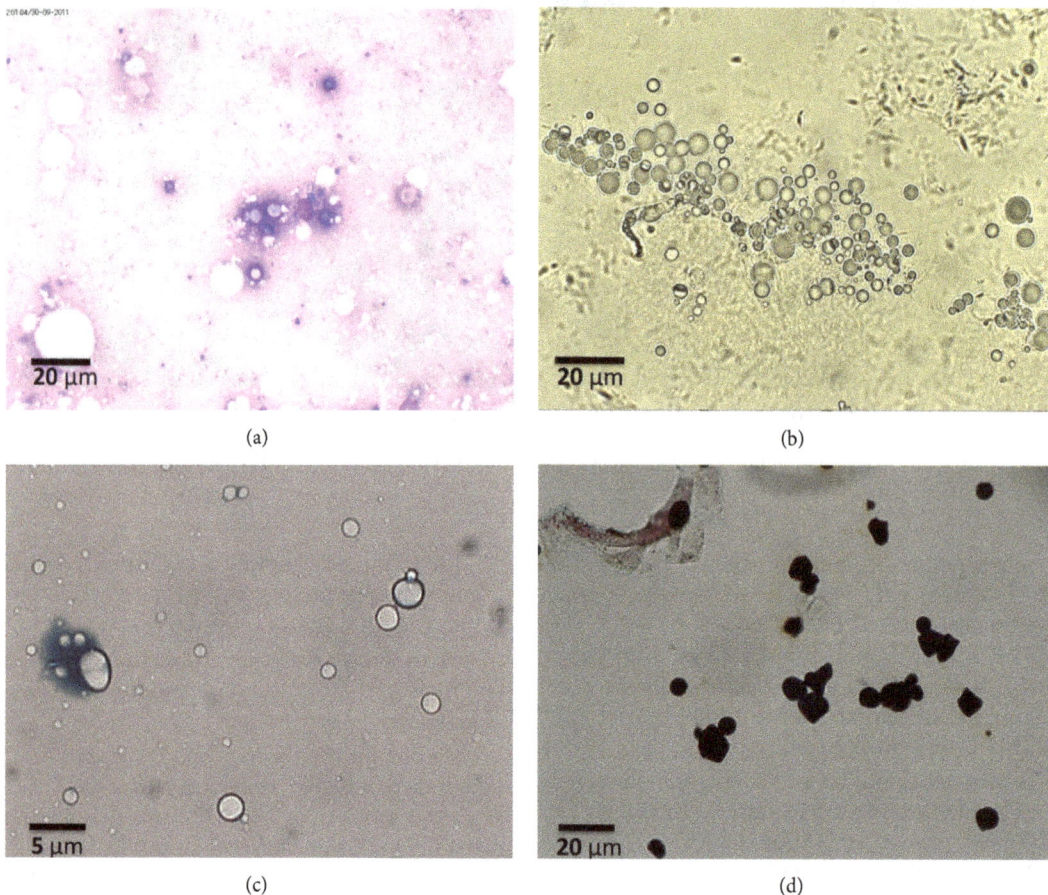

FIGURE 8: Multiple budding yeast-like cells derived from Case 2 stained by Giemsa (×200, (a)), in 5% KOH mount (×200, (b)), in 5% KOH plus lactophenol cotton blue (×400, (c)), and stained with GMS (×200, (d)).

macroscopy and photography without histopathologic and molecular biological data [23]. Furthermore, some lacaziosis-like diseases have been recorded in dolphins in Japanese waters [24]; however, those cases were also diagnosed by photographic images. Therefore, the present cases are the first of lacaziosis from the Pacific Ocean to be diagnosed

according to the definition recommended by Kiszka et al. [22] as follows: lacaziosis-like disease is very similar to lobomycosis but lacking a histologic diagnosis.

The serum cross-reaction in the immunodiffusion test with *P. brasiliensis* antigen and positive immune-staining with *P. brasiliensis* antisera have previously been reported as characteristics of lacaziosis [30]. The slightly positive reaction in the immunodiffusion test with *P. brasiliensis* antigen and the positive results upon immune-staining were matched to Brazilian human lacaziosis.

Establishing a diagnosis of lacaziosis requires clinical data, cytologic observation, histopathologic techniques, immunological methods, and detection of species-specific genes because of the difficultly of culture [2, 3, 8, 10]. Furthermore, it seems very unlikely that cutaneous lesions of cauliflower-like eczema in dolphins would be recognized as lacaziosis outside of endemic areas. In such cases, molecular biological techniques are useful.

In general, identification of fungal species is made on the basis of the internal transcribed spacer (ITS)-1-5.8S-ITS-2 regions of ribosomal RNA (ITS rRNA) gene sequences with more than 98 to 99% diversity between species or at least 95% even in a fungal species with higher intraspecies diversity [31]. However, we failed to detect the ITS rRNA gene from the dolphins' samples in the present study and could not compare to those from the Atlantic Ocean [20].

Interestingly, Esperón et al. reported that the ITS region of the ribosomal RNA sequence derived from dolphins living in the Atlantic Ocean was more related to *P. brasiliensis* than to *L. loboi* [20]. The preset cases also showed a close relationship of the genotype of the *gp43* to *P. brasiliensis*. Further study may confirm that the genotypes of lacaziosis out of Amazon areas.

The virulence of lacaziosis endemic in Japanese waters remains unknown; however, the disease seems to be virulent among dolphins since the animals that have spent a period in the same tribe suffered lacaziosis caused by identical genotype. They might be infected by contact or receive the pathogen simultaneously, and/or endemic in the tribe.

Lacaziosis sometimes causes immune disorders in dolphins [32]. Although we could not evaluate immune markers, the present animals suffered fatal outcomes caused by systemic bacterial infections or cardiac and respiratory problems, indicating that they were suffering from severe immune disorders.

Japan is a maritime nation. Many people in Japan have contact with the sea and marine products: not only fishermen but also the general public through swimming, fishing, boating, and visiting the marine aquarium. Therefore, we speculate that some latent human cases of lacaziosis may exist in our country.

## 4. Conclusions

We diagnosed 2 cases of lacaziosis in bottlenose dolphins on the basis of clinical, cytologic, histologic, serologic, and molecular biological data and confirmed that the causative agent at the present cases was a different genotype of *L. loboi* from Amazon area.

## Conflict of Interests

The corresponding author, Ayako Sano, declared that there is no conflict of interests submitted to the University of the Ryukyus no. H24-763.

## Acknowledgments

This study was supported in part by the Special Research Fund for Emerging and Re-emerging Infections of the Ministry of Health, Welfare and Labor (Grant no. H-21-Shinkou-004). The authors express their thanks to Ms. Michiko Murata (Azabu University) for technical support on the preliminary sequencing of *gp43*.

## References

[1] P. R. Taborda, V. A. Taborda, and M. R. McGinnis, "*Lacazia loboi* gen. nov., comb. nov., the etiologic agent of lobomycosis," *Journal of Clinical Microbiology*, vol. 37, no. 6, pp. 2031–2033, 1999.

[2] M. Ramos-E-Silva, F. Aguiar-Santos-Vilela, A. Cardoso-De-Brito, and S. Coelho-Carneiro, "Lobomycosis. Literature review and future perspectives," *Actas Dermo-Sifiliograficas*, vol. 100, no. 1, pp. 92–100, 2009.

[3] S. Talhari and C. Talhari, "Lobomycosis," *Clinics in Dermatology*, vol. 30, no. 4, pp. 420–424, 2012.

[4] R. Vilela, P. S. Rosa, A. F. F. Belone, J. W. Taylor, S. M. Diório, and L. Mendoza, "Molecular phylogeny of animal pathogen *Lacazia loboi* inferred from rDNA and DNA coding sequences," *Mycological Research*, vol. 113, no. 8, pp. 851–857, 2009.

[5] A. Fialho, "Blastomicose du tipo, "JorgeLobo"," *O Hospital, (Rio De Janeiro)*, vol. 14, article 903, 1938.

[6] D. Borelli, "*Aspergillus*, sorpresas en micopatologia," *Dermatologia Venezolana*, vol. 1, article 286, 1958.

[7] R. Vilela, L. Mendoza, P. S. Rosa et al., "Molecular model for studying the uncultivated fungal pathogen *Lacazia loboi*," *Journal of Clinical Microbiology*, vol. 43, no. 8, pp. 3657–3661, 2005.

[8] K. L. Horner and G. J. Raugi, "Lobomycosis on MedScape," 2012, http://emedicine.medscape.com/article/1092451-overview.

[9] W. C. Symmers, "A possible case of Lobo's disease acquired in Europe from a bottle-nosed dolphin (*Tursiops truncatus*)," *Bulletin de la Societe de Pathologie Exotique et de ses Filiales*, vol. 76, no. 5, pp. 777–784, 1983.

[10] A. Paniz-Mondolfi, C. Talhari, L. Sander Hoffmann et al., "Lobomycosis: an emerging disease in humans and delphinidae," *Mycoses*, vol. 55, no. 4, pp. 298–309, 2012.

[11] E. Papadavid, M. Dalamaga, I. Kapniari et al., "Lobomycosis: a case from Southeastern Europe and review of the literature," *Journal of Dermatological Case Reports*, vol. 6, no. 3, pp. 65–69, 2012.

[12] T. K. Rumi and R. A. Kapkaev, "Keloidal blastomycosis (Lobo's disease)," *Vestnik Dermatologii i Venerologii*, no. 11, pp. 41–43, 1988.

[13] P. C. Simões-Lopes, G. S. Paula, F. M. Xavier, and A. C. Scaramelo, "First case of lobomycosis in bottlenose dolphin from southern Brazil," *Marine Mammal Sciences*, vol. 9, no. 3, pp. 329–331, 1993.

[14] G. A. De Vries and J. J. Laarman, "A case of Lobo's disease in the dolphin *Sotalia guianensis*," *Aquatic Mammals*, vol. 1, pp. 1–8, 1973.

[15] G. Migaki, M. G. Valerio, B. Irvine, and F. M. Garner, "Lobo's disease in an atlantic bottle-nosed dolphin," *Journal of the American Veterinary Medical Association*, vol. 159, no. 5, pp. 578–582, 1971.

[16] D. K. Caldwell, M. C. Caldwell, and J. C. Woodard, "Lobomycosis as a disease of the Atlantic bottlenosed dolphin (*Tursiops truncatus* Montagu, 1821)," *American Journal of Tropical Medicine and Hygiene*, vol. 24, no. 1, pp. 105–114, 1975.

[17] J. S. Reif, M. S. Mazzoil, S. D. McCulloch et al., "Lobomycosis in Atlantic bottlenose dolphins from the Indian River Lagoon, Florida," *Journal of the American Veterinary Medical Association*, vol. 228, no. 1, pp. 104–108, 2006.

[18] D. S. Rotstein, L. G. Burdett, W. McLellan et al., "Lobomycosis in offshore bottlenose dolphins (*Tursiops truncatus*), North Carolina," *Emerging Infectious Diseases*, vol. 15, no. 4, pp. 588–590, 2009.

[19] D. F. Cowan, "Lobo's disease in a bottlenose dolphin (*Tursiops truncatus*) from Matagorda Bay, Texas," *Journal of Wildlife Diseases*, vol. 29, no. 3, pp. 488–489, 1993.

[20] F. Esperón, D. García-Párraga, E. N. Bellière, and J. M. Sánchez-Vizcaíno, "Molecular diagnosis of lobomycosis-like disease in a bottlenose dolphin in captivity," *Medical Mycology*, vol. 50, no. 1, pp. 106–109, 2012.

[21] J. P. Schroeder, "Apparent toxicity of ketoconazole for *Tursiaps truncatus* during treatment of lobomycosis," in *Proceedings of the IAAAM 14th Annual Conference and Workshop*, Long Beach, Calif, USA, May 1983.

[22] J. Kiszka, M.-F. Van Bressem, and C. Pusineri, "Lobomycosis-like disease and other skin conditions in Indo-Pacific bottlenose dolphins *Tursiops aduncus* from the Indian Ocean," *Diseases of Aquatic Organisms*, vol. 84, no. 2, pp. 151–157, 2009.

[23] B. Bedrinana-Romano, B. Best, C. Brownell et al., "Report of the workshop on cetacean skin diseases," *The Journal of Cetacean Research and Management*, vol. 11, supplement, pp. 503–514, 2009.

[24] M. F. Van Bressem, M. Shirakihara, and M. Amano, "Cutaneous nodular disease in a small population of Indo-Pacific bottlenose dolphins, *Tursiops aduncus*, from Japan," *Marine Mammal Science*, vol. 29, no. 3, pp. 525–532.

[25] I. F. G. Hampton, G. C. Whittow, J. Szekerczes, and S. Rutherford, "Heat transfer and body temperature in the atlantic bottlenose dolphin, *Tursiops truncatus*," *International Journal of Biometeorology*, vol. 15, no. 2–4, pp. 247–253, 1971.

[26] G. D. Bossart, T. H. Reidarson, L. A. Dierauf, and D. A. Duffield, "Clinical pathology," in *CRC Handbook of Marine Mammal Medicine*, L. A. Dierauf and F. M. D. Gulland, Eds., Chapter 19, pp. 383–436, CRC Press, Washington, DC, USA, 2nd edition, 2001.

[27] A. Sano, K. Yokoyama, M. Tamura et al., "Detection of *gp43* and ITS1-5.8S-ITS2 ribosomal RNA genes of *Paracoccidioides brasiliensis* in paraffin-embedded tissue," *Nihon Ishinkin Gakkai Zasshi*, vol. 42, no. 1, pp. 23–27, 2001.

[28] A. Takayama, E. N. Itano, A. Sano, M. A. Ono, and K. Kamei, "An atypical *Paracoccidioides brasiliensis* clinical isolate based on multiple gene analysis," *Medical Mycology*, vol. 48, no. 1, pp. 64–72, 2010.

[29] P. S. Cisalpino, R. Puccia, L. M. Yamauchi, M. I. N. Cano, J. F. Da Silveira, and L. R. Travassos, "Cloning, characterization, and epitope expression of the major diagnostic antigen of *Paracoccidioides brasiliensis*," *Journal of Biological Chemistry*, vol. 271, no. 8, pp. 4553–4560, 1996.

[30] Z. P. Camargo, R. G. Baruzzi, S. M. Maeda, and M. C. Floriano, "Antigenic relationship between *Loboa loboi* and *Paracoccidioides brasiliensis* as shown by serological method," *Medical Mycology*, vol. 36, no. 6, pp. 413–417, 1998.

[31] S. A. Balajee, A. M. Borman, M. E. Brandt et al., "Sequence-based identification of *aspergillus*, *fusarium*, and *mucorales* species in the clinical mycology laboratory: where are we and where should we go from here?" *Journal of Clinical Microbiology*, vol. 47, no. 4, pp. 877–884, 2009.

[32] J. S. Reif, M. M. Peden-Adams, T. A. Romano, C. D. Rice, P. A. Fair, and G. D. Bossart, "Immune dysfunction in Atlantic bottlenose dolphins (*Tursiops truncatus*) with lobomycosis," *Medical Mycology*, vol. 47, no. 2, pp. 125–135, 2009.

# 5

# Magnetic Resonance Imaging of Bacterial Meningoencephalitis in a Foal

**Judit Viu,[1] Lara Armengou,[1] Cristian de la Fuente,[2] Carla Cesarini,[1] Sònia Añor,[2] and Eduard Jose-Cunilleras[1]**

[1] Servei de Medicina Interna Equina, Departament de Medicina i Cirugia Animals, Facultat de Veterinària, Universitat Autònoma de Barcelona, Bellaterra, 08193 Barcelona, Spain
[2] Servei de Neurologia i Neurocirurgia, Departament de Medicina i Cirugia Animals, Facultat de Veterinària, Universitat Autònoma de Barcelona, Bellaterra, 08193 Barcelona, Spain

Correspondence should be addressed to Lara Armengou, lara.armengou@uab.es

Academic Editors: L. Arroyo and C. Cantile

Magnetic resonance imaging (MRI) in equidae suffering meningoencephalitis (ME) has not been described. The objective of this paper is to describe brain MRI findings in a foal with bacterial ME. A five-month-old, 200 kg bwt Arabian filly was referred with a history of abnormal mental status and locomotion. The filly was recumbent and obtunded, and pupillary light reflexes were sluggish, and oculocephalic movements were normally present. Ophthalmic examination revealed bilateral optic neuritis. Hematology revealed leukocytosis and neutrophilia. Cerebrospinal fluid analysis showed neutrophilic pleocytosis with intracellular bacteria. On brain MRI, there were multifocal cortical areas of mild hyperintensity on T2-weighted images (T2WI) affecting both hemispheres. The lesions had ill-delineated margins, and there was loss of differentiation between gray and white matter. Diffuse hyperintensity was also identified in the left cerebellar cortex on T2WI. Neither mass effect nor cerebral midline shift were identified. On FLAIR images, the lesions were also hyperintense and, in some areas, they seemed to coalescence to form diffuse cortical areas of hyperintensity. The MRI findings described were similar to the MRI features described in cases of humans and small animals with ME. Brain MRI can be a useful diagnostic tool in foals and small-sized equidae with intracranial disease.

## 1. Introduction

Magnetic resonance imaging (MRI) is a very useful imaging technique in human neurology since the eighties. The use of MRI in veterinary medicine is very common in small animals, specially in those with neurological disease, but the use in horses is less frequent. The most common application of MRI in equine medicine is in the diagnosis of muscular or skeletal problems. The use of MRI in equine neurology is restricted due to limitations of size and weight-bearing capacity of most MRI units. However, due to the smaller size and lower weight of foals, MRI has been used in these animals and the findings reported for several cases of neonatal equine neurological disorders. Nevertheless, to the authors' knowledge, there are no reports describing the MRI lesions of bacterial meningoencephalitis (ME) in foals. This paper describes these lesions and demonstrates how MRI can be extremely useful in the diagnosis of ME in foals.

## 2. Case Details

A five-month-old, 200 kg bwt Arabian filly was referred to the *Unitat Equina* of the *Hospital Clínic Veterinari de la UAB* for evaluation of abnormal mental status and generalized profound weakness. The filly had began to show signs of progressive lethargy a week prior to admission, that progressed to right thoracic limb paresis and inability to stand at 12 hours before referral. According to the referring veterinarian, the filly was born at term but it showed confusion and inability to nurse. Five mares and their foals as well as the filly's dam lived together and none of them showed any neurological or physical alterations. All animals were in regular vaccination and deworming programs.

Physical examination on admission revealed that the filly was recumbent and markedly obtunded. Its body condition and hair coat were normal. No swollen joints or wounds were observed. Mild tachycardia (60 bpm) and tachypnea (48 bpm) were detected, and gastrointestinal sounds were decreased. Body temperature was within normal limits (37.6°C), and no cervical stiffness or painful areas were detected on palpation. On neurological examination, pupillary reflexes were sluggish bilaterally, and oculocephalic movements were normally present. No other alterations were detected in cranial nerve or spinal reflex evaluation. Proprioception tests could not be performed due to recumbency. The results of the neurological examination were consistent with an intracranial lesion affecting diffusely the cerebral hemispheres. Ophthalmological examination revealed papillary congestion with mild peripapillar exudates in both eyes and uveitis with small amounts of fibrin in the anterior chamber of the left eye.

Radiographs of the cervical vertebrae and skull were apparently normal. Thoracic radiographs revealed an alveolar pattern consistent with subclinical pneumonia. Hematology and plasma biochemistry performed upon admission revealed mildly increased blood lactate concentration (3.2 mmol/L, reference value <2 mmol/L), [1] marked leukocytosis (20,110 cells/$\mu$L, reference value 5,400–14,300 cells/$\mu$L) [1] and neutrophilia (16,210 cells/$\mu$L, reference value 2,200–8,600 cells/$\mu$L) [1], and normal values of packed cell volume, total plasma protein, and fibrinogen concentrations. Plasma sodium, potassium, and chloride concentrations were within normal limits, and no alterations were detected in acid-base status. Increased creatine kinase (CK 6782 IU/L, reference range 60–266 IU/L) [1] and aspartate transaminase (AST 512 IU/L reference range 280–520 IU/L) [1] activities were also detected.

Cerebrospinal fluid (CSF) was obtained under general anesthesia from the atlanto-occipital space, and an MRI study of the brain was performed under the same anesthesia with a 0.2 T open permanent magnet (VetMR; Esaote, Genoa, Italy). The foal was premedicated with romifidine (0.03 mg/kg IV) and butorphanol (0.03 mg/kg IV). The anaesthesia was induced with diazepam (0.05 mg/kg IV) and thiobarbital (4 mg/kg IV) and maintained in lateral recumbency with isoflurane in 100% oxygen. Total anesthetic time was 2 hours. For MRI, the foal was kept in left lateral recumbency with the neck extended and the head against a linear coil. Transverse spin-echo T1-weighted images (T1WI; TR = 590 ms, TE = 26 ms, slice thickness = 6 mm, interslice gap = 0.6 mm), transverse and sagittal T2-weighted images (T2WI; TR = 3090 ms, TE = 80 ms, slice thickness = 6 mm, interslice gap = 0.6 mm), and transverse FLAIR images (TR = 7860 ms, TE = 90 ms, TI = 1500 ms, slice thickness = 6 mm, interslice gap = 0.6 mm) were obtained. In addition, transverse T1WI were acquired after intravenous (iv) injection of gadopentate dimeglumine (Magnevist, Bayer Schering Pharma, Berlin, Germany.) (0.1 mmol/kg). The mean obtention time for each sequence was 15 minutes, and the total scanning time was one hour and a half. MR

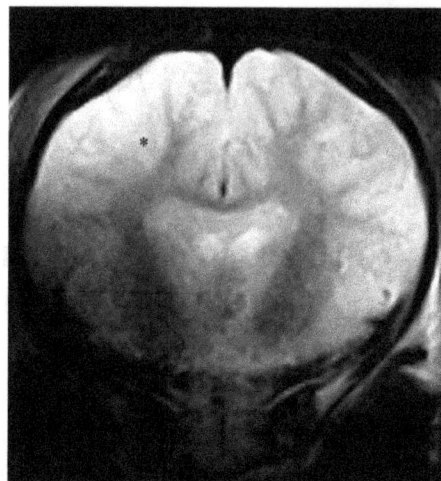

Figure 1: Transverse T2-weighted image at the level of rostral diencephalon showing a cortical area of mild hyperintensity with loss of differentiation between gray and white matter in the right hemisphere (*).

images were loaded and evaluated with a Medical Imaging Software (OsiriX, open source software; http://www.osirix-viewer.com, Macintosh platform). MRI showed multifocal cortical areas of mild hyperintensity on T2WI affecting both hemispheres. The lesions had diffuse margins, and there was loss of differentiation between gray and white matter. Although both hemispheres were affected, the lesions were more severe in the cortical gray matter of the frontal and parietal lobes of the right hemisphere (Figure 1). Diffuse hyperintensity also was identified affecting the left cerebellar cortex on T2WI. Neither mass effect nor cerebral midline shift was identified. On precontrast T1WI, the lesions were isointense to normal gray matter (Figure 2). On FLAIR images the lesions were hyperintense and, in some areas, they tended to coalescence to form diffuse cortical areas of hyperintensity. Some cortical areas that had normal appearance in T1WI and T2WI showed high signal intensity on FLAIR images (Figure 3). These changes were more evident in the parietal and temporal lobes of the right cerebral hemisphere, where diffuse FLAIR hyperintensity was detected. Due to cerebrospinal fluid signal suppression, areas of mild periventricular hyperintensity were more easily identified on FLAIR images than on T2WI. On postcontrast T1WI, only mild gyral enhancement was seen in both frontal lobes. Most lesions did not enhance after contrast administration. Ther was no meningeal enhancement either. The MR imaging findings were considered consistent with either an infectious-inflammatory process (encephalitis), or a multifocal vascular (ischemic) condition affecting the cerebral and cerebellar cortices.

Analysis of CSF revealed normal total protein concentration (76.5 mg/dL, reference range 10–120 mg/dL) [1] and neutrophilic pleocytosis (15 cells/$\mu$L, reference range 0–7 cells/$\mu$L) [1], with intracytoplasmic bacillus identified on cytology. Blood and CSF cultures were not performed

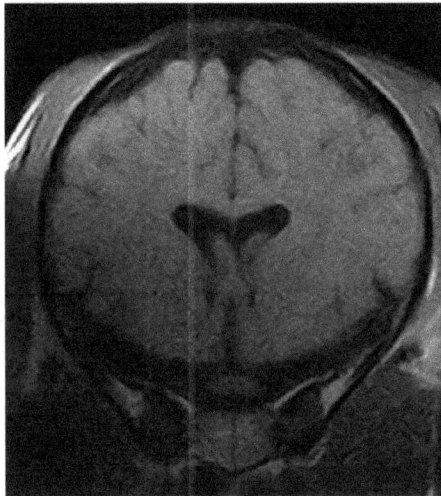

FIGURE 2: Transverse T1-weighted image at the level of rostral diencephalon showing isointensity of the lesion identified on T2-weighted and FLAIR images.

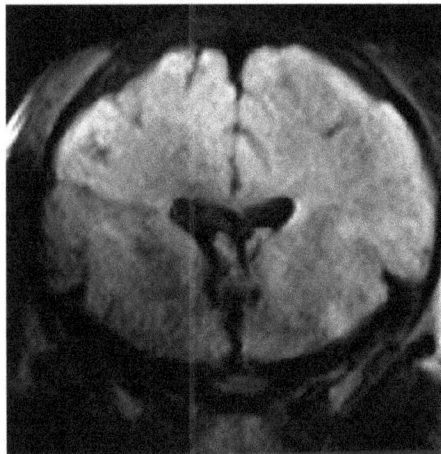

FIGURE 3: Transverse FLAIR image at the level of rostral diencephalon showing multiple hyperintense areas in the cerebral cortex of both hemispheres.

because of lack of availability of a microbiology laboratory at that time.

Based on history, clinicopathological findings, and diagnostic test results, a presumptive diagnosis of ME including bilateral optic neuritis was given, with associated diagnosis of left eye uveitis, pneumonia, and mild myositis.

The foal received iv and oral antimicrobials (sulfadiazine-trimethoprim and rifampin, resp.). Intravenous sodium-rich crystalloid (Lactated Ringer's plus 10 mL/L of 7.5% NaCl) and iv colloidal solutions (6% hydroxyethyl starch) were administered according to the animal requirements. Intranasal oxygen supplementation, iv 2% dimethyl sulfoxide solution, and iv flunixin meglumine were also administered. Topical ocular therapy consisting of broad spectrum antibiotic and nonsteroidal anti-inflammatory drugs (NSAIDs) was applied. Once the foal recovered from general

anesthesia, it began to show hyperexcitability, intention tremors, and vestibular signs. After 12 hours of treatment, the filly's mental status improved and at 24 hours after treatment initiation, it was able to stand up for short periods of time. Paresis of the right thoracic limb was consistently observed when the filly was standing.

Radiographs of the right thoracic limb showed no evident alterations. After a week of treatment, hematology and plasma muscle enzyme activities normalized, but the animal still showed paresis of the right thoracic limb upon discharge from the hospital. Systemic antimicrobial and NSAID treatments were continued for two weeks after leaving the hospital.

Oral communication with the referring veterinarian confirmed full recovery by the time medical therapy was interrupted without persistence of neurological or orthopedic signs.

## 3. Discussion

Bacterial meningitis is an uncommon condition in mature horses. In adult horses, the condition has been related to infectious diseases involving the head and [2, 3] trauma or common variable immunodeficiency [4]. In young horses, *Streptococcus equi equi* meningoencephalomyelitis [5], *S. equi equi* abscessation [2, 6], and intracranial *Rhodococcus equi* abscessation [7] have been described. ME has been identified as a complication in 8–10% of septicemic foals [8, 9]. Cytological CSF findings in foals with meningitis usually include neutrophilic pleocytosis and increased protein concentration; however, normal or moderately increased values have also been reported in few cases. [10] The CSF obtained in the foal herein reported had a normal protein concentration with a mild neutrophilic pleocytosis and evidence of intracellular bacteria on cytology. The mild alterations found on CSF analysis were probably due to the predominance of encephalitis over meningitis, and perhaps the presence of nonexudative lesions found mainly in the brain parenchyma. Normal CSF analysis cannot completely rule out inflammatory central nervous system (CNS) disease in veterinary cases [11]. Because of this, MRI is highly recommended in cases of suspected inflammatory brain disease to improve the diagnostic yield [12, 13].

The MRI study was performed using a low-magnetic field unit (0.2 T) designed for small animal imaging. Because of this, positioning of our patient and coil selection were limited. In addition, low field MRI is time consuming if high-resolution images, small slice thickness, and large regions, of study are desired. In order to minimize anesthetic time, temporal resolution (minimum acquisition time to achieve diagnostic images prevailing over high resolution images) was elected. So large slice thickness/interslice gap and small image matrixes were selected to improve signal-noise ratio and reduce acquisition time. Lesion morphology, topography, and magnetic resonance signal characteristics observed in this case were similar to the MRI features described in humans and small animals with meningoencephalitis, although these patterns are not pathognomonic [14, 15]. In the case reported herein, the lesions were mildly hyperintense on T2WI but they were better visualized and delineated in the FLAIR images. FLAIR sequences have been advocated as a very useful MRI technique to detect inflammatory brain lesions due its high sensitivity over T2WI [16, 17]. In addition, periventricular white matter involvement is well depicted due to CSF signal suppression on FLAIR images. These features were also observed in this case and allowed better assessment of lesion extension. Paramagnetic contrast enhancement was mild and only observed in lesions affecting both frontal lobes, showing a gyral pattern. This contrast enhancement pattern has also been described in human infectious ME but it is not disease-specific [14]. Although meningeal contrast uptake is not always present in confirmed cases of meningitis in other species [15], the absence of meningeal, either dural or leptomeningeal, contrast enhancement strongly suggested brain parenchyma involvement rather than meningeal involvement.

Cerebellar lesions were also detected on the MRI study. However, the filly presented mild vestibulocerebellar signs only for a few hours in the postanesthetic period. The lack of clinical evidence of vestibulocerebellar signs on initial presentation could be explained by a predominance of diffuse bilateral hemispheric signs causing a profoundly obtunded mental status and hiding other concomitant neurolocalizations. Another possible explanation is a drug-related exacerbation of vestibulocerebellar signs in the postanesthetic period. Although there are not many studies in the literature about the effect of sedatives or anesthetic agents on the neurologic status of patients with CNS disorders, it has been postulated that some anesthetic agents could induce worsening of neurologic signs, specially vestibulocerebellar signs [18].

Bacterial meningitis is a disease difficult to diagnose and usually carries a poor prognosis. To the authors' knowledge, there are no previous descriptions of the MRI findings in horses with bacterial ME. The similarity of the herein reported findings to those observed in bacterial ME cases in other species leads to consider MRI as a very helpful diagnostic tool in foals.

## References

[1] K. T. T. Corley and J. Stephen, "Appendix," in *The Equine Hospital Manual*, T. T. Corley and J. Stephen, Eds., pp. 654–689, Blackwell, 1st edition, 2008.

[2] J. J. Smith, P. J. Provost, and M. R. Paradis, "Bacterial meningitis and brain abscesses secondary to infectious disease processes involving the head in horses: seven cases (1980–2001)," *Journal of the American Veterinary Medical Association*, vol. 224, no. 5, pp. 739–742, 2004.

[3] E. Mitchell, M. O. Furr, and H. C. McKenzie, "Bacterial meningitis in five mature horses," *Equine Veterinary Education*, vol. 18, no. 5, pp. 249–255, 2006.

[4] A. Pellegrini-Masini, A. I. Bentz, I. C. Johns et al., "Common variable immunodeficiency in three horses with presumptive bacterial meningitis," *Journal of the American Veterinary Medical Association*, vol. 227, no. 1, pp. 114–122, 2005.

[5] C. Finno, N. Pusterla, M. Aleman et al., "Streptococcus equi meningoencephalomyelitis in a foal," *Journal of the American Veterinary Medical Association*, vol. 229, no. 5, pp. 721–724, 2006.

[6] A. Pellegrini-Masini and L. C. Livesey, "Meningitis and Encephalomyelitis in Horses," *Veterinary Clinics of North America*, vol. 22, no. 2, pp. 553–589, 2006.

[7] J. C. Janicek, J. Kramer, J. R. Coates, J. C. Lattimer, A. M. LaCarrubba, and N. T. Messer, "Intracranial abscess caused by Rhodococcus equi infection in a foal," *Journal of the American Veterinary Medical Association*, vol. 228, no. 2, pp. 251–253, 2006.

[8] B. D. Brewer and A. M. Koterba, "Bacterial isolates and susceptibility patterns in foals in a neonatal intensive care unit," *Compendium on Continuing Education for the Practicing Veterinarian*, vol. 12, pp. 1773–1781, 1990.

[9] A. M. Koterba, B. D. Brewer, and F. A. Tarplee, "Clinical and clinicopathological characteristics of the septicaemic neonatal foal: review of 38 cases," *Equine Veterinary Journal*, vol. 16, no. 4, pp. 376–382, 1984.

[10] M. O. Furr, "Bacterial infections of the central nervous system," in *Equine Neurology*, M. O. Furr and S. Reed, Eds., pp. 187–194, Wiley-Blackwell, 1st edition, 2008.

[11] K. G. Braund, *Clinical Neurology in Small Animals: Localization, Diagnosis and Treatmen*, International Veterinary Information Service Ithaca, Ithaca , NY, USA, 2002.

[12] A. A. Bohn, T. B. Wills, C. L. West, R. L. Tucker, and R. S. Bagley, "Cerebrospinal fluid analysis and magnetic resonance imaging in the diagnosis of neurologic disease in dogs: a retrospective study," *Veterinary Clinical Pathology*, vol. 35, no. 3, pp. 315–320, 2006.

[13] A. Splendiani, E. Puglielli, R. De Amicis, S. Necozione, C. Masciocchi, and M. Gallucci, "Contrast-enhanced FLAIR in the early diagnosis of infectious meningitis," *Neuroradiology*, vol. 47, no. 8, pp. 591–598, 2005.

[14] O. Kastrup, I. Wanke, and M. Maschke, "Neuroimaging of infections," *NeuroRx*, vol. 2, no. 2, pp. 324–332, 2005.

[15] S. Hecht and W. H. Adams, "MRI of brain disease in veterinary patients part 2: acquired brain disorders," *Veterinary Clinics of North America—Small Animal Practice*, vol. 40, no. 1, pp. 39–63, 2010.

[16] K. Tsuchiya, S. Inaoka, Y. Mizutani, and J. Hachiya, "Fast fluid-attenuated inversion-recovery MR of intracranial infections," *American Journal of Neuroradiology*, vol. 18, no. 5, pp. 909–913, 1997.

[17] G. B. Cherubini, S. R. Platt, S. Howson, E. Baines, D. C. Brodbelt, and R. Dennis, "Comparison of magnetic resonance imaging sequences in dogs with multi-focal intracranial disease: PAPER," *Journal of Small Animal Practice*, vol. 49, no. 12, pp. 634–640, 2008.

[18] G. D. Thal, M. D. Szabo, M. Lopez-Bresnahan, and G. Crosby, "Exacerbation or unmasking of focal neurologic deficits by sedatives," *Anesthesiology*, vol. 85, no. 1, pp. 21–25, 1996.

# 6

# *Klossiella equi* Infection in an Immunosuppressed Horse: Evidence of Long-Term Infection

**Lora R. Ballweber,[1] Deanna Dailey,[2] and Gabriele Landolt[3]**

[1] *Veterinary Diagnostic Laboratory, College of Veterinary Medicine and Biomedical Sciences, Colorado State University, Fort Collins, CO 80523-1644, USA*

[2] *Cell and Molecular Biology Graduate Program, College of Veterinary Medicine and Biomedical Sciences, Colorado State University, Fort Collins, CO 80523-1005, USA*

[3] *Department of Clinical Sciences, College of Veterinary Medicine and Biomedical Sciences, Colorado State University, 300 West Drake Road, Fort Collins, CO 80523-1678, USA*

Correspondence should be addressed to Lora R. Ballweber, lora.ballweber@colostate.edu

Academic Editors: J. Orós, I. Pires, and D. M. Wong

A 13-year-old quarter horse gelding presented with a history of hematuria of approximately 1-year duration, anemia, weight loss over the previous six months, and bilateral nasal discharge of 2-week duration. It was determined that hematuria was most likely caused by the coccidian parasite *Klossiella equi*. Additional case workup suggested a diagnosis of pituitary pars intermedia dysfunction. Confirmatory testing was declined by the owners and the horse was discharged on medical therapy. Despite initial improvement after discharge, the horse developed unresolving sinusitis approximately 1 year later and was euthanized. Necropsy confirmed the presence of an adenoma of the pars intermedia of the pituitary gland, supporting the initial diagnosis. Additional findings included multiple developmental stages of *K. equi* present in the kidneys. This finding demonstrates infections with *K. equi* can be chronic in nature and supports the association of increased severity of klossiellosis and impaired immune function.

## 1. Introduction

*Klossiella equi* is the only known renal coccidian parasite of equines [1–8]. Although first described in 1946, very little is known about this parasite. Schizogony occurs within Bowman's capsule and the proximal convoluted tubles while gametogony and sporogony occur within the loop of Henle and distal convoluted tubles [3, 5, 6, 9, 10]. Mode of transmission has not been identified but is thought to be through ingestion of sporulated sporocysts passed in urine [4, 9]. The duration of infection has not been determined, although, as a coccidian it has been proposed that infections would be self-limiting [7]. There is no known effective treatment.

*Klossiella equi* has been reported in various areas of the world but the prevalence is unknown. Attempts to define the prevalence ante mortem have met with difficulties in recovery of sporocysts in urine samples [7]; thus, prevalence has been primarily based on histological examination of the kidneys taken at necropsy. Using this, 6/47 horses in Australia [7], 2/8 donkeys in Kenya [6], 8/14 burros residing in the US but born in Mexico [1], and 5/40 ponies and 3/14 burros in the US [9] have been found to be infected. Thus, the prevalence appears to vary considerably. In addition to horses, ponies, donkeys, and burros, *K. equi* has also been reported from zebras [8].

*Klossiella equi* is usually considered to be an incidental finding [1, 6, 8], although it has been associated with renal tubular nephrosis and nephritis in immunocompromised animals [4, 5, 7]. Thus, there may be an association between severity of infection with *K. equi* and impaired immune function.

## 2. Case Presentation

A 13-year-old quarter horse gelding was admitted to the Colorado State University (CSU) Veterinary Teaching Hospital (VTH) with a history of hematuria of approximately 1-year duration, anemia, weight loss over the previous six months, and bilateral nasal discharge of 2-week duration. Urethroscopy and cystoscopy performed by the referring veterinarian revealed macroscopic pigmenturia originating from the left ureter. No other abnormalities were detected. The horse was treated (duration unknown) with antimicrobials consisting of sulfadiazine/trimethoprim (30 mg/kg PO BID) and ceftiofur (2.2 mg/kg IM SID) for presumed urinary tract infection, which did not resolve the hematuria.

Upon presentation at the VTH, the horse was quiet, alert, and responsive. His body weight was 454 kg with a body condition score of 4/9. Physical examination demonstrated normal vital signs, bilateral mucopurulent nasal discharge, and an enlarged right submandibular lymph node. Rebreathing examination and rectal palpation revealed no abnormalities. Complete blood count and biochemical profile revealed the presence of a lymphopenia ($0.7 \times 10^3/\mu L$ reference range $1.5-4.0 \times 10^3/\mu L$), macrocytic erythrocytopenia (red blood cell count: $5.7 \times 10^6/\mu L$ reference range $6.5-10.5 \times 10^6/\mu L$; mean corpuscular volume: 61 fL reference range 42–52 fL), and hyperglycemia (239 mg/dL reference range 70–135 mg/dL). Quantitative serum immunoglobulin test indicated that IgM was decreased (31 mg/dL reference range 89–151 mg/dL) with a compensatory increase in IgG and IgA (IgG: 3863 mg/dL reference range 984–1684 mg/dL; IgA: 658 mg/dL reference range 67–239 mg/dL).

Endoscopy of the lower urinary tract showed no structural abnormalities within the urethra or bladder; however, the urine present in the bladder was red in color. Urine was observed flowing from both ureteral openings, with urine exiting from the right ureter straw colored and urine from the left ureter red in color. The bladder and both ureters were catheterized (endoscopically guided) and urine collected. Glucosuria (100 mg/dL) was evident in all 3 urine samples; hematuria (200–500 red blood cells/high-power field) and mild proteinuria were present in the urine from the left ureter and bladder. Coccidian sporocysts (Figure 1) were found in the urine sediment in all 3 samples and on centrifugal flotation with Sheather's sugar solution (1.27 sp. g.). Sporocysts measured $15.0-17.5 \times 7.5-12.5\,\mu m$ (average $= 16.25 \times 10.25\,\mu m$), contained 8–12 sporozoites and were morphologically identical to *K. equi* [4, 7]. Bacterial culture of both ureter samples resulted in no growth. Ultrasonographic evaluation of the kidneys showed a mildly enlarged left kidney with normal shape and corticomedullary distinction.

An upper airway endoscopic examination revealed mucopurulent exudate in both nasal passages, which appeared to originate from the sinus openings; examination of the guttural pouches, ethmoids, and upper trachea did not reveal any abnormalities. Radiographs of the maxillary sinuses and tooth roots showed an irregular wavy surface to the occlusion surfaces of the upper and lower dental arcades. Moreover, a gap was evident between the fourth premolar and first molar bilaterally, with an increased lucency along the caudal border of the fourth premolar (108) and the rostral border of the first molar (109) on the right side, with sclerosis of the alveolar bone surrounding these teeth. Lastly, there was evidence of fluid in the right rostral and caudal maxillary sinuses. An oral examination confirmed the presence of a

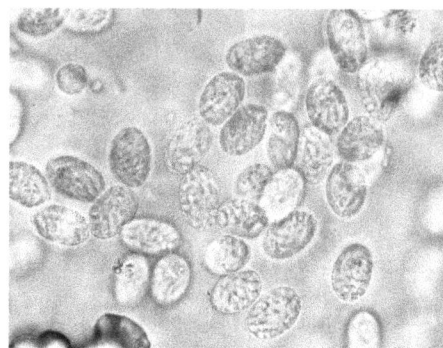

FIGURE 1: Sporocysts of *Klossiella equi* found on centrifugal flotation of urine with Sheather's sugar solution (1.27 sp. g.).

wave mouth and bilateral diastemata between the upper fourth premolars (108, 208) and first molars (109, 209), as well as the presence of periodontal disease.

The findings of hyperglycemia, glucosuria, and evidence of chronic infections (sinusitis and hematuria) in a >7-year old horse are consistent with pituitary pars intermedia dysfunction (PPID) [11] and testing recommended. Although the dexamethasone suppression test (DST) is the most widely accepted and recommended test for the diagnosis of PPID in horses, the owners declined this procedure but did consent to resting ACTH concentration. Determination of the resting ACTH level is considered to be a good alternative to the DST when the latter is inconclusive or not an option [11]. A blood sample was collected which showed baseline endogenous ACTH level to be elevated (63 pg/mL reference range 18–25 pg/mL), a finding consistent with PPID [11]. Recommendations were made regarding the treatment of the dental abnormalities, the sinusitis, the presumed PPID, and the *K. equi* infection. The owners elected to pursue medical therapy consisting of administration of a nonsteroidal anti-inflammatory drug (phenylbutazone, 4.4 mg/kg PO once daily for 3 days, followed by 2.2 mg/kg PO once daily for 10 days), an antibiotic (sulfadiazine/trimethoprim, 30 mg/kg PO twice daily for 2 weeks), as well as an antiprotozoal agent (pyrimethamine, 1 mg/kg PO once daily for 2 weeks). The horse was discharged from the VTH with a guarded prognosis.

Over the next several months, follow-up reports by the referring veterinarian indicated that the horse did well on the treatment with improvement in appetite and resolution of the macroscopic hematuria. However, approximately 1 year after the initial evaluation at the VTH, the horse developed bilateral facial swelling. In addition, a focal area of skin necrosis and swelling developed over the right mandible that drained mucopurulent exudate. Antibiotic treatment by the referring veterinarian resulted in improvement in clinical signs; however, as complete resolution was not achieved, the owners elected to euthanize the horse. The carcass of the animal was submitted to the CSU Veterinary Diagnostic Laboratory for necropsy.

Gross necropsy revealed firm, bilateral swelling of the maxillary sinuses and a focal area of erosion on the right

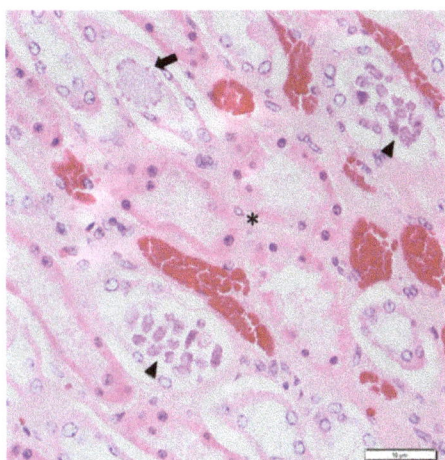

FIGURE 2: Multiple stages of *Klossiella equi* are found multifocally expanding tubular epithelial cells (schizont, arrow; sporocysts, arrowheads). Occasional tubular necrosis is present (asterick). (HE).

mandible. Subcutaneous tissue in this area was hyperemic and swollen but a draining tract could not be identified. Examination of the teeth showed multiple periodontal fistulas with extension into the maxillary sinuses. There was severe bilateral maxillary sinus impaction with abundant feed material and purulent exudate and chronic bilateral suppurative sinusitis of the frontal sinuses. The lungs showed focally extensive chronic fibrinous sclerosing bronchopneumonia. The pituitary gland was approximately 2.5–3 times its normal size, with a focal nodular area of hemorrhage ($\sim$1.5 cm diameter) and histologic features consistent with an adenoma of the pars intermedia. There was gross and histologic evidence of compression of the pars distalis and the overlying brain stem.

Grossly, the kidneys were normal in appearance; however, multiple developmental stages consistent with *K. equi* were found within the tubular epithelium (Figure 2). There was occasional scattered tubular ectasia and/or tubular necrosis, which was sometimes associated with the presence of parasites. There were also occasional small interstitial lymphoplasmacytic inflammatory infiltrates with rare interstitial fibroplasia, consistent with mild, chronic interstitial nephritis. Urine was not present in the bladder; thus, evaluation for sporocyst shedding could not be done.

## 3. Discussion

Postmortem examination of this horse confirmed the presence of an adenoma of the pars intermedia of the pituitary gland, supporting the presumed diagnosis of PPID made one year prior. PPID is a chronic disease of aged horses [11]. Typical clinical signs include hirsutism, hyperhidrosis, muscle loss, chronic or recurrent laminitis, chronic infections, delayed wound healing, and possibly polyuria/polydipsia. Commonly observed infections include chronic respiratory tract infections, sinusitis, skin diseases, and hoof abscesses. Recently, an increased susceptibility to endoparasites (i.e.,

small strongyles), resulting from impairment of the immune system, has been suggested [12]. Likewise, a relationship between severity of infection with *K. equi* and impaired immune function has been proposed [4, 5, 7] which is consistent with the findings of the present case.

It has been suggested that infections with *K. equi* would likely be self-limiting [7]. However, with evidence of infection spanning a year in the present case, it appears klossiellosis can be chronic in nature, at least in animals with impaired immune function. Whether this represents long-term infection or multiple reinfection events cannot be determined at this time.

The clinical sign primarily responsible for the initial referral to the VTH was unresolving hematuria despite antibiotic treatment for a presumed urinary tract infection. Hematuria has rarely been reported in *K. equi* infections [10]; however, it seems reasonable that hematuria could be a result of the epithelial cell damage caused by developing parasites.

It appears that equids with PPID or other immunosuppressive disorders are at a higher risk of chronic klossiellosis, which should be considered when evaluating these animals. Ante mortem diagnosis of klossiellosis depends on the detection of sporocysts in urine, which can be problematic. Sporocysts do not sediment readily in undiluted urine and flotation in salt solutions results in rupture of the sporocysts [7]. In the present case, sporocysts were successfully concentrated from undiluted urine by flotation with Sheather's sugar solution (1.27 sp. g.). Thus, it is suggested that sedimentation of diluted urine sample [7] or centrifugal flotation in sugar (present case) be performed when attempting to detect *K. equi* sporocysts in urine.

## Conflict of Interests

The authors declare that they have no conflict of interests.

## Acknowledgments

The authors wish to thank David Manuelito for assitance with case management during the initial hospital stay; they also thank the staff of both the Clinical Pathology Laboratory and the Veterinary Diagnostic Laboratory at the College of Veterinary Medicine and Biomedical Sciences for providing laboratory findings.

## References

[1] H. A. Hartman, "The protozoan parasite, Klossiella equi, in the Mexican burro," *American Journal of Veterinary Research*, vol. 22, pp. 1126–1128, 1961.

[2] K. S. Todd, H. S. Gosser, and D. P. Hamilton, "*Klossiella equi* Baumann, 1946 (Sporozoa: Eucoccidiorida) from an Illinois horse," *Veterinary Medicine/Small Animal Clinician*, vol. 72, no. 3, pp. 443–448, 1977.

[3] R. J. Austin and K. H. Dies, "*Klossiella equi* in the kidneys of a horse," *Canadian Veterinary Journal*, vol. 22, no. 5, pp. 159–161, 1981.

[4] C. R. Reinemeyer, R. M. Jacobs, and G. N. Spurlock, "A coccidial sporocyst in equine urine," *Journal of the American*

*Veterinary Medical Association*, vol. 182, no. 11, pp. 1250–1251, 1983.

[5] W. I. Anderson, C. A. Picut, and M. E. Georgi, "*Klossiella equi* induced tubular nephrosis and interstitial nephritis in a pony," *Journal of Comparative Pathology*, vol. 98, no. 3, pp. 363–366, 1988.

[6] D. N. R. Karanja, T. A. Ngatia, and J. G. Wandera, "Donkey klossiellosis in Kenya," *Veterinary Parasitology*, vol. 59, no. 1, pp. 1–5, 1995.

[7] G. P. Reppas and G. H. Collins, "*Klossiella equi* infection in horses; sporocyst stage identified in urine," *Australian Veterinary Journal*, vol. 72, no. 8, pp. 316–318, 1995.

[8] W. K. Suedmeyer, E. Restis, and B. T. Beerntsen, "*Klossiella equi* infection in a Hartmann's Mountain zebra (*Equus zebra hartmannae*)," *Journal of Zoo and Wildlife Medicine*, vol. 37, no. 3, pp. 420–423, 2006.

[9] J. M. Vetterling and D. E. Thompson, "*Klossiella equi* Baumann, 1946 (Sporozoa: Eucoccidia: Adeleina) from equids," *Journal of Parasitology*, vol. 58, no. 3, pp. 589–594, 1972.

[10] P. K. Gathumbi, V. Varma, and C. W. Wells, "Pathological and ultrastructural features of *Equine Klossiellosis*," *The Kenya Veterinarian*, vol. 21, pp. 45–48, 2001.

[11] D. McFarlane and R. E. Toribio, "Pituitary pars intermedia dysfunction (equine cushing's disease)," in *Equine Internal Medicine*, S. M. Reed, W. M. Bayly, and D.C. Sellon, Eds., pp. 1262–1270, Elsevier, St. Louis, Mo, USA, 3rd edition, 2010.

[12] D. McFarlane, G. M. Hale, E. M. Johnson, and L. K. Maxwell, "Fecal egg counts after anthelmintic administration to aged horses and horses with pituitary pars intermedia dysfunction," *Journal of the American Veterinary Medical Association*, vol. 236, no. 3, pp. 330–334, 2010.

# 7

# Persistent Hypercalcemia and Hyperparathyroidism in a Horse

**Claudia Cruz Villagrán,[1] Nicholas Frank,[1] James Schumacher,[1] and Danielle Reel[2]**

[1] Department of Large Animal Clinical Sciences, University of Tennessee College of Veterinary Medicine, 2407 River Drive, Knoxville, TN 37996, USA
[2] Department of Biomedical and Diagnostic Sciences, University of Tennessee College of Veterinary Medicine, 2407 River Drive, Knoxville, TN 37996, USA

Correspondence should be addressed to Claudia Cruz Villagrán; ccruz@utk.edu

Academic Editor: Lysimachos G. Papazoglou

A 27-year-old, American Quarter Horse gelding was evaluated for anorexia, lethargy, a swelling on the right, cranial aspect of the neck, and signs of esophageal obstruction. Serum biochemical analyses revealed hypophosphatemia, total and ionized hypercalcemia, and hemoconcentration. Sonographic examination of the neck revealed a 1.7 cm diameter mass within the right lobe of the thyroid. The serum concentration of intact parathyroid hormone (iPTH) was increased. The right lobe of the thyroid was excised with the horse sedated. The mass within that lobe was determined, by histological examination, to be a parathyroid adenoma. Despite excision of the mass, serial blood analyses revealed persistent hypercalcemia, hypophosphatemia, and increased iPTH. Anorexia and lethargy resolved, and follow-up communication with the owner and referring veterinarian one year later indicated that the horse was clinically stable.

## 1. Case Presentation

A 27-year-old, 500 kg, American Quarter Horse gelding, kept as a pet, was presented to the University of Tennessee Veterinary Medical Center with signs of esophageal obstruction for 12 hours, including hypersalivation, frequent stretching of the neck, and signs of discomfort. The horse, along with other pasture mates, had been treated for cantharidin toxicity 2 years previously. It was housed in a stall and had free access to pasture. Its diet consisted of orchard grass hay provided *ad libitum*, 800 g oats, and 300 g complete pelleted feed containing 0.8% calcium (% of dry matter), 0.4% phosphorus, and 14% crude protein, fed twice daily. The horse had been vaccinated and dewormed regularly by the referring veterinarian.

When presented, the horse was dull, tachycardic (80 bpm), and dehydrated (6% on the basis of tacky mucosal membranes). Respiratory rate and temperature were normal. The packed cell volume was 0.48 L/L (reference interval, 0.28–0.44 L/L), and total solids were 8.2 g/dL (range, 6–8 g/dL) when measured with a refractometer. The horse's body condition score was 4/9 [1]. No cardiac arrhythmias,

murmurs, or abnormal lung sounds were auscultated. No abnormalities were detected during palpation of abdominal viscera performed *per rectum*, and a nasogastric tube was inserted into the stomach without resistance. The absence of two maxillary cheek teeth and the presence of malocclusion and mild enamel points were observed during examination of the horse's oral cavity, but no evidence of severe periodontal disease was found. Palpation of the neck revealed a firm, mobile, subcutaneous mass in the right, cranial aspect of the neck, thought to be the right lobe of the thyroid gland.

The primary problems identified included lethargy, tachycardia, dehydration, poor dentition, and a mass on the neck. Causes of lethargy considered were inflammation, electrolyte imbalance, and neurologic, renal, GI, respiratory, and endocrine disease. The lethargy and anorexia were most likely related to the underlying disease. Causes of tachycardia considered were pain, stress, endotoxemia, electrolyte and metabolic imbalances, hypovolemia, anemia, endotoxemia, and cardiopathy. Causes of dehydration considered were profuse sweating, decreased water intake, renal failure, hemorrhage, and GI disease. Although esophageal obstruction was the presenting complaint, this problem had resolved before or

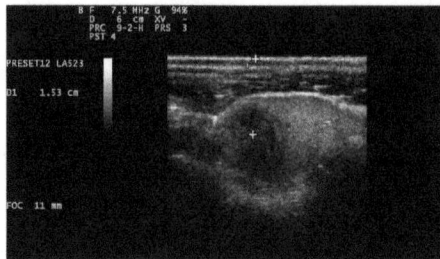

FIGURE 1: Transverse ultrasonographic image of the right lobe of the thyroid gland showing a 1.7 cm diameter, hypoechoic, circular mass within the thyroid gland. Image obtained with a 7.5 MHz, linear probe.

soon after arrival and was attributed to poor dentition. At this point, further diagnostic tests were conducted to determine the cause of the identified problems.

Abnormalities on CBC and plasma biochemical analyses included a mature ($10.92 \times 10^3/\mu L$; reference interval, $2.6$–$5.5 \times 10^3/\mu L$) and immature ($0.94 \times 10^3/\mu L$; $0$–$0.1 \times 10^3/\mu L$) neutrophilia without toxic changes, slightly increased plasma concentration of creatinine (2.1 mg/dL; 0.9–1.7 mg/dL), hypophosphatemia (1.0 mg/dL; 1.9–4.1 mg/dL), total hypercalcemia (18.4 mg/dL; 11.3–13.2 mg/dL), and ionized hypercalcemia (10.5 mg/dL; 5–7 mg/dL). Results of a urine dipstick test on a free-catch urine sample were normal. The horse was administered polyionic fluid therapy intravenously by continuous rate infusion at 60 mL/kg/day for 2 days after first administering a 10-L bolus.

On day 2, urine obtained through a urinary catheter inserted aseptically into the bladder had a specific gravity of 1.025. Fluid therapy was discontinued at the end of day 2 because the horse was euhydrated (PCV, 0.36 L/L; TS, 7 g/dL) and because the horse's urine had a normal specific gravity. Results of urinalysis were normal. Ultrasonographic examination of the mass on the neck revealed a 1.7 cm diameter, hypoechoic, circular mass of homogeneous density contained within the right lobe of the thyroid gland (Figure 1). The left lobe of the thyroid gland had a normal appearance. No ultrasonographic abnormalities were observed during thoracic, transabdominal, and transrectal examinations. The left kidney appeared to be normal in size when it was palpated *per rectum*, and both kidneys appeared to be normal in size, based on their ultrasonographic appearance. An attempt to obtain an ultrasound-guided, fine-needle aspirate of the mass contained within the right lobe of the thyroid gland was unsuccessful. During radiographic examination of the skull, the density of the dental alveoli appeared to be normal, and no signs of apical dental infection were observed. No abnormalities were observed during radiographic examination of the thorax. Administration of omeprazole (1 mg/kg, PO, q24 h) was initiated after mild hyperemia of the nonglandular mucosa of the stomach was observed during gastroscopy. Ionized serum calcium, measured daily, remained increased. The serum concentration of iPTH (14.1 pmol/L; reference < 4 pmol/L [2]. Diagnostic Center for Population and Animal Health laboratory, Michigan State University) was increased, and the serum concentration of 1,25-di-hydroxyvitamin

$D_3$ was within normal range (17 nmol/L; 10–25 nmol/L). Parathyroid hormone-related protein (PTHrP) could not be measured because the immunoassay reagent was not available at the time.

On day 3, calculation of fractional clearance of electrolytes in the urine revealed low fractional clearance of calcium (0.55%; 5.3–14.5%), which was attributed to increased reabsorption of calcium from the renal tubules in response to increased serum concentration of PTH. Fractional clearance of sodium (0.36%; reference < 1%) and phosphorous (0.9%; reference < 1%) was normal [3]. Serum urea nitrogen (12 mg/dL) and creatinine (1.9 mg/dL) concentrations had decreased, suggesting that the azotemia present when the horse was presented was prerenal. Although these analyses did not support a diagnosis of glomerular or tubular renal failure, a certain degree of renal insufficiency was still considered to be a possible cause of the horse's anorexia given its previous exposure to cantharidin. Administration of trimethoprim-sulfamethoxazole (20 mg/kg PO q12 h) was initiated, after the horse received extensive dental work because of concerns that this dental work may have caused bacteria to shed into the circulation and also because of concerns that the horse may have aspirated feed during the episode of choke.

The horse was determined to be suffering from primary hyperparathyroidism on the basis of the increased serum iPTH concentration, hypercalcemia, hypophosphatemia, low fractional clearance of calcium, clinical signs, and ultrasonographic findings. Lethargy persisted, but appetite and water consumption improved. The horse was discharged on day 4, and the owner was instructed to continue administering omeprazole (1 mg/kg, PO q24 h) for 4 days and trimethoprim-sulfamethoxazole (20 mg/kg, PO, q12 h) for 5 days.

Ten days after discharge, the horse was readmitted to undergo excision of the right lobe of the thyroid gland and the suspected parathyroid adenoma contained within it. The horse had a lower body condition score (3/9) and appeared dull. Results of serum biochemical analyses revealed total (17 mg/dL; 11.3–13.2 mg/dL) and ionized hypercalcemia (9.64 mg/dL; 5–7 mg/dL), hypophosphatemia (1.7 mg/dL; 1.9–4.1 mg/dL), and a mild hypertriglyceridemia (88 mg/dL; 10–77 mg/dL) consistent with a negative energy balance and release of lipids into the circulation. Results of PCV (0.48 L/L) and TS (7 g/dL) indicated that the horse was euhydrated. Serum urea nitrogen (15 mg/dL) and creatinine (2 mg/dL) remained stable.

To remove the right lobe of the thyroid with the horse standing, the horse was sedated with detomidine hydrochloride (0.02 mg/kg, IV) and butorphanol tartrate (0.01 mg/kg, IV). The right cranial portion of the neck was prepared for aseptic surgery, and the proposed site of incision over the palpable right lobe of the thyroid was desensitized by subcutaneous injection of 2% mepivacaine hydrochloride. A 5 cm, longitudinal, cutaneous incision was created over the right lobe of the thyroid gland, which was exposed by sharply dividing the overlying *cutaneous colli* muscle. Traction was placed on the gland with a suture of 0 polypropylene inserted through the gland. The lobe was separated from surrounding

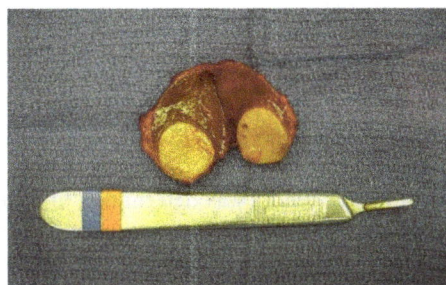

FIGURE 2: Right thyroid lobe excised from the horse. Note the circular parathyroid adenoma.

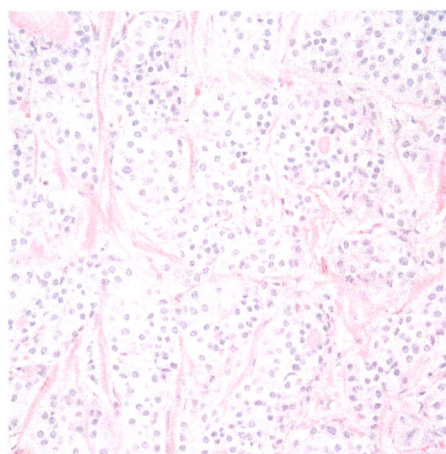

FIGURE 3: Histologic section of neoplasm within the right thyroid lobe excised from the horse. Hematoxylin and eosin, 20x.

fascia and removed after the thyroid artery and vein at the cranial aspect of the gland were ligated with 2-0 polydioxanone sutures and divided. The cutaneous colli muscle and subcutaneous tissue were apposed separately with 2-0 polydioxanone suture placed in a simple-continuous pattern, and the cutaneous incision was closed with staples. The horse was administered firocoxib (0.27 mg/kg, IV, loading dose; 0.09 mg/kg, IV, q24 h for subsequent doses) for 3 days. Staples were removed 12 days after surgery.

Gross examination of the right lobe of the thyroid gland revealed a circular, well-delineated, 1.7 cm diameter, white mass (Figure 2). Polygonal to cuboidal cells arranged in packets with fine, fibrovascular stroma and low mitotic activity were observed during histologic examination of the mass (Figure 3). The nuclei of these cells had stippled chromatin with moderate amounts of pale, foamy to granular cytoplasm. The immunohistochemical antibody for PTH was ineffective on the parathyroid gland tissue from this horse, but the neoplastic cells stained strongly for chromogranin A (Figure 4) and did not stain for calcitonin or thyroglobulin. These findings confirmed the presence of a neuroendocrine tumor, most likely a parathyroid adenoma based on the clinical signs and high concentrations of iPTH and ionized calcium. The tissue surrounding the mass was compressed thyroid tissue.

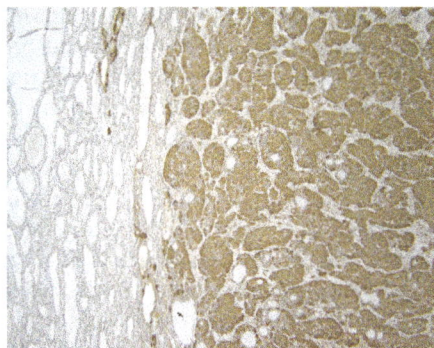

FIGURE 4: Chromogranin A immunostain on parathyroid tissue. There is diffuse strong cytoplasmic staining of the neoplastic cells. Adjacent thyroid follicles are negative for immunostaining of chromogranin A.

Ten days after partial thyroidectomy, the serum concentrations of iPTH (10.3 pmol/L; reference < 4 pmol/L) and ionized calcium (9.64 mg/dL; 5–7 mg/dL) remained increased. The horse's clinical appearance and demeanor were normal, and its appetite gradually increased. The horse was discharged 19 days after surgery. The owner was instructed to observe the horse for signs of synchronous diaphragmatic flutter in case the horse's serum concentration of calcium decreased leading to this complication. Bags containing 50 g of calcium carbonate powder (limestone) were provided to the owner to administer orally to the horse if this complication developed.

When the horse was examined 30 days after discharge, its serum concentrations of iPTH (23.9 pmol/L; reference < 4 pmol/L) and ionized calcium (8.28 mg/dL; 5–7 mg/dL) remained increased, suggesting the presence of other neoplastic or hyperplastic parathyroid glands or MEN-like syndrome [4]. At 60 days after discharge, serum concentrations of thyroid hormones, total $T_3$ and $T_4$, were decreased from concentrations considered to be normal ($T_3$, 0.18 ng/L; reference, 0.5–1.5 ng/L and $T_4$, <1.7 ng/L; 3.65–26 ng/L), and ionized hypercalcemia was still present (9.8 mg/dL; 5–7 mg/dL). Serum urea nitrogen (16 mg/dL) and creatinine (2.1 mg/dL) had remained stable. After cautioning the owner about the danger of inducing hypovolemia, renal failure, and shock by administering furosemide to a dehydrated horse, the owner was instructed to administer furosemide for 14 days (0.5 mg/kg, PO q12 h) to promote diuresis and calciuresis and to supplement the horse's diet with levothyroxine sodium (24 mg total, PO, q24h; Thyro-L, Vet-A-Mix, Inc., Shenandoah, IA) indefinitely.

The owner indicated during a telephone conversation, conducted one year after the presumed parathyroid adenoma and right lobe of the thyroid gland were removed, that the horse's appetite and attitude were normal. Intact PTH and concentrations of electrolytes in the serum were not measured.

## 2. Discussion

Primary hyperparathyroidism is a rare disease of the horse caused by parathyroid neoplasia or hyperplasia [5, 6]. Other causes of increased concentration of iPTH include nutritional and renal secondary hyperparathyroidism and production of PTHrP from MEN [2, 6–8]. PTH is closely involved in calcium homeostasis, and its secretion from the chief cells of the parathyroid glands is regulated by a negative feedback mechanism that involves serum concentrations of calcium, PTH, and 1,25-di-hydroxyvitamin D [2]. Serum concentrations of magnesium and PTH are also codependent but in a more complex manner [9]. The effects of PTH on various target cells include enhanced reabsorption of calcium by the renal tubules, increased absorption of calcium from the small intestine, decreased reabsorption and increased excretion of phosphorous from the renal tubules, increased excretion of phosphorus from the salivary glands, and increased synthesis of 1,25-di-hydroxyvitamin D by the kidney [2, 6]. The equine parathyroid glands, usually 1 or sometimes 2 on each side of the neck, are located adjacent to or within each lobe of the thyroid gland, but their number and location vary among horses [10, 11]. In humans, single or multiple adenomas can arise in each parathyroid gland, and multiple parathyroid glands can be affected [12].

Differential diagnoses for hypercalcemia in the horse include chronic renal failure, hypervitaminosis D, nutritional secondary hyperparathyroidism (including consumption of oxalates in forage), primary hyperparathyroidism, hypercalcemia of malignancy, and multiple endocrine neoplasia-(MEN-) like syndrome [4–6, 13, 14]. The clinical history and laboratory and ultrasonographic findings made hypervitaminosis D, chronic renal failure, and nutritional secondary hyperparathyroidism less likely to be the cause of this horse's hypercalcemia.

Malignant neoplasms secrete an exaggerated amount of PTHrP, which can imitate several functions of PTH due to molecular similarities between these 2 peptides (i.e., 6 of the first 7 amino acids are identical between them) [15]. Dogs and cats suffering from hypercalcemia of malignancy have a high serum concentration of PTHrP, but their serum concentration of iPTH is normal or low, unless the malignancy is a functional parathyroid adenocarcinoma [8]. Despite our inability to rule out hypercalcemia due to malignancy elsewhere in this horse, the persistently high iPTH and the improvement on clinical signs even after a year later do not support a diagnosis of hypercalcemia caused by malignancy. Primary hyperparathyroidism and MEN-like syndrome remained as likely causes for the hypercalcemia.

Chronic renal failure was initially considered as a cause of hypercalcemia in this case because the horse had been exposed to cantharidin 2 years previously. Cantharidin irritates the gastrointestinal and urinary tracts directly and can result in colic, renal failure, shock, and death [16]. Fractional excretion of sodium, an indicator of renal tubular function, was found to be normal. Other tests of renal function were not performed, but serum urea nitrogen and creatinine concentrations decreased in response to fluid therapy and remained constant after its discontinuation.

Clinical signs of hyperparathyroidism in horses include lethargy, generalized weakness, lameness, and enlarged facial bones [5, 17–19]. Weakness is attributed to increased extracellular calcium because calcium concentration plays a role in the onset of action potentials, primarily in neurons and smooth and cardiac myocytes. Hypercalcemia raises the resting membrane potential causing, in humans, clinical manifestations of depression of the central and peripheral nervous system, anorexia, muscular weakness, and constipation [20, 21].

The horse in this report was determined to have hypercalcemia and hyperparathyroidism 30 days after surgery. The horse remained anorexic and dull for several days after surgery, and this was attributed to persistent hypercalcemia [17, 19]. We can find no reports describing the amount of time required for calcium concentrations to return to normal in horses after a functional parathyroid adenoma is removed. Humans that have had one or more parathyroid glands removed are expected to experience a decrease in the concentration of serum calcium after 4 days, and dogs undergoing a similar procedure are expected to show a similar decrease after 7 days [22, 23]. Persistent hypercalcemia can also occur after one or more parathyroid glands of dogs are removed, and when this occurs, the presence of ectopic, active parathyroid tissue, hyperplasia of parathyroid tissue, or an adenoma of one or more of the remaining parathyroid glands is suspected [8, 22].

Radiographic assessment of the skull revealed no resorption of facial or alveolar bone, a predominant sign of *osteodystrophia fibrosa*, which can result from hyperparathyroidism. The long bones of this horse were not radiographed to detect osteopenia because of economic reasons. Although osteopenia caused by hyperparathyroidism preferentially affects facial bones, other bones could have been affected. The clinician should also be aware of the timing between detection of hyperparathyroidism and radiological assessment.

The diagnosis of primary hyperparathyroidism in this horse was based on clinical signs, the presence of elevated serum concentrations of iPTH and total and ionized calcium, hypophosphatemia, and low fractional excretion of calcium. Hypophosphatemia with hyperphosphaturia is typical of primary hyperparathyroidism. PTH prevents the reabsorption of phosphorus from the brush border membrane of the proximal tubule by inhibiting the sodium-phosphate cotransporter, resulting in enhanced renal phosphorus excretion [24]. With a low phosphorus intake, however, the body is able to maximize phosphorus conservation by being resistant to the action of PTH in the kidney [25]. Renal phosphorus excretion in this horse was normal. Our most logical explanation for the hypophosphatemia is that the horse had decreased intake of phosphorus due to prolonged anorexia, but phosphorus was maximally conserved in the face of hyperparathyroidism by mechanisms that enhanced renal reabsorption of phosphorus, attenuating the phosphaturic action of PTH. Hyperphosphaturia would possibly have been detected if the horse had had a normal appetite at the time that fractional excretion of electrolytes was examined.

Histological and immunohistochemical analyses of the tissue excised from the horse contrasted. The absence of staining for calcitonin and thyroglobulin ruled out thyroid neoplasia. The presence of strong, diffuse staining for chromogranin A indicated that the mass was of neuroendocrine origin, suggesting parathyroid origin, based on clinical signs and an increased concentration of iPTH [26]. We could not confirm this, however, because the monoclonal rat anti-human PTH antibody did not stain the mass. Possibilities for lack of staining may include species-specific issues and the fact that the tumour was originated from tissue other than a parathyroid gland.

Treatment of horses for primary hyperparathyroidism requires excision of the neoplastic parathyroid gland. Excision is sometimes challenging because the location and number of parathyroid glands vary among horses, making locating and removing the affected gland or glands difficult [5, 18, 19]. Preoperative scintigraphy may help locate parathyroid tissue [27]. In a retrospective study of dogs suffering from hyperparathyroidism, parathyroidectomy of the affected glands, ultrasound-guided, percutaneous, radiofrequency-induced heat ablation, or chemical ablation using ethanol resulted in a 94, 90, and 72% success rate, respectively, in resolving hypercalcemia [22, 28].

Calcimimetic drugs, which act as activators of the calcium-sensing receptors in the parathyroid gland and other tissues, thereby reducing the release of PTH, are used to treat humans for hyperparathyroidism secondary to chronic kidney disease [17, 23]. Additionally, bisphosphonates are administered to prevent bone resorption and to lower the serum concentration of calcium [23]. We can find no reports describing the use of calcimimetic or bisphosphonate drugs to treat horses for hyperparathyroidism, but treatment with these drugs might prevent bone resorption caused by it. Regardless, because the horse in this report had no signs of excessive resorption of the bone, we administered neither of these medications.

Levothyroxine sodium was administered after the concentrations of serum thyroid hormones were found to be low 60 days after the right lobe of the thyroid gland was excised. Levothyroxine sodium has been administered to humans suffering from hypothyroidism because it returns the concentrations of thyroid hormones to normal. Administering levothyroxine sodium to healthy horses for 48 weeks increased the total concentration of $T_4$ without causing adverse effects on health [29]. No changes to the diet of this horse were recommended because the phosphorous-calcium ratio of the diet was appropriate.

Removing the presumed parathyroid adenoma within the right lobe of the thyroid gland failed to resolve the hypercalcemia in this horse, and iPTH concentrations were still increased when a follow-up examination was performed one month after surgery. We suspected, therefore, that multiple parathyroid adenomas were present in this horse. MEN-like syndrome was also possible. The absence of clinical signs associated with hyperparathyroidism one month after surgery was also difficult to explain. Absence of clinical signs associated with hyperparathyroidism after excision of neoplastic parathyroid tissue has been reported previously in a mule [19] and in humans [23]. We assumed the horse had absence of clinical signs of disease because it had adapted to the hypercalcemia or because it had responded to the treatments administered at our hospital. Humans can develop high serum concentrations of calcium associated with asymptomatic primary hyperparathyroidism, and excision of the

affected gland is delayed until the concentration of calcium becomes so high that it results in symptoms by exerting negative effects on neurological, renal, and musculoskeletal functions [23].

This report describes the clinical signs and diagnosis of primary hyperparathyroidism, detection of a neuroendocrine tumour of unknown origin within the thyroid gland, and surgical management of the horse. A unique aspect of this case is the resolution of clinical signs associated with hyperparathyroidism after surgery, despite the persistence of increased concentrations of serum iPTH and iCa. Presence of a second parathyroid adenoma or MEN-like syndrome was highly suspected. Additional diagnostic and treatment options were declined by the owner because clinical signs of hyperparathyroidism resolved.

## Conflict of Interests

The authors declare that there is no conflict of interests regarding the publication of this paper.

## References

[1] D. R. Henneke, G. D. Potter, J. L. Kreider, and B. F. Yeates, "Relationship between condition score, physical measurements and body fat percentage in mares," *Equine veterinary journal*, vol. 15, no. 4, pp. 371–372, 1983.

[2] R. E. Toribio, "Disorders of the endocrine system," in *Equine Internal Medicine*, S. M. Reed, W. M. Bayly, and D. Sellon, Eds., pp. 1248–1311, WB Saunders, Philadelphia, Pa, USA, 3rd edition, 2009.

[3] J. E. Cunilleras, "Abnormalities of body fluids and electrolytes in equine athletes," in *Equine Sports Medicine and Surgery*, vol. 914, Saunders, Philadelphia, Pa, USA, 2004.

[4] S. E. Germann, M. Rütten, S. B. Derungs, and K. Feige, "Multiple endocrine neoplasia-like syndrome in a horse," *Veterinary Record*, vol. 159, no. 16, pp. 530–532, 2006.

[5] N. Frank, J. F. Hawkins, L. L. Couëtil, and J. T. Raymond, "Primary hyperparathyroidism with osteodystrophia fibrosa of the facial bones in a pony," *Journal of the American Veterinary Medical Association*, vol. 212, no. 1, pp. 84–86, 1998.

[6] J. R. Peauroi, D. J. Fisher, F. C. Mohr, and S. L. Vivrette, "Primary hyperparathyroidism caused by a functional parathyroid adenoma in a horse," *Journal of the American Veterinary Medical Association*, vol. 212, no. 12, pp. 1915–1918, 1998.

[7] N. A. Benders, K. Junker, T. Wensing, T. S. G. A. M. van den Ingh, and J. H. van der Kolk, "Diagnosis of secondary hyperparathyroidism in a pony using intact parathyroid hormone radioimmunoassay," *Veterinary Record*, vol. 149, no. 6, pp. 185–187, 2001.

[8] P. J. Bergman, "Paraneoplastic hypercalcemia," *Topics in Companion Animal Medicine*, vol. 27, no. 4, pp. 156–158, 2012.

[9] T. Vetter and M. J. Lohse, "Magnesium and the parathyroid," *Current Opinion in Nephrology and Hypertension*, vol. 11, no. 4, pp. 403–410, 2002.

[10] L. Krook and J. E. Lowe, "Nutritional secondary hyperparathyroidism in the horse, with a description of the normal anatomy of the normal equine parathyroid gland," *Veterinary Pathology*, supplement 1, pp. 1–98, 1964.

[11] International Committee on Veterinary Gross Anatomy Nomenclature, "Glandulae endocrinae," in *Nomina Anatomica Veterinaria*, pp. 64–65, Editorial Committee, 5th edition, 2012.

[12] N. W. Thompson, F. E. Eckhauser, and J. K. Harness, "The anatomy of primary hyperparathyroidism," *Surgery*, vol. 92, no. 5, pp. 814–821, 1982.

[13] M. H. Barton, P. Sharma, B. E. LeRoy, and E. W. Howerth, "Hypercalcomia hypercalcemia and high serum parathyroid hormone-related protein concentration in a horse with multiple myeloma," *Journal of the American Veterinary Medical Association*, vol. 225, no. 3, pp. 409–376, 2004.

[14] R. E. Toribio, C. W. Kohn, K. M. Rourke, A. L. Levine, and T. J. Rosol, "Effects of hypercalcemia on serum concentrations of magnesium, potassium, and phosphate and urinary excretion of electrolytes in horses," *The American Journal of Veterinary Research*, vol. 68, no. 5, pp. 543–554, 2007.

[15] K.-D. Schlüter, "PTH and PTHrP: similar structures but different functions," *News in Physiological Sciences*, vol. 14, no. 6, pp. 243–248, 1999.

[16] R. G. Helman and W. C. Edwards, "Clinical features of blister beetle poisoning in equids: 70 cases (1983–1996)," *Journal of the American Veterinary Medical Association*, vol. 211, no. 8, pp. 1018–1021, 1997.

[17] A. A. Khan, "Medical management of primary hyperparathyroidism," *Journal of Clinical Densitometry*, vol. 16, no. 1, pp. 60–63, 2013.

[18] J. R. Joyce, K. R. Pierce, W. M. Romane, and J. M. Baker, "Clinical study of nutritional secondary hyperparathyroidism in horses," *Journal of the American Veterinary Medical Association*, vol. 158, no. 12, pp. 2033–2042, 1971.

[19] D. Wong, B. Sponseller, K. Miles, T. Butt, and K. Kersh, "Failure of technetium Tc 99m sestamibi scanning to detect abnormal parathyroid tissue in a horse and a mule with primary hyperparathyroidism," *Journal of Veterinary Internal Medicine*, vol. 18, pp. 589–593, 2004.

[20] E. M. Brown and R. J. Macleod, "Extracellular calcium sensing and extracellular calcium signaling," *Physiological Reviews*, vol. 81, no. 1, pp. 239–297, 2001.

[21] J. E. Hall, "Parathyroid hormone, calcitonin, calcium and phosphate metabolism, vitamin D, bone and teeth," in *Guyton and Hall Textbook of Medical Physiology*, J. E. Hall, Ed., pp. 955–972, WB Saunders, Philadelphia, Pa, USA, 12th edition, 2011.

[22] R. W. Nelson, "Disorders of the parathyroid gland," in *Small Animal Internal Medicine*, R. W. Nelson and G. C. Couto, Eds., pp. 715–723, Mosby-Elsevier, 4th edition, 2009.

[23] J. E. Witteveen, S. van Thiel, J. A. Romijn, and N. A. Hamdy, "Hungry bone syndrome: still a challenge in the post-operative management of primary hyperparathyroidism: a systematic review of the literature," *European Journal of Endocrinology*, vol. 168, no. 3, pp. R45–53, 2013.

[24] H. Murer, A. Werner, S. Reshkin, F. Wuarin, and J. Biber, "Cellular mechanisms in proximal tubular reabsorption of inorganic phosphate," *The American Journal of Physiology—Cell Physiology*, vol. 260, no. 5, pp. C885–C899, 1991.

[25] T. J. Berndt, J. D. Pfeifer, F. G. Knox, S. A. Kempson, and T. P. Dousa, "Nicotinamide restores phosphaturic effect of PTH and calcitonin in phosphate deprivation," *The American Journal of Physiology*, vol. 242, no. 5, pp. F447–F452, 1982.

[26] L. Luts, A. Bergenfelz, J. Alumets, and F. Sundler, "Parathyroid function and histology in patients with parathyroid adenoma: correlation of clinical and morphologic findings," *World Journal of Surgery*, vol. 21, no. 5, pp. 553–563, 1997.

[27] J. E. Tomlinson, A. L. Johnson, M. W. Ross et al., "Successful detection and removal of a functional parathyroid adenoma in a pony using Technetium Tc 99m Sestamibi scintigraphy," *Journal of Veterinary Internal Medicine*, vol. 28, no. 2, 2014.

[28] L. Rasor, R. Pollard, and E. C. Feldman, "Retrospective evaluation of three treatment methods for primary hyperparathyroidism in dogs," *Journal of the American Animal Hospital Association*, vol. 43, no. 2, pp. 70–77, 2007.

[29] N. Frank, B. R. Buchanan, and S. B. Elliott, "Effects of long-term oral administration of levothyroxine sodium on serum thyroid hormone concentrations, clinicopathologicvariables, and echocardiographic measurements in healthy adult horses," *The American Journal of Veterinary Research*, vol. 69, no. 1, pp. 68–75, 2008.

# 8

# A Case Report of Avian Polyomavirus Infection in a Blue Fronted Parrot (*Amazona aestiva*) Associated with Anemia

**Natalia Azevedo Philadelpho, Marta B. Guimarães, and Antonio J. Piantino Ferreira**

*Department of Pathology, School of Veterinary Medicine, University of São Paulo, Avenida Prof. Orlando Marques de Paiva 87, 05508-900 São Paulo, SP, Brazil*

Correspondence should be addressed to Antonio J. Piantino Ferreira; ajpferr@usp.br

Academic Editor: Carlos Gutierrez

An adult Blue Fronted Amazon parrot (*A. aestiva*) presenting with emesis, apathy, undigested seed in feces, and severe anemia was treated for approximately 2 months. Upon radiographic examination, an enlarged kidney was the only alteration. PCR for avian *Bornavirus, Circovirus*, and Polyomavirus was performed for the feces and blood. The results were positive for APV in both samples and negative for the other viruses. After 6 months, the feces from the same animal were negative for APV. Because the animal was positive for APV in both the feces and the blood, it is likely that these clinical symptoms were due to Polyomavirus infection. Severe anemia is an unusual clinical sign of Polyomavirus, and this study aims to identify novel differential diagnostic criteria for the disease.

## 1. Introduction

The Polyomavirus, one of the most important viruses in psittacines, is a highly infectious virus [1], reaching almost 100% infection rates in indoor aviaries. The disease has been described in North America, Europe, South Africa, Asia, and Australia [2–4] and is more common in budgerigars (*Melopsittacus undulatus*), lovebirds (*Agapornis* sp.), ringnecks (*Psittacula krameri*), conures (*Aratinga* spp., *Nandayus nenday*, and *Pyrrhura* spp.), and macaws (*Ara* spp.) [4, 5]. However, the disease has also been described in passerines and Falconiformes [6, 7]. There are few reports in Amazon parrots worldwide and no description of APV in this species in Brazil. The aim of this report is to describe a possible clinical sign of APV in Amazon parrot.

## 2. Case Presentation

A Blue Fronted Amazon parrot (*A. aestiva*) aged 2 years and 4 months was presented at the Avian Clinic of the School of Veterinary Medicine and Animal Science of the University of São Paulo (FMVZ-USP) for emergency evaluation after three days of anorexia and apathy and one day of emesis. The bird was housed in a cage alone and was fed commercial pellet feed, sunflower seeds, fruits, and vegetables. On physical examination, the bird was in molt, with good pectoral muscle conformation, mild dehydration, and pale mucous membranes. Melena and polyuria were also observed. Treatment was initiated with enrofloxacin (IM 15 mg/kg Baytril 5%, Bayer), iron (20 mg/kg Ferrodex, Tortuga), vitamin B (3 mg/kg Vitamin B1, Labovet), and fluid (crystalloid solution 20 mL/kg, Equiplex).

The bird returned on day 3, with no improvement in its clinical condition. Undigested seeds and fat in the feces were observed; however, there was no blood present. Because the animal was dehydrated and possibly anemic, no blood work was performed. Radiographic examination revealed an enlarged kidney and mildly dilated crop (Figure 1). On the same day, feces samples were collected for polymerase chain reaction (PCR) for avian *Bornavirus, Circovirus*, and Polyomavirus. Due to the presence of fat in the feces, oral pancreatin (2 g/kg, compounded drug) and nystatin (300,000 IU/kg, Micostatin, Bristol) were prescribed.

There was no improvement on day 7, and the animal was anemic, dehydrated, dyspneic, and still presenting with emesis, delayed emptying of the crop, and undigested seeds

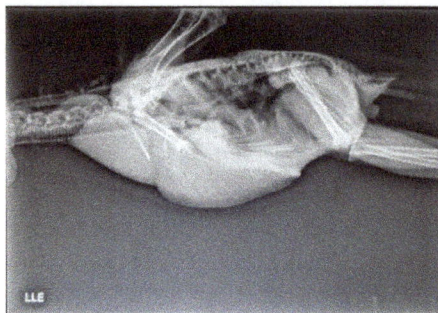

FIGURE 1: Radiographic image showing enlarged kidney and mildly dilated crop.

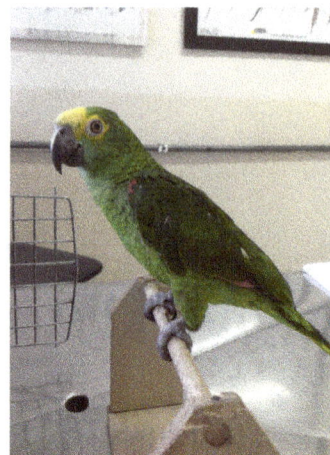

FIGURE 2: Blue Fronted Amazon parrot six months after the clinical presentation, with no clinical signs.

in the feces. For two days (days 8 and 9), the bird was unable to perch, staying at the bottom of the cage. The feces still had fat, but there was no blood. Because the animal was apathetic and anemic, a hematocrit test was performed, with a result of 33%. Thus, we administered IM metoclopramide (0.5 mg/kg, Noprosil, Isofarma) and fluid (crystalloid solution 20 mL/kg, Equiplex, and colloidal solution 10 mL/kg, Voluven).

The following day (day 10), the animal had another emesis episode and was brought to the clinic. The bird received enrofloxacin, nystatin, and food through a gavage needle for three days. At day 14, the bird was slightly more active, and blood was collected for complete blood work and a drop of blood was sent for viral testing (Bornavirus, Circovirus, and Polyomavirus). Emesis and undigested seeds in the feces were still present. Fluid therapy with colloidal solution was again performed and the bird was given sucralfate SID (25 mg/kg, Sucrafilm, Sigma Pharma), thymomodulin, an immunostimulant that modulates maturation and function of T-lymphocytes and enhances the function of mature lymphocytes (2 mg/kg, Leucogen, Aché), and vitamins. Hemogram results showed a severe nonregenerative, normocytic, normochromic anemia, with a hematocrit of 14% with discreet anisocytosis, polychromasia, and severe leucopenia, with no morphological alterations in the white blood cells. This anemia indicates decreased erythropoiesis. PCR results were positive for APV in the blood and feces and negative for Circovirus and PaBV, confirming an active Polyomavirus infection.

On day 20, the bird started eating, was more active, and had no episodes of emesis, although it presented movements similar to emesis. Enrofloxacin treatment and nystatin treatment were suspended, but metoclopramide, sucralfate, immunostimulant, and vitamins were maintained. After seven days, the animal returned with a better appetite and was more active. Nystatin, vitamin, and immunostimulant were administered for another 10 days.

One month after the initial presentation, the bird started to vocalize and had a normal appetite. A hematocrit was performed with a result of 51%, indicating the normalization of the hematological disorders. All medications were suspended, and the animal was discharged. After 6 months, the bird returned for a routine check-up (Figure 2). Feces were collected for PCR and were negative for APV.

## 3. Discussion

The Polyomavirus is a highly infectious psittacine virus [1], reaching almost 100% infection rates in indoor aviaries. The disease has been described in North America, Europe, South Africa, Asia, and Australia [2, 3] and is more common in budgerigars (Melopsittacus undulatus) [4], lovebirds (Agapornis sp.), ring-necks (Psittacula krameri), conures (Aratinga spp., Nandayus nenday, and Pyrrhura spp.), and macaws (Ara spp.) [5]. However, the disease has also been described in passerines [6] and Falconiformes [7].

There are few reports on Amazon parrots worldwide and no description of APV in this species in Brazil. Because clinical signs are not specific and are present in several differential diagnoses, investigation of Polyomavirus by the veterinarian is often neglected. However, there is also a reduced incidence of differential laboratory diagnosis of this disease compared with other viral infections in parrots. Thus, the prevalence of this disease in Brazil is unknown.

Clinical signs for APV are variable, depending on the species and the age. Death without any premonitory signs of the disease is reported in fledglings of various Psittaciformes [8], but abnormal feathers, skin discoloration, and abdominal distension are the most common clinical presentations [5, 9]. Other clinical signs include apathy, polyuria, diarrhea, dyspnea, weight loss, hemorrhage, and regurgitation [1, 4, 5, 10].

In the Amazon parrot, most infections are asymptomatic, and the few case reports are usually concomitant with Circovirus. As a result, few clinical signs of Polyomavirus are described in Amazon parrots, such as sudden death, depression, anorexia, weight loss, delayed crop empting, regurgitation, diarrhea, dehydration, subcutaneous hemorrhages, ataxia, and paralysis [8]. The possibility of chronic infections of psittacine birds with APV indicates the existence of an APV-positive subpopulation inside the population of captive psittacine birds that have subclinical infections that could serve as a viral reservoir [8].

All clinical signs presented in this paper are compatible with APV; however, severe resulting in a 14% hematocrit during viremia is a novel symptom compared to reports in the literature. The hematocrit observed was 14%, with reduced hemoglobin and red blood cells, anisocytosis, and polychromasia, forming nonregenerative normocytic, normochromic anemia, indicating decreased erythropoiesis. Anemia can be caused by an acute or chronic kidney lesion due to lower production of erythropoietin, a hormone regulating the production of blood cells [11]. There are no case reports of avian Polyomavirus infection in the bone marrow, and unfortunately we did not perform a cytological evaluation of the bird bone marrow. However, a viral infection in the bone marrow cannot be discarded.

In this report, the animal had polyuria, clear signal kidney disease, and active infection by APV virus, commonly found in the renal parenchyma. Commonly, viral infections lead to anemia, a hemolytic process arising as a result of the body's immune response. Thus, one can consider the possibility of anemia caused by a nephropathy generated or exacerbated by viral infection. In psittacine birds with enlarged kidneys and other minor changes, glomerulopathy with a positive PAS (periodic acid-Schiff) reaction may indicate infection with avian Polyomavirus [12]. The PAS reaction in Polyomavirus occurs due to the, sometimes massive, deposition of immune complexes [12]. With the improvement of clinical signs and support care, anemia was resolved within a month after treatment.

Phalen et al. [1] reported the apparent thrombocytopenia in blood smears from a breeder with an APV infection. They indicated the possibility of this thrombocytopenia as the cause of hemorrhage resulting from the disease. The cause of the thrombocytopenia was not detected; however, these authors suggested the possibility of a viral thrombolysis or an induction of a disseminated vascular coagulation. Nevertheless, in this report, there was no change in the thrombocytes, but the blood count was performed only 14 days after the onset of viral presentation. Thus, there is the possibility of a normalization of this symptom because the bird showed early clinical improvement.

Although anemia is not commonly described, one should take into account that most of the birds die without clinical signs, and thus, it is not possible to perform additional tests such as blood work. Considering the commonly observed symptoms, such as hematuria and subcutaneous petechia [1], the possibility that anemia also occurs in other birds cannot be disregarded. It is known that, in non-psittacine species, general hemorrhage is described [10], which obviously can lead to mild anemia or even to severe anemia. In addition, infectious agent can cause nonregenerative, normocytic anemia. Birds tend to develop anemia due to the lack of erythropoiesis very fast and maybe due to the short erythrocyte half-life [11].

In addition to the severe anemia, another hematological alteration was observed. Severe leukopenia without alterations in the other white cells, which is common in acute viral infections, was an interesting finding. According to the hemogram, there were no obvious signs of a bacterial infection that could be acting in conjunction with APV.

Acute APV in adult Amazon parrots has been described and is frequently caused by immunosuppression, usually associated with concomitant Psittacine Beak and Feather Disease Virus (PBFDV) infection [4]. Considering this possibility, we also tested the feces and blood for both PBFDV and ABV (avian Bornavirus, an agent that normally causes emesis and undigested seeds in the feces) by PCR, and the bird was negative for both viruses. It is probable that another underlying cause could have led to immunosuppression and the appearance of the clinical symptoms, such as stress associated with changes in the weather, diet, or breeding.

The transmission may have occurred in several ways, even by contact with contaminated ectoparasites [13]. A major problem of this disease is the difficulty of diagnosis due to the nonspecific symptoms and transmission by asymptomatic animals. The virus is shed in the feces, skin desquamation, and fomites [14]. It is suggested that viremia precedes cloacal virus shedding, because viremia has always been detected prior to or concurrent with cloacal virus shedding. The duration between the onset of viremia and the onset of cloacal virus shedding appears to be only a few days in a typical infection [1]. Another factor that plays an important role in the spread of avian viral diseases is the lack of epizootic control of imported birds [3]. This clinical report documents a two-year-and-four-month-old A. aestiva, positive for APV in the feces and blood by PCR, presenting with emesis, undigested seeds in the feces, and severe anemia. Considering that the duration of the disease progression in this case, one month, corroborates with the literature [1, 4] as well as with the positive PCR results in both the feces and the blood, there is strong evidence that the clinical signs were related to APV. This is important due to the small amount of reports of infection in this species and the severe anemia, a symptom rarely described in APV infections. To the authors' knowledge, this is the first report of APV described in the Blue Fronted parrot in the country, and thus, we aim to alert clinicians of birds to a new clinical sign to include in the differential diagnosis.

## Conflict of Interests

The authors declare that there is no conflict of interests regarding the publication of this paper.

## Acknowledgment

This work was supported by a grant received from Conselho Nacional de Desenvolvimento Científico e Tecnológico (CNPq Grant no. 453920/2014-4). Antonio J. Piantino Ferreira is a recipient of CNPq fellowships-1B.

## References

[1] D. N. Phalen, C. S. Radabaugh, R. D. Dahlhausen, and D. K. Styles, "Viremia, virus shedding, and antibody response during natural avian polyomavirus infection in parrots," *Journal of the American Veterinary Medical Association*, vol. 217, no. 1, pp. 32–36, 2000.

[2] C.-M. Hsu, C.-Y. Ko, and H.-J. Tsai, "Detection and sequence analysis of avian polyomavirus and psittacine beak and feather

disease virus from psittacine birds in Taiwan," *Avian Diseases*, vol. 50, no. 3, pp. 348–353, 2006.

[3] T. Piasecki and A. Wieliczko, "Detection of beak and feather disease virus and avian polyomavirus DNA in psittacine birds in Poland," *Bulletin of the Veterinary Institute in Pulawy*, vol. 54, no. 2, pp. 141–146, 2010.

[4] M. Szweda, A. KoŁodziejska, J. Szarek, and I. Babińska, "Avian polyomavirus infections in Amazon parrots," *Medycyna Weterynaryjna*, vol. 67, no. 3, pp. 147–150, 2011.

[5] D. N. Phalen, "Avian polyomavirus: my thoughts," *American Federation of Aviculture Watchbird*, vol. 10, pp. 28–39, 1998.

[6] G. Rossi, E. Taccini, and C. Tarantino, "Outbreak of avian polyomavirus infection with high mortality in recently captured Crimson's seedcrackers (*Pyrenestes sanguineus*)," *Journal of Wildlife Diseases*, vol. 41, no. 1, pp. 236–240, 2005.

[7] R. Johne and H. Müller, "Avian polyomavirus in wild birds: genome analysis of isolates from Falconiformes and Psittaciformes," *Archives of Virology*, vol. 143, no. 8, pp. 1501–1512, 1998.

[8] M. Rahaus and M. H. Wolff, "A survey to detect subclinical polyomavirus infections of captive psittacine birds in Germany," *Veterinary Microbiology*, vol. 105, no. 1, pp. 73–76, 2005.

[9] A. Ramis, K. S. Latimer, X. Gibert, and R. A. Campagnoli, "A concurrent outbreak of psittacine beak and feather disease virus, and avian polyomavirus infection in budgerigars (*Melopsittacus undulatus*)," *Avian Pathology*, vol. 27, no. 1, pp. 43–50, 1998.

[10] S. L. Lafferty, A. M. Fudge, R. E. Schmidt, G. V. Wilson, and D. N. Phalen, "Avian polyomavirus infection and disease in a green aracaris (*Pteroglossus viridis*)," *Avian Diseases*, vol. 43, no. 3, pp. 577–585, 1999.

[11] T. W. Campbell, "Hematology in birds," in *Veterinary Hematological and Clinical Chemistry*, M. Thrall, D. Barker, and T. Campbell, Eds., pp. 238–277, Lippincott Williams & Wilkins, 2004.

[12] H. Gerlach, F. Enders, M. Casares, H. Müller, R. Johne, and T. Hänichen, "Membranous glomerulopathy as an indicator of avian polyomavirus infection in psittaciformes," *Journal of Avian Medicine and Surgery*, vol. 12, no. 4, pp. 248–254, 1998.

[13] J. Potti, G. Blanco, J. Á. Lemus, and D. Canal, "Infectious offspring: how birds acquire and transmit an avia polyomavirus in the wild," *PLoS ONE*, vol. 2, no. 12, Article ID e1276, 2007.

[14] B. Ritchie, *Avian Viruses: Function and Control*, Wingers Publishing, Lake Worth, Fla, USA, 1995.

# 9

# The Use of a Cutting Balloon for Dilation of a Fibrous Esophageal Stricture in a Cat

**Alexander E. Gallagher and Andrew J. Specht**

*Department of Small Animal Clinical Sciences, College of Veterinary Medicine, University of Florida, Gainesville, FL 32608, USA*

Correspondence should be addressed to Alexander E. Gallagher; gallaghera@ufl.edu

Academic Editors: C. Hyun, F. Mutinelli, L. G. Papazoglou, and S. Stuen

Esophageal strictures are uncommon in cats with causes including medications, ingestion of caustic substances, or gastroesophageal reflux under anesthesia. Bougienage and balloon dilation are the main treatments for strictures but have variable success rates. This paper describes the novel use of a cutting balloon for dilation of a fibrous stricture in a cat that was previously refractory to treatment with traditional balloon dilation.

## 1. Introduction

Esophageal strictures are uncommon in cats and dogs and are generally the consequence of esophagitis caused by gastroesophageal reflux secondary to anesthesia, esophageal foreign bodies, persistent vomiting, or esophageal retention of certain medications such as tetracyclines and clindamycin [1–3]. Strictures occur when the esophagitis extends into the submucosa or muscularis resulting in a fibroproliferative reaction. Clinical signs including regurgitation, ptyalism, and dysphagia typically appear within 7–10 days of the inciting event.

Bougienage and balloon dilation are the most common nonsurgical techniques for treatment of strictures. Balloon dilation has been purported to offer an advantage due to the generation of only radial stretch forces without the concurrent longitudinal shear stress generated by bougienage, but retrospective studies in humans and a recent study in dogs have not shown any difference in clinical outcome [4–6]. The use of perendoscopic multiquadrant electrocautery has been reported for use in annular or recurrent strictures [7, 8]. Using an electrosurgical unit, three to four equidistant incisions are made in the fibrous ring followed by balloon dilation. The created incisions provide weak areas restricting the trauma of dilation to these sites and sparing the rest of the tissue [7]. Melendez et al. [8] noted an apparent benefit in decreasing the number of balloon procedures required using

this technique. In this paper, we describe the use of a cutting balloon to create incisions for treatment of a refractory fibrous stricture in a cat.

## 2. Case Presentation

A 12-year-old female spayed Ragdoll cat was evaluated for a 3-week history of vomiting, retching, and ptyalism. Four weeks prior to presentation, the cat was evaluated at another hospital for periocular erythema and edema. Due to suspected tooth root abscessation, the cat was anesthetized and the left maxillary third premolar extracted. An unknown oral antibiotic was prescribed. One week prior to presentation, the cat was seen at a second hospital for vomiting. Examination identified prolapse of the left third eyelid with mild corneal edema. Results of a biochemistry panel, complete blood count, and total T4 were unremarkable. Bacitracin-neomycin-polymyixin B ophthalmic ointment was prescribed.

Physical examination at initial presentation (day 1) identified a body temperature of 39.9°C, body weight of 2.4 kg, and a body condition score of 3 out of 9. General examination was unremarkable. Ophthalmic examination identified a superficial corneal ulcer in the left eye. Routine topical treatment for the ulcer was prescribed. Initial differentials for the clinical signs included true vomiting due to primary gastrointestinal disease or regurgitation due to esophageal disease. Diagnostics on day 1 included abdominal radiographs which revealed diffuse small intestinal adynamic ileus without obstruction and abdominal ultrasound which revealed mildly decreased renal size bilaterally and mineralization of the left adrenal gland.

On day 2, an esophagram was performed fluoroscopically and a focal circumferential area of stricture was noted at the level of C5 (Figure 1). Esophagoscopy (Fujinon EG-270N5 and EG-250WR5 gastroscopes, Fujinon Inc., Wayne, NJ) was performed on day 3 and confirmed a circumferential stricture in the proximal esophagus narrowing the lumen to 2 mm in diameter. Balloon dilation (CRE esophageal balloon dilation catheter, Boston Scientific, Natick, MA) was performed and resulted in a severe, deep esophageal mucosal tear. Thoracic radiographs did not identify evidence of perforation, and the owner declined gastrostomy tube placement. Conservative treatment included partial parenteral nutrition, cefazolin (21.4 mg/kg i.v. q8 h), buprenorphine (0.01 mg/kg p.o. q8 h), famotidine (1 mg/kg IV q12 h), and IV fluids.

On day 8, repeat esophagoscopy revealed the previous tear to be nearly healed and recurrent stricture. The area of stricture was balloon dilated to 6 mm with only mild mucosal tearing. Partial parenteral nutrition was discontinued, and the patient was discharged from the hospital. Home medications included ranitidine (2 mg/kg PO q12 h) and sucralfate suspension (250 mg PO q8 h).

The cat presented on day 12 for reexamination. The owner reported that the cat had done well at home eating a canned food diet mixed with water. No clinical signs were noted. Esophagoscopy revealed complete mucosal healing and recurrent stricture to a lumen diameter of 4 mm. During the examination, a fibrous band of tissue extending approximately 70% of the circumference was noted at the stricture site. The stricture was serially dilated to 8 mm with minimal mucosal tearing. When dilated to 9 mm, a longitudinal, focal, and deep mucosal tear developed with persistence of the fibrous, band and no further dilation was attempted. The cat was discharged with instructions to continue the ranitidine and sucralfate at home.

On day 23, the cat presented for reexamination. The owner noted that the cat did well at home for 7 days after balloon dilation but began gagging and drooling on the 8th day. Esophagoscopy showed the same appearance to the stricture as on day 12 with the same results noted after balloon dilation to 9 mm. The owner was instructed to continue ranitidine and sucralfate upon discharge. At followup by telephone on day 29, the owner reported that the cat was eating the canned food with water without any clinical signs. Due to financial constraints, the owner elected not to return for re-examination unless clinical signs returned.

The cat presented on day 53 with a 2-week history of intermittent episodes of gagging while eating. The owner had been noncompliant by stopping all medications 2 weeks prior. Esophagoscopy revealed findings similar to the previous 2 examinations (Figure 2(a)). Due to the persistence of the fibrous band, an 8 mm cutting balloon (CB, cutting balloon peripheral, 8.0 mm × 2.0 cm × 135 cm; Boston Scientific, Natick, MA) was used for the initial dilation. The CB was passed

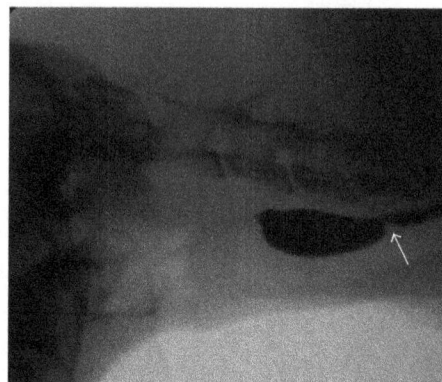

FIGURE 1: Fluoroscopic image from an esophagram performed in a cat with a history of vomiting, retching, and ptyalism. A focal circumferential area of stricture is noted at the level of C5 (white arrow) with dilation of the esophagus orad to the lesion.

adjacent to the endoscope and inflated to 10 atmospheres (rated burst pressure) with pressure maintained for 1 minute. At the end of the minute, the CB was withdrawn from the stricture area prior to deflation. The deflated CB was rotated and replaced across the stricture, and the process repeated until obvious scoring of the fibrous band was noted (Figure 2(b)). The stricture was subsequently serially dilated to 10 mm with mild, superficial, and diffuse mucosal tearing and disruption of the fibrous band (Figures 2(c) and 2(d)). The cat was prescribed sucralfate suspension (250 mg PO q8 h) at discharge.

At re-examination on day 60, the owner reported that the cat was eating canned food with water well at home with no clinical signs. Esophagoscopy showed mild stricture recurrence with a lumen diameter of approximately 7 mm (Figure 3). The CB was used to dilate the stricture as before followed by dilation with a balloon catheter to approximately 11 mm with mild, superficial, and diffuse mucosal tearing. The cat was discharged with instructions to continue the sucralfate for 4 weeks. Further esophagoscopic evaluation was declined by the owner due to financial constraints. At telephone followup on days 90 and 143, the owner reported that the cat was eating a canned food diet mixed with a small volume of water well and no clinical signs were reported.

The cat presented for unrelated issues one year later. No clinical signs of esophageal disease had recurred, and the cat was eating a canned food diet with a small volume of water added. Esophagoscopy was repeated. At the site of previous stricture, there remained a band of fibrous tissue involving approximately 50% of the circumference. The lumen diameter was estimated to be 9 mm. The rest of the esophagus appeared normal.

## 3. Discussion

The CB was first designed by Barath et al. in 1991 as a novel approach to angioplasty and features three to four atherotomes, or microsurgical blades, that are fixed at equidistant

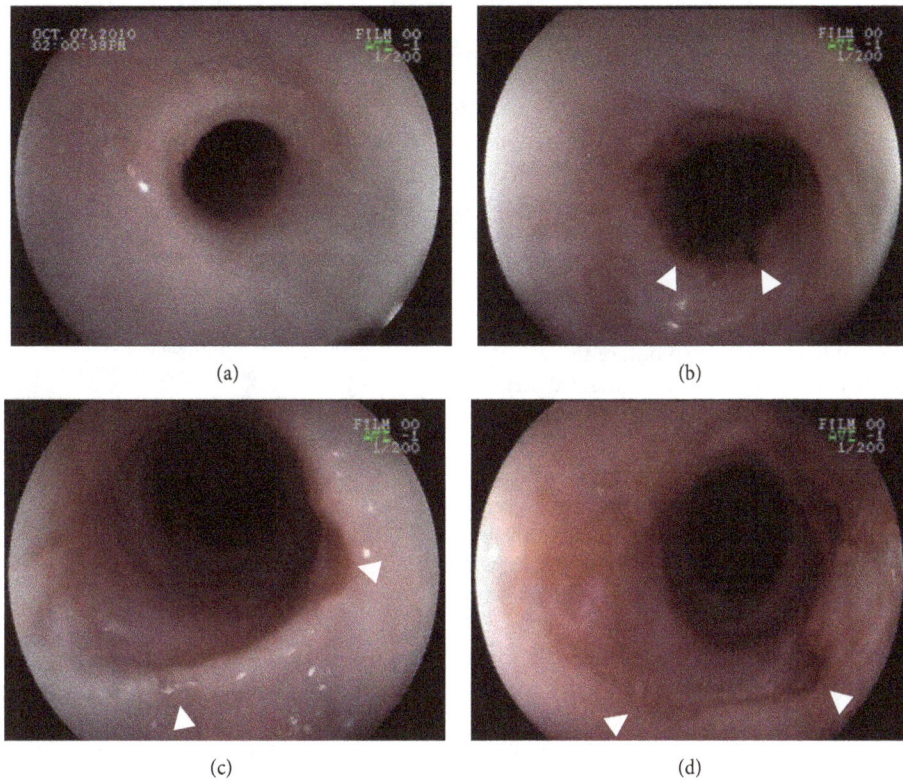

(a)

(b)

(c)

(d)

FIGURE 2: Endoscopic appearance of the esophageal stricture at re-examination on day 53 after 4 previous dilations. A band of fibrous tissue is present at the site of stricture extending from 7 o'clock to 2 o'clock resulting in a lumen diameter of 4 mm (a). After initial dilation with an 8 mm cutting balloon, multiple defects (white arrowheads) are noted in the fibrous band, now at 3 o'clock to 9 o'clock (b). Subsequent serial dilations with conventional dilation balloons resulted in further disruption of the fibrous band at these defects (c) and more diffuse mucosal tearing resulting in a lumen diameter of 10 mm (d).

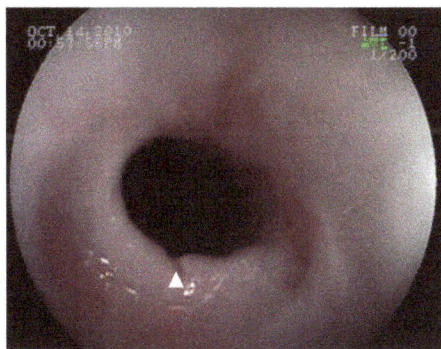

FIGURE 3: Endoscopic appearance of the esophageal stricture at re-examination on day 60, one week after cutting balloon dilation. Note the persistent defect in the fibrous band (white arrowhead).

points longitudinally along the circumference of a noncompliant balloon [9]. The blades are used to score lesions during dilation allowing for easier angioplasty at lower pressures to decrease the risk of a neoproliferative response and restenosis [10]. While CBs were originally designed for use in blood vessels, they have also been used to dilate strictures in the ureter, urethra, biliary system, trachea, and lungs in humans [11–15].

In 2004, Wilkinson and MacKinlay described the use of a CB in the dilation of a chronic esophageal stricture caused by ingestion of a caustic substance in a 14-year-old boy [16]. During the first two attempts to dilate to 8 mm with a conventional balloon, wasting of the balloon could not be abolished. On the third attempt, the stricture was dilated to 8 mm using a CB which required several inflations of the balloon with rotation and retraction/advancement of the deflated balloon to completely abolish wasting. Over a six-month period, the stricture was serially dilated to 20 mm using conventional balloons without complications.

Recently, the use of CBs in valvuloplasty for severe sub-aortic stenosis in dogs was reported [17]. To the authors' knowledge, the use of CBs in esophageal strictures in cats or dogs has not been reported. The cat in this paper had a partial annular fibrotic ring. During initial dilation attempts with a conventional balloon catheter, a focal deep mucosal tear occurred without disruption of the annular ring limiting the degree of dilation that could be achieved and resulting in recurrence of the stricture within 14 days. The use of the CB resulted in the scoring of the fibrotic ring in multiple sites. Subsequent dilation with a conventional balloon caused breakdown of the fibrotic ring at the sites of scoring. This resulted in milder mucosal tearing that was distributed around the circumference of the lesion allowing for dilation of the stricture to a larger diameter. The procedure was considered successful as the cat was noted to be free of clinical signs one year after the last procedure and eating a normal canned food diet.

It is possible that the improved outcome in this case was due to the repeated dilations alone. However, after the 2nd and 3rd dilations, the fibrotic ring persisted and resulted in a focal deep mucosal tear during dilation. After initial dilation with the CB, this fibrotic ring was disrupted allowing for radial stretch of the stricture around the circumference of the lesion, resulting in dilation to a larger diameter using conventional balloons. Better owner compliance with medications may also have contributed to the improved outcome.

A limiting factor for the use of CBs in esophageal strictures may be cost. The CB used in this case costs $866 but was donated after a one-time use for valvuloplasty in a dog. Prior to first use in this case, the CB was cleaned and gas sterilized. The atherotomes were still sharp enough to score the lesion during both dilations, but it is unknown what effect repeat sterilizations or use may have. It is possible that a CB may be used for multiple procedures which would help reduce the cost per procedure. In addition, if use of a CB can reduce the total number of dilations that need to be performed, then the total cost of treatment may be reduced.

In conclusion, the use of a CB for esophageal stricture has only been reported once in the human literature and has not been reported in the veterinary literature. This paper illustrates the potential benefits of CB in dilation of recurrent strictures associated with a fibrotic band that is resistant to dilation by conventional balloon catheters. Further evaluation to determine if the use of CBs can reduce the need for repeat dilations should be considered.

## Conflict of Interests

The authors declare that there is no conflict of interests with respect to their authorship or publication of this paper. There was no financial support provided.

## References

[1] J. A. Beatty, N. Swift, D. J. Foster, and V. R. D. Barrs, "Suspected clindamycin-associated oesophageal injury in cats: five cases," *Journal of Feline Medicine and Surgery*, vol. 8, no. 6, pp. 412–419, 2006.

[2] A. J. German, M. J. Canon, C. Dye et al., "Oesophageal strictures in cats associated with doxycycline therapy," *Journal of Feline Medicine and Surgery*, vol. 7, no. 1, pp. 33–41, 2005.

[3] M. S. Leib, H. Dinnel, D. L. Ward, M. E. Reimer, T. L. Towell, and W. E. Monroe, "Endoscopic balloon dilation of benign esophageal strictures in dogs and cats," *Journal of Veterinary Internal Medicine*, vol. 15, no. 6, pp. 547–552, 2001.

[4] S. A. Bissett, J. Davis, K. Subler, and L. A. Degernes, "Risk factors and outcome of bougienage for treatment of benign esophageal strictures in dogs and cats: 28 cases (1995–2004)," *Journal of the American Veterinary Medical Association*, vol. 235, no. 7, pp. 840–850, 2009.

[5] M. Guelrud, "Management of benign esophageal strictures," September 2010, http://www.uptodate.com/.

[6] S. J. Spechler, "AGA technical review on treatment of patients with dysphagia caused by benign disorders of the distal esophagus," *Gastroenterology*, vol. 117, no. 1, pp. 233–254, 1999.

[7] M. Gualtieri, "Esophagoscopy," *Veterinary Clinics of North America*, vol. 31, no. 4, pp. 605–630, 2001.

[8] L. D. Melendez, D. C. Twedt, E. A. Weyrauch et al., "Conservative therapy using balloon dilation for intramural, inflammatory esophageal strictures in dogs and cats: a retrospective study of 23 cases. [1987–1997]," *European Journal of Comparative Gastroenterology*, vol. 3, no. 1, pp. 31–36, 1998.

[9] P. Barath, M. C. Fishbein, S. Vari, and J. S. Forrester, "Cutting balloon: a novel approach to percutaneous angioplasty," *American Journal of Cardiology*, vol. 68, no. 11, pp. 1249–1252, 1991.

[10] M. S. Lee, V. Singh, T. J. Nero, and J. R. Wilentz, "Cutting balloon angioplasty," *Journal of Invasive Cardiology*, vol. 14, no. 9, pp. 552–556, 2002.

[11] E. Atar, G. N. Bachar, G. Bartal et al., "Use of peripheral cutting balloon in the management of resistant benign ureteral and biliary strictures," *Journal of Vascular and Interventional Radiology*, vol. 16, no. 2, pp. 241–245, 2005.

[12] M. Cejna, "Cutting balloon: review on principles and background of use in peripheral arteries," *CardioVascular and Interventional Radiology*, vol. 28, no. 4, pp. 400–408, 2005.

[13] W. E. A. Saad, "Percutaneous management of postoperative anastomotic biliary strictures," *Techniques in Vascular and Interventional Radiology*, vol. 11, no. 2, pp. 143–153, 2008.

[14] J. H. Shin, H. Y. Song, J. H. Kim et al., "Cutting balloon treatment for recurrent benign bronchial strictures," *American Journal of Roentgenology*, vol. 190, no. 2, pp. W130–W132, 2008.

[15] E. Yildirim, T. Cicek, O. Istanbulluoglu, and B. Ozturk, "Use of cutting balloon in the treatment of urethral stricture: a novel technique," *CardioVascular and Interventional Radiology*, vol. 32, no. 3, pp. 525–528, 2009.

[16] A. G. Wilkinson and G. A. MacKinlay, "Use of a cutting balloon in the dilatation of caustic oesophageal stricture," *Pediatric Radiology*, vol. 34, no. 5, pp. 414–416, 2004.

[17] M. K. Schmidt, A. H. Estrada, H. W. Maisenbacher et al., "Combined cutting balloon and high pressure balloon valvuloplasty for dogs with severe subaortic stenosis," *Journal of Veterinary Internal Medicine*, vol. 24, p. 693, 2010.

# 10

# Gastrointestinal Stromal Tumor in the Cecum of a Horse

### S. Stephan,[1] S. Hug,[2] and M. Hilbe[1]

[1] Institute of Veterinary Pathology, Vetsuisse Faculty, University of Zurich, 8057 Zurich, Switzerland
[2] Department of Equine Medicine, Vetsuisse Faculty, University of Zurich, 8057 Zurich, Switzerland

Correspondence should be addressed to S. Stephan, sara.stephan@laposte.net

Academic Editors: J. Carmalt, C. Hyun, J. S. Munday, and F. Mutinelli

Gastrointestinal stromal tumors (GISTs) are defined as specific CD117-(Kit, stem cell factor receptor) expressing tumors of the gastrointestinal (GI) tract. They are believed to originate from the interstitial pacemaker cells of Cajal (ICC) or their progenitor cells. In horses only a few cases of GISTs are described in the literature. In the present paper the macroscopical, histological, immunohistochemical, and ultrastructural features of an equine cecal GIST are described.

## 1. Case History

A 24-year-old, 540 kg, warm-blood gelding was referred to the Internal Medicine Section of the Equine Department at the Vetsuisse Faculty of Zurich with colic. The horse was regularly vaccinated and dewormed. The horse had suffered from colic the previous week and had lost a lot of weight over the past few months. Five years before, the horse had undergone a colic surgery, where 5 meters of the small intestine had to be removed and an end-to-end anastomosis was performed. Since then it had been without clinical signs. On initial examination at the Vetsuisse Faculty of Zurich, the horse had a poor general condition. After rectal palpation, an impaction of the cranial colon ascendens was suspected and the horse was treated with dipyrone (25 mg/kg iv) and paraffinum liquidum as well as intravenous fluids. The next day the impaction was still present and the horse was treated further with hyperinfusion, moderate exercise, and was fasted. On the third day the gelding had recovered temporarily, but then relapsed and developed colic again. This time the medical treatment consisted of dipyrone (25 mg/kg iv), butylscopolamine (60 mg iv), and xylazine (120 mg iv). A hematological and biochemical blood examination, abdominocentesis, gastroscopy, and an ultrasonographic examination of the abdomen were initiated. The hematological blood examination showed a slight leukocytosis (9,400/μL; 4,700–8,200); the other parameters were within reference values. The biochemistry was unremarkable. The abdominal fluid was increased, yellow colored, and turbid with an increased cell count of 15,825/μL, specific gravity 1019, and protein 19 g/L. The cytological evaluation of the abdominal fluid showed a slight suppurative inflammation without neutrophilic degeneration. The gastroscopy showed no abnormal findings. On the ultrasonographic examination of the abdomen, two large heterogeneous solid masses of approximately 10 to 15 cm and 5 cm in diameter located in the mid and right caudal aspect of the abdomen most likely associated with the cecal wall could be seen. The suspected diagnosis of the cecal masses was a neoplasia (malignant lymphoma or carcinoma) and as a differential diagnosis an abscess formation or a granuloma. The horse was euthanized because of the poor prognosis and a necropsy was performed.

## 2. Necropsy Findings

Necropsy revealed two masses in the external cecal wall. One mass of approximately 10 × 10 × 8 cm was attached by a small stalk of about 1,5 cm in diameter approximately 10 cm distant to the apex region of the cecum located between the medial and ventral taenia of the cecum (Figure 1). The mass was oval shaped with a multilobulated surface and a red-beige-brown marmorated cross-section. The mass was soft, partially cystic, and of brittle consistency, separated by multifocal necrosis and hemorrhage (Figure 2). The second mass was of transmural (5 × 5 × 8 cm) and intraluminal (4 × 4 × 3 cm) growth, located in the corpus region of the cecum between the medial and lateral taenia. The nodule was of firm

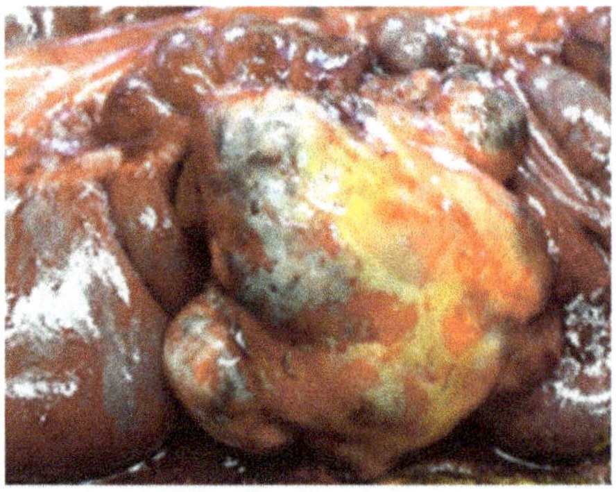

FIGURE 1: Necropsy revealed an approximately $10 \times 10 \times 8$ cm neoplastic mass attached by a small stalk to the external cecal wall.

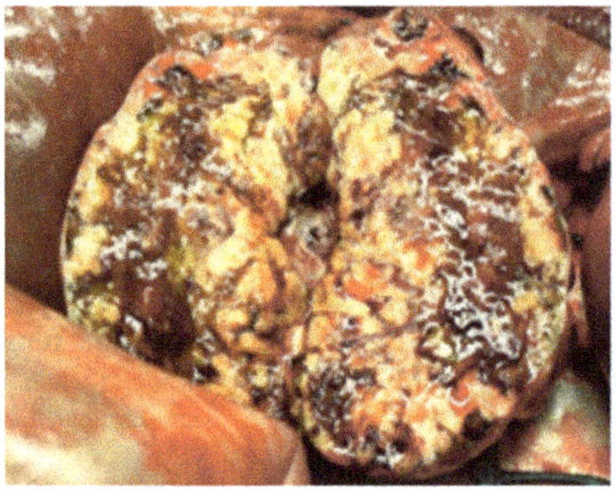

FIGURE 2: Cross-section: brittle consistency, red-beige mottled with multifocal necrosis/hemorrhage.

texture and of whitish color with central necrosis. Additional diagnostic finding consisted of an encapsulated foreign body (piece of wire) of 5 cm length located in the cranial part of the duodenum with secondary fistula formation. The other internal organs showed no macroscopic changes.

## 3. Histologic, Immunohistochemical, and Electron Microscopic Findings

Tissue samples of the cecum, the jejunum, the liver, and the tumor were fixed in 4% buffered-formalin processed conventionally and embedded in paraffin. Sections of about $2$-$3\,\mu$m were cut and stained with hematoxylin-eosin (HE) and periodic-acid-Schiff (PAS) and evaluated with light microscopy.

Histological examination revealed that the mass consisted of well-demarcated densely cellular tissue arranged in interlacing fascicles or in a storiform pattern with abundant fibrovascular tumor stroma and moderate mucinous matrix. The muscle layer of the cecal wall surrounded the extraluminal tumor part. Multifocal acute hemorrhages, edema, and necrosis were visible. Tumor cell populations showed slight-to-moderate anisocytosis and anisokaryosis without mitosis. In the present case the tumor population was of mixed cell type with about 5% epithelioid cells and about 95%

spindle cells. Cells of epithelioid morphology were round-to-polygonal-shaped with well-defined cell borders, round-to-oval nuclei, loosely arranged chromatin, and moderate eosinophilic cytoplasm. Spindle-shaped cells had indistinct cell borders, oval nuclei with dispersed granular heterochromatin, 1 to 2 small nucleoli, and scant fibrillar cytoplasm (Figures 3 and 4). The inflammatory response was slight and mainly composed of lymphocytes, few neutrophils, and some hemosiderin-loaded macrophages. Multifocal in between the cell groups and strands, some hyaline brightly bulked eosinophilic material could be found. These structures were PAS-positive aggregates of extracellular collagen bundles known as skeinoid fibers [1, 2]. Additionally a severe focal-extensive subacute to chronic lymphohistiocytic duodenitis with formation of moderate fibroangioblastic granulation tissue due to a foreign body could be diagnosed as an incidental finding.

Immunohistochemical staining was performed for CD117, vimentin, "alpha smooth muscle actin (SMA)," desmin, S100, "neuron specific enolase (NSE)," and Melan A. All sections, except for CD117 and desmin, were pretreated with a citrated (pH 6) buffer for 20 minutes at 98°C by heating in a microwave oven. Section for desmin was pretreated in the same buffer only for 5 minutes at 98°C, and section for CD117 was pretreated with an alkaline buffer (pH 9) for 20 minutes at 98°C. For vimentin, SMA, desmin, S100, NSE, and melan A, the Detection-kit ChemMate from DAKO was used. For CD117 the OUM-kit from Roche was applied and performed on the discovery machine. Additionally, in all sections, endogenous peroxidase reaction was blocked with peroxidase-blocking solution (DAKO S2023). Antibodies from DAKO against the following antigens were used in the DAKO Autostainer (DAKO AG Switzerland): CD117 (rabbit, dilution 1 : 400, DAKO A4502), vimentin (mouse, dilution 1 : 100, DAKO M7020), SMA (prediluted mouse, DAKO N1584), desmin (prediluted mouse, DAKO N1526), S100 (prediluted rabbit, DAKO N1573), NSE (mouse, dilution 1 : 150, DAKO M087301), and Melan A (mouse, dilution 1 : 10, DAKO M719601). All antibodies were diluted with dilution buffer from DAKO (S2022). The sections were incubated with streptavidin-peroxidase conjugate and reacted with the substrate-chromogen 3-amino-9-ethylcarbazole (AEC, Detection-kit DAKO K 5003) at room temperature and counterstained with hematoxylin. Positive and negative controls were included. The neoplastic cells had moderate diffuse positive red intracytoplasmic granular staining for vimentin, showed strong diffuse pancytoplasmic homogenous to slight granular positive staining for CD117 (Figure 5), and were diffusely slight to moderate positive for NSE. In contrast, the tumor was negative for desmin, S100, and Melan A (Table 1).

For electron microscopy, one millimeter cubes of formalin-fixed and paraffin-embedded tumor locations were selected and further fixed in 2,5% glutaraldehyde in 0,1 M natriumphosphat buffer (pH 7,4). Postfixation was performed with 1% osmium tetroxide buffered in natriumphosphat. After dehydration in graded ethanol series, followed by propylenoxide, the samples were embedded in Epon resin. Ultrathin sections were stained with 2% uranyl acetate and

TABLE 1: Slight staining (+), moderate staining (++), strong staining (+++), no reaction (−).

| ICH | Results |
|---|---|
| CD117 | +++ |
| Vimentin | +++ |
| SMA | − |
| Desmin | − |
| S100 | − |
| NSE | ++ |

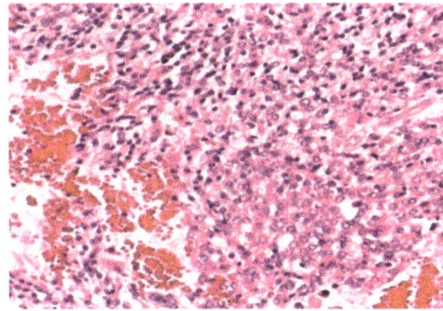

FIGURE 4: The distinction between epithelioid type (lower side right) and spindle cell type (upper side left) (HE).

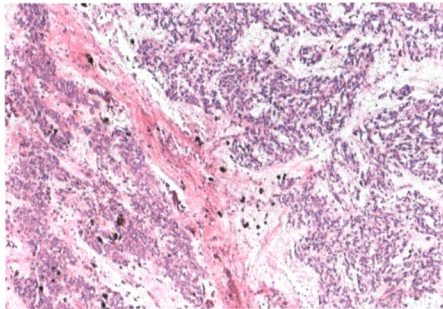

FIGURE 3: Predominant spindle-shaped tumor cells with a fascicular pattern. Spaces between tumor cell trabeculae are filled with erythrocytes, siderophages and collagenous (skeinoid fibers) as well as mucinous matrix (HE).

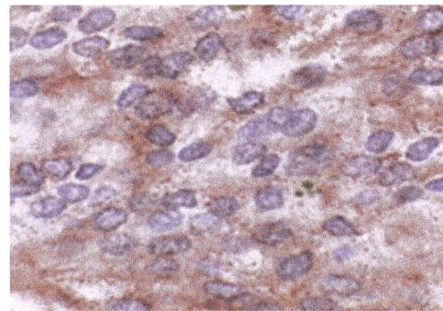

FIGURE 5: All tumor cells showed strong diffuse red pancytoplasmic homogenous to slight granular positive staining for CD117 (c-kit).

lead acetate. Samples were examined on a Philips CM 10 transmission electron microscope.

The tumor had a pleomorphic cell population with indistinct cell borders. The cells had round-to-elongated nuclei with marked nuclear lobulation and low-to-moderate peripheral packed chromatin. The cytoplasm contained variable swollen and dilatated mitochondria, low-to-moderate perinuclear smooth endoplasmic reticulum, and few neurosecretory granules (150 nm) which displayed an ultrastructural feature of neuronal differentiation. Foci of intermediate filaments and arrays of microtubules were detected. Furthermore, tumor cells were embedded in an amorphous matrix and were separated by moderate dense collagen fibers, interpreted as interstitial skeinoid fibers.

## 4. Discussion

GISTs are rather uncommon tumors in horses. To the author's knowledge, there are only five publications between 2001 and 2010 reporting on 15 GISTs in 14 horses. A former study in France could show that thoroughbred horses (13,43%) and horses older than 10 years (23,90%) were significantly more often affected by tumors in general and that the most frequent tumors were benign (adenomas, lipomas) [3]. Of the malignant tumors, the alimentary lymphoma is the most common intestinal neoplasia in horses, followed by adenocarcinoma and leiomyosarcoma most likely located in the small intestine, mainly in Arabian horses [4]. GISTs have been described for decades in humans and more recently

in dogs, nonhuman primates, horses, and rodents (rat and guinea pig) [5–9]. They are the most common primary nonlymphoid mesenchymal tumors of the GI tract with presumed histogenetic origin from the interstitial cells of Cajal (ICC) or of their pluripotent stem cells (precursor-cell-hypothesis). Both are Kit-positive cells [10, 11]. Kit is a transmembrane receptor tyrosine kinase encoded by the c-kit protooncogene and is nearly consistently expressed in all GISTs [12]. In addition, the embryonic isoform of smooth muscle myosin heavy chain is expressed in both GISTs and ICCs what supports the origin from ICCs [13]. Previously, these tumors were often misdiagnosed on morphologic basis as leiomyoma/-sarcomas, or schwannomas. Electron microscopic findings have demonstrated that most human GISTs derive from primitive mesenchymal cells that undergo either neurogenic, myogenic, dual, or no differentiation [14]. In the present case, without c-kit-staining, the tumor would have been diagnosed as a neuroendocrine tumor at histological level showing characteristics of neurogenic differentiation (NSE +). Ultrastructural studies revealed that a subgroup of GISTs seems to derive from the enteric plexi and is therefore called plexosarcoma or gastrointestinal autonomic nerve tumor (GANT) [15]. Most equine GISTs seem to be incidental findings at postmortem examination, but a few caused clinical signs like weight loss, chronic bleeding, anemia, and recurrent colic [5, 16]. GIST development can be associated with gain-of-function mutations of c-kit, a protooncogene in humans that may lead to autophosphorylation, cellular proliferation, and reduction of apoptosis [17]. Actually, in horses no genetic investigations for GIST mutations are described in the literature. This would be important if therapies targeting the c-kit tyrosine kinase receptor, already available in human medicine, could be applied in horses. For tumor grading, the most consistent histologic features applied to predict malignancy are tumor size and mitotic index. Fletcher et al. in 2002 classified human GISTs into 4 risk categories: very low risk, low risk, intermediate risk, and high risk based on tumor size and mitotic counting [21]. Applying the human classification, the present tumor would be categorized into a high-risk tumor because of a size of >10 cm and no mitotic figures. Other criteria of malignancy were present in this tumor-like marked cellular pleomorphism, pronounced anisokaryosis, invasiveness, hemorrhage, and necrosis, but it still remains difficult to provide an accurate prognosis for animals [8]. The location of the tumor may also be an important prognostic factor in human GISTs where a significant difference in site-specific survival could be shown. The survival curve was very good for GISTs located in the stomach. In contrast, small-bowel tumors showed a much poorer prognosis [18]. In horses it depends primarily on the degree of expansive tumor growth that may result in intestinal obstruction and colic. In the present case, the tumor was located in the apex and corpus region of the cecum. In a recent study from Hafner et al. in 1998, most of nine GISTs from seven horses investigated were also located in the distal region of the cecum. Thus, the cecum appears to be a common location in horses and dogs [5, 8, 16]. Curiously, human GISTs occur more often in the stomach followed by the small intestine [19], and it is interesting to note that five of seven GISTs in nonhuman primates have also been found in the stomach [6]. In addition the present tumor was of multiple incidence, which is in contrast to a recent study where almost all equine GISTs were solitary and without detected metastasis in necropsy [16]. However multiple tumors have been described in old horses, dogs, and cats, but metastases were rare [14]. Thus it is difficult to decide whether multifocal tumors may be interpreted as metastasis or multiple tumor formation. Metastatic GISTs are described in the literature. In a previous study metastatic nodules were found in the liver, the spleen, the femur, and the bone marrow of a F344 rat [7] and widespread abdominal metastasis were diagnosed in a rhesus macaque [20]. Typical of malignant human GISTs is intra-abdominal spread and distant metastases most commonly to the liver followed by the lung and the bone [18]. Furthermore, vimentin expression is correlated with a light microscopic diagnosis of malignancy. Thus immunohistochemical staining for vimentin may be useful in more accurately defining tumors of questionable malignant behavior [8]. GISTs that are considered as tumors of malignant behavior need to be surgically removed. Segmental resection or complete en bloc resection is the standard treatment in human and equine medicine. Inoperable or metastatic human GISTs are treated with imatinib mesylate a competitive inhibitor of c-kit (CD117) [21]. Tumors without CD117 expression but with similar morphologic features are called GIST-like tumors [22]. There was no immunohistochemistry performed on CD34 (hematopoietic progenitor cell antigen), commonly

immunopositive in human GISTs and in ICCs, because the antibody did not stain equine control tissue in a recent study [16]. Besides, in a nonhuman primate none of the neoplastic cells were immunoreactive for CD34 [7]. The SMA positivity of human GISTs is about 30–40% and is correlated with a more favorable prognosis in gastric and small intestine tumors. In contrast, desmin is rare in human GISTs of all sites [23]. In the present case, the staining was negative for both implying no myogenic differentiation of the tumor cells. This is in accordance to previous studies on equine GISTs [5, 16]. As human GISTs, equine tumors occur in mature adults and more often in mares [5], but case numbers are limited. Finally in the present case, the foreign body located in the cranial part of the duodenum might also have caused digestion disturbance and recurrent colic, so that we cannot explain whether the foreign body, the GIST, or both had caused the clinical signs. In summary, the tumor presented here was diagnosed as a GIST because of positive expression of CD117 and vimentin, immunonegativity for desmin, and variable staining features for SMA, S100, and NSE depending on the tumor differentiation. Immunohistochemical and ultrastructural features suggested a tumor of the neural type according to the classification from Rosai in 1996 [24]. This study demonstrated once more the necessity of immunohistochemical staining of c-kit to support the diagnosis of a GIST.

## Conflict of Interests

The authors declared that they had no conflict of interests with respect to their authorship or the publication of this paper.

## Funding

The authors declared that they received no financial support for their research and/or authorship of this paper.

## Acknowledgments

The authors thank the whole laboratory staff of the Institute of Veterinary Pathology of the Vetsuisse Faculty of Zurich for excellent technical work. They are also grateful to the Department of Equine Medicine of the Vetsuisse Faculty of Zurich for providing clinical and laboratory findings.

## References

[1] K. W. Min, "Small intestinal stromal tumors with skeinoid fibers: clinicopathological, immunohistochemical, and ultrastructural investigations," *American Journal of Surgical Pathology*, vol. 16, no. 2, pp. 145–155, 1992.

[2] S. Matsukuma, M. Doi, M. Suzuki, K. Ikegawa, K. Sato, and N. Kuwabara, "Numerous eosinophilic globules (skeinoid fibers) in a duodenal stromal tumor: an exceptional case showing smooth muscle differentiation," *Pathology International*, vol. 47, no. 11, pp. 789–793, 1997.

[3] C. Laugier, N. Doux, C. George et al., "Prévalence de la pathologie tumorale dans un effectif de 1 771 chevaux autopsiés," *Pratique Vétérinaire Equine*, vol. 143, pp. 21–35, 2004.

[4] S. D. Taylor, N. Pusterla, B. Vaughan, M. B. Whitcomb, and W. D. Wilson, "Intestinal neoplasia in horses," *Journal of Veterinary Internal Medicine*, vol. 20, no. 6, pp. 1429–1436, 2006.

[5] F. Del Piero, B. A. Summers, J. F. Cummings, G. Mandelli, and E. A. Blomme, "Gastrointestinal stromal tumors in equids," *Veterinary Pathology*, vol. 38, no. 6, pp. 689–697, 2001.

[6] Y. R. Bommineni, E. J. Dick, and G. B. Hubbard, "Gastrointestinal stromal tumors in a baboon, a spider monkey, and a chimpanzee and a review of the literature," *Journal of Medical Primatology*, vol. 38, no. 3, pp. 199–203, 2009.

[7] H. Fujimoto, M. Shibutani, K. Kuroiwa et al., "A case report of a spontaneous gastrointestinal stromal tumor (GIST) occurring in a F344 rat," *Toxicologic Pathology*, vol. 34, no. 2, pp. 164–167, 2006.

[8] R. G. Larock and P. E. Ginn, "Immunohistochemical staining characteristics of canine gastrointestinal stromal tumors," *Veterinary Pathology*, vol. 34, no. 4, pp. 303–311, 1997.

[9] H. Bielefeldt-Ohmann, D. H. Barouch, A. M. Bakke, A. G. Bruce, M. Durning, and R. Grant, "Intestinal stromal tumors in a simian immunodeficiency virus-infected, simian retrovirus-2 negative rhesus macaque (Macaca mulatta)," *Veterinary Pathology*, vol. 42, no. 3, pp. 391–396, 2005.

[10] L. G. Kindblom, H. E. Remotti, F. Aldenborg, and J. M. Meis-Kindblom, "Gastrointestinal pacemaker cell tumor (GIPACT): gastrointestinal stromal tumors show phenotypic characteristics of the interstitial cells of Cajal," *The American Journal of Pathology*, vol. 152, no. 5, pp. 1259–1269, 1998.

[11] M. Miettinen, J. M. Monihan, M. Sarlomo-Rikala et al., "Gastrointestinal stromal tumors/smooth muscle tumors (GISTs) primary in the omentum and mesentery: clinicopathologic and immunohistochemical study of 26 cases," *The American Journal of Surgical Pathology*, vol. 23, no. 9, pp. 1109–1118, 1999.

[12] H. Joensuu, C. Fletcher, S. Dimitrijevic, S. Silberman, P. Roberts, and G. Demetri, "Management of malignant gastrointestinal stromal tumours," *The Lancet Oncology*, vol. 3, no. 11, pp. 655–664, 2002.

[13] S. Sakurai, T. Fukasawa, J. M. Chong, A. Tanaka, and M. Fukayama, "Embryonic form of smooth muscle myosin heavy chain (SMemb/MHC-B) in gastrointestinal stromal tumor and interstitial cells of Cajal," *The American Journal of Pathology*, vol. 154, no. 1, pp. 23–28, 1999.

[14] K. W. Head, J. M. Cullen, P. R. Dubielzig et al., *Histological Classification of Tumors of the Alimentary System of Domestic Animals*, vol. 10 of *International Histological Classification of Tumors of Domestic Animals*, WHO, Armed Forces Institute of Pathology, Washington, DC, USA, 2003.

[15] G. Isimbaldi, M. Santangelo, G. Cenacchi et al., "Gastrointestinal autonomic nerve tumor (Plexosarcoma): report of a case with fine needle aspiration biopsy and histologic, immunocytochemical and ultrastructural study," *Acta Cytologica*, vol. 42, no. 5, pp. 1189–1194, 1998.

[16] S. Hafner, B. G. Harmon, and T. King, "Gastrointestinal stromal tumors of the equine cecum," *Veterinary Pathology*, vol. 38, no. 2, pp. 242–246, 2001.

[17] S. Hirota, K. Isozaki, Y. Moriyama et al., "Gain-of-function mutations of C-kit in human gastrointestinal stromal tumors," *Science*, vol. 279, no. 5350, pp. 577–580, 1998.

[18] T. S. Emory, L. H. Sobin, L. Lukes, D. H. Lee, and T. J. O'Leary, "Prognosis of gastrointestinal smooth-muscle (stromal) tumors: dependence on anatomic site," *The American Journal of Surgical Pathology*, vol. 23, no. 1, pp. 82–87, 1999.

[19] M. Miettinen and J. Lasota, "Gastrointestinal stromal tumors—definition, clinical, histological, immunohistochemical, and molecular genetic features and differential diagnosis," *Virchows Archiv*, vol. 438, no. 1, pp. 1–12, 2001.

[20] M. Banerjee, L. J. Lowenstine, and R. J. Munn, "Gastric stromal tumors in two rhesus macaques (Macaca mulatta)," *Veterinary Pathology*, vol. 28, no. 1, pp. 30–36, 1991.

[21] C. D. M. Fletcher, J. J. Berman, C. Corless et al., "Diagnosis of gastrointestinal stromal tumors: a consensus approach," *Human Pathology*, vol. 33, no. 5, pp. 459–465, 2002.

[22] M. V. C. De Silva and R. Reid, "Gastrointestinal stromal tumors (GIST): C-kit mutations, CD117 expression, differential diagnosis and targeted cancer therapy with imatinib," *Pathology and Oncology Research*, vol. 9, no. 1, pp. 13–19, 2003.

[23] M. Miettinen and J. Lasota, "Gastrointestinal stromal tumors: review on morphology, molecular pathology, prognosis, and differential diagnosis," *Archives of Pathology and Laboratory Medicine*, vol. 130, no. 10, pp. 1466–1478, 2006.

[24] J. Rosai, "Stromal tumors," in *Ackerman's Surgical Pathology*, J. Rosai, Ed., vol. 8, pp. 691–693, Mosby, St. Louis, Mo, USA, 1996.

# 11

# Metastasis of a Prostatic Carcinoma along an Omental Graft in a Dog

**Terry M. Jacobs,[1] Bruce R. Hoppe,[1] Cathy E. Poehlmann,[1] Marie E. Pinkerton,[2] and Milan Milovancev[3,4]**

[1] Park Pet Hospital, 7378 N. Teutonia Avenue, Milwaukee, WI 53209, USA

[2] Department of Pathobiological Sciences, School of Veterinary Medicine, University of Wisconsin, 2015 Linden Drive, Madison, WI 53706, USA

[3] Wisconsin Veterinary Referral Center, Waukesha, WI 53188, USA

[4] Department of Small Animal Surgery, College of Veterinary Medicine, Oregon State University, 267 Magruder Hall, Corvallis, OR 97331, USA

Correspondence should be addressed to Terry M. Jacobs; petfxr@wi.rr.com

Academic Editors: S. M. Abutarbush, C. Hyun, R. M. Santos, and S. Stuen

An 11-year-old male American Bulldog was presented for hematuria and tenesmus. It had been treated for chronic bacterial prostatitis with abscessation two years earlier and underwent castration and a prostatic omentalization procedure. There was no histologic evidence of prostatic neoplasia at that time. On physical examination, an enlarged prostate was found by rectal palpation, and it was characterized with ultrasonography and computed tomography. Surgical biopsies were obtained, and histopathology identified prostatic adenocarcinoma. It received carprofen and mitoxantrone chemotherapy in addition to palliative radiation therapy; it was euthanized six weeks later due to a progression of clinical signs. Necropsy findings included marked localized expansion of the prostatic tumor and dissemination of prostatic carcinoma cells throughout the peritoneal cavity along the omental graft with infiltration onto the serosal surfaces of most abdominal viscera and fat. This case represents a previously unreported potential complication of the omentalization procedure wherein carcinoma cells from a prostatic tumor that independently arose after omentalization may have metastasized along the surgically created omental graft.

## 1. Introduction

The surgical treatment of canine prostate abscesses was revolutionized by the application of an intracapsular prostatic omentalization technique first reported by White and Williams in 1995 [1]. In this procedure, an omental graft is tunneled through the parenchyma of the prostate after digitally breaking down any loculated abscesses and is sutured to the prostate. The omentum provides vascular and lymphatic drainage to cavitated sites of infection within the prostate gland. Along with systemic antibiotic therapy, prostatic omentalization has enabled the successful management of many refractory cases of prostatitis in dogs. No long-term complications have been reported with this technique.

Prostatic carcinoma in dogs is generally an aggressive malignancy characterized by local invasiveness and early metastasis to regional lymph nodes, liver, lung, and bone [2–5]. Clinical signs are variable but typically include hematuria, stranguria, urinary incontinence, tenesmus, and pain, which may be localized if skeletal metastasis has occurred. The presence of an enlarged prostate in a neutered male dog may indicate malignancy; however, the prostate is not enlarged in all cases of prostatic carcinoma [4]. Radiography, ultrasonography, and computed tomography (CT) are useful imaging techniques to assess the prostate for the disease and to evaluate for evidence of metastasis. Diagnosis is confirmed by cytologic or histologic examination of prostatic fluid or tissue that is frequently obtained under ultrasonic guidance or by surgical biopsy. Oftentimes, the diagnosis is made at an advanced stage of the disease; therefore, the prognosis is guarded. Treatment options include surgery, radiotherapy, and chemotherapy [6–8]. Attempts at partial or complete

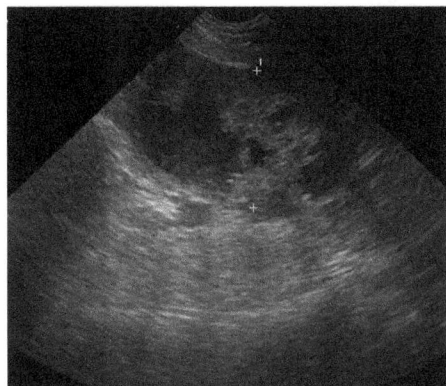

FIGURE 1: Sagittal ultrasound image of the prostate gland taken on initial presentation. Note the marked prostatomegaly with large cavitary areas containing hyperechogenic fluid within the gland.

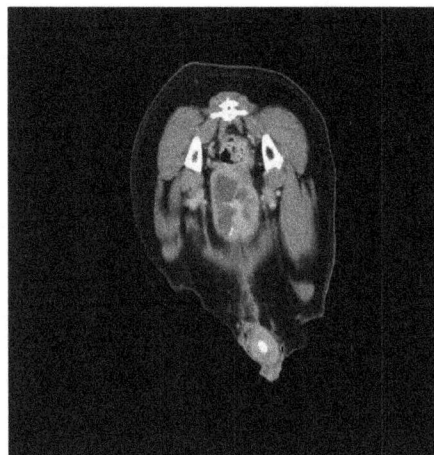

FIGURE 2: CT image of the prostate gland obtained prior to chemotherapy and radiotherapy. Note the prostatic enlargement and mineralization.

prostatectomy in dogs are usually avoided due to the risk of traumatizing neurovascular structures during dissection around the trigone of the bladder which may result in urinary incontinence or less commonly avascular necrosis [9]. Radiotherapy has the potential to achieve temporary local tumor control, but complications can include acute signs of urethritis and colitis or later the occurrence of urethral or colonic stricture and bladder fibrosis [10–12].

Chemotherapy utilizing mitoxantrone and cyclooxygenase inhibitors (COX-2) is frequently considered the most appropriate treatment option for both localized and metastatic diseases; however, limited responses are usually obtained, and median survival times are measured in months [6–8]. This report describes the occurrence of prostatic carcinoma with metastasis along an omental graft in a dog that had an omentalization procedure performed for a prior episode of bacterial prostatitis and abscessation.

## 2. Case Report

An 11-year-old castrated male American Bulldog was examined for signs of recent onset of hematuria with dyschezia. It had a chronic history of recurrent urinary tract infections with hematuria, prostatomegaly, and bacterial prostatitis and was treated repeatedly with appropriate antibiotics. The dog underwent castration 20 months prior to presentation; however, the prostate enlargement was not resolved. Ongoing signs of hematuria led to reevaluation two months later. Abdominal radiographs and ultrasonography identified prostatomegaly with multiple dilated cystic cavities within the prostate gland (Figure 1). During abdominal exploratory surgery, both lobes of the prostate gland were distended with multiple cystic cavities containing brown, cloudy fluid. Prostatic biopsies from four sites were obtained, and omentalization of the prostate gland was performed as previously described. Histology revealed severe lymphoplasmacytic prostatitis with regions of hemorrhage, necrosis, and fibrosis and no evidence of neoplasia. No further episodes of hematuria or urinary tract infection were observed for the next 18 months.

At presentation, firm symmetric prostatomegaly with tenderness was found on rectal palpation. Urinalysis revealed

hematuria and proteinuria, and no bacteria grew on aerobic culture. The results of a complete blood cell count and serum biochemistry profile were unremarkable. Abdominal radiographs showed an enlarged prostate; spondylosis along the spine was noted; however, no evidence of bone metastasis was seen. Ultrasonography identified two small cystic cavities and focal hyperechoic regions within the parenchyma of the prostate as well as mineralization along the wall of the urinary bladder. Celiotomy was performed, and the prostate gland was examined. The omental graft was observed to be intact, entering and exiting the cranioventral aspect of the prostate gland, which was enlarged with mildly distorted contours but no obvious masses. There were no cystic calculi present and no appreciable thickening of the wall of the urinary bladder. Biopsies were taken from the urinary bladder and from two sites within the right lobe of the prostate. Aerobic and anaerobic cultures of the prostate yielded no growth. Histological examination of the bladder tissue revealed cystitis with mineralization. The prostatic tissue sample identified medium to large moderately pleomorphic polygonal epithelial cells with considerable variation in cell and nuclear size, a large nucleolus, and frequent mitoses. The histologic diagnosis was prostatic adenocarcinoma. Staging was undertaken utilizing three-view thoracic radiographs and CT scanning of the chest and abdomen. No significant abnormalities were found in the chest. Prostatomegaly and mild iliac lymphadenopathy were found on the CT scan (Figure 2) along with mild mineralization of the prostate, bladder, and renal pelvis.

Treatment options were discussed with the owners, and chemotherapy with palliative tomotherapy was selected. Carprofen (Rimadyl; Pfizer, Exton, PA) (4 mg/kg P.O. $q$ 24 hr) and mitoxantrone (Mitoxantrone Injection; Hospira, Lake Forest, IL) (5 mg/m$^2$ IV once) were administered. One week later, the first of the four planned doses of coarsely fractioned radiotherapy directed at the prostate gland, 6.5 Gray (Gy), was given under general anesthesia. Appropriate analgesic, antiemetic, and antidiarrheal medications were provided as needed. The dog experienced a febrile neutropenia (494/$\mu$L)

(a)

(b)

(c)

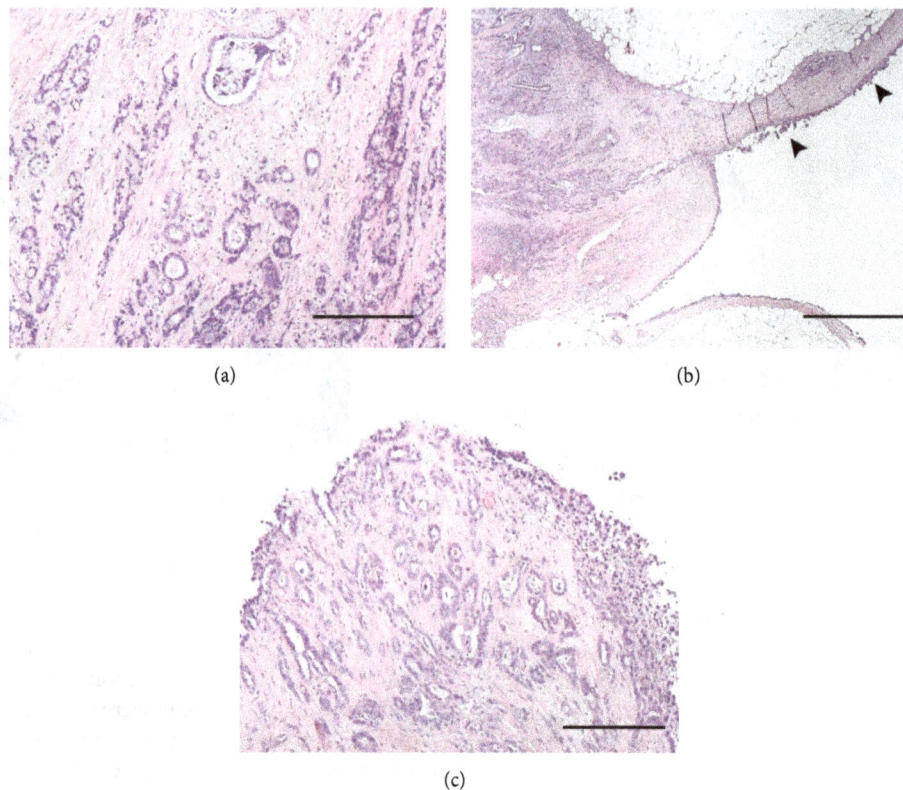

FIGURE 3: (a) Prostate gland: prostatic adenocarcinoma. Note the neoplastic cells arranged in nests and variably sized acinar structures amidst a dense fibrovascular stroma. Hematoxylin and eosin stain. Bar = 200 $\mu$m. (b) Omentum: note the metastatic spread of prostatic adenocarcinoma cells on the serosal surfaces forming small papillary fronds (arrowheads) and within the omental adipose tissue (carcinomatosis). Hematoxylin and eosin stain. Bar = 1000 $\mu$m. (c) Omentum: note the metastasis of prostatic adenocarcinoma cells on the serosal surface. Hematoxylin and eosin stain. Bar = 200 $\mu$m.

one week after mitoxantrone was given that responded to supportive intravenous fluids and broad-spectrum antibiotics; the mitoxantrone was then discontinued. A methicillin-resistant Staphylococcus intermedius urinary tract infection developed and was resolved with chloramphenicol (50 mg/kg P.O. q 8 hrs for 7 days). Three additional radiation treatments of 6.5 Gy with tomotherapy were completed, to a total dose of 26 Gy, over the next four weeks. The radiotherapy was well tolerated, but signs of tenesmus and abdominal discomfort persisted. One month after the final radiation treatment, progressive signs of dyschezia, hematochezia, anorexia, weight loss, and abdominal pain developed. The patient was euthanized three months after the diagnosis of prostatic carcinoma, and a complete necropsy was performed.

Postmortem examination revealed that all gross pathology was confined to the abdominal cavity. The prostate gland was enlarged (5 × 5 × 4 cm) with a markedly irregular surface and bilateral cystic cavities up to 2.5 cm diameter containing brown fluid and nodular tissue and surrounded by firmly adhered adipose tissue containing multiple white firm nodules. The prostatic urethra was patent but narrowed. The caudal and midabdominal fat was firm and variably infiltrated with white nodules; no peritoneal effusion was present. One kidney had an uneven capsular surface and foci of cortical thinning (infarctions), and the spleen had an irregular capsular depression. Sections of lung, liver, kidney, spleen, abdominal fat, and the entire prostate and urinary bladder were submitted in neutral buffered formalin and processed routinely for histology. On histological examination, the prostate gland contained a poorly demarcated, unencapsulated, and invasive mass composed of cuboidal to columnar cells arranged in variably sized, disorganized tubules, acini, and nests separated by a dense fibrovascular stroma, with 2–4 mitotic figures observed per ten high-power (400x) fields (Figure 3(a)).

In the kidney sample, subacute renal infarctions were associated with interstitial/intravascular nests of similar neoplastic cells. The neoplastic cells were also found within the splenic capsular depression, along many serosal surfaces, and within bands of scirrhous tissue throughout the abdominal fat, including the omentum (Figures 3(b) and 3(c)).

No metastatic sites were discovered in the liver or lung. The urinary tract had lymphoplasmacytic cystitis and pyelonephritis. The pathologic diagnosis was prostatic adenocarcinoma with metastasis to the spleen, kidney, abdominal fat including omentum, and serosal surfaces (carcinomatosis).

## 3. Discussion

Based on necropsy studies, the incidence of prostatic carcinoma in dogs is estimated to be 0.2%–0.6% [4, 13]. It is seen most often in older, castrated dogs, and while its pathogenesis is unknown, canine prostatic carcinomas are thought to originate from ductal epithelium in an androgen-independent process [13–15]. Recent molecular studies suggest that many prostatic tumors are transitional cell carcinomas arising from the prostatic urothelium [14, 16]. In contrast, prostate cancer is very common in older men, and its carcinogenesis is believed to be a multistep process involving androgens in the malignant transformation of acinar cells with inflammation and sexually transmitted diseases identified as risk factors [17]. Dogs with prostatic carcinoma typically have a high-grade malignancy, and the disease is generally multicentric at the time of diagnosis [6, 7]. A metastatic rate of 80% was found in one necropsy study of canine prostatic carcinomas, most commonly to lymph nodes, lung, and bone with rarer spread to the liver, colon, kidney, heart, adrenal gland, brain and spleen [15]. Direct extension of the tumor may occur, cranially into the urinary bladder, caudally into the urethra, or dorsally into the lumbar vertebrae [6, 8]. Regional metastasis to lumbosacral or iliac lymph nodes occurs frequently, and many dogs have a considerable pain during defecation due to lymphadenopathy and prostatomegaly [4, 6]. Radiographically, the finding of prostatomegaly with mineralization or bony reaction of the ventral surface of the caudal lumbar vertebrae is suspicious for prostatic carcinoma [18]. Surgical treatment of dogs with prostatic carcinoma is rarely recommended; however, selected cases have benefited from transurethral partial prostatectomy, urethral stenting, and/or tube cystotomy [9, 19–21]. Protocols for radiotherapy of dogs with prostate tumors are currently being investigated, but few reports have been published. A recent pilot study utilizing coarsely fractioned radiotherapy along with piroxicam and mitoxantrone for the treatment of dogs with transitional cell carcinoma of the bladder found that doses of 5.75 Gy were well tolerated and largely ameliorated clinical urinary signs [22]. Tomotherapy, a newly emerging technology, combines precise three-dimensional helical CT imaging with intensity-modulated radiotherapy (IMRT) to try to contour the radiation field to conform to the shape of the tumor [23]. Chemotherapy with piroxicam or other nonsteroidal anti-inflammatory drugs (NSAIDs) and mitoxantrone has become a standard of care for dogs with prostatic carcinomas based largely on studies showing partial efficacy in the management of transitional cell carcinomas of the urinary bladder [22, 24]. A recent study demonstrated the expression of COX-2 in nearly 90% of dog prostatic carcinomas, and a statistically significant survival advantage in 16 dogs given NSAIDs (14 treated with piroxicam and 2 treated with carprofen) compared with untreated controls [25].

In this case report, prostatic omentalization was successful in treating the dog's prostatic abscess two years prior to presentation; however, on subsequent biopsy nearly two years later, prostatic carcinoma had developed. Although chronic inflammation is considered a risk factor for human prostate cancer [17, 26, 27], this process remains uninvestigated in

veterinary medicine. Metastasis of prostatic cancer can occur by hematogenous or lymphatic routes as well as by direct attachment of tumor cells onto the peritoneal lining. There are rare reports of human prostatic carcinomas metastasizing to the omentum [28, 29]. Carcinomatosis is the seeding of a body cavity by malignant carcinoma cells, sometimes leading to a malignant effusion. Carcinomatosis in dogs most often is associated with ovarian or gastrointestinal neoplasia; however, one study reported evidence of carcinomatosis in 15% of dogs with prostate tumors [14]. Transitional cell carcinomas of the bladder are recognized for their ability to seed the abdomen during aspiration or surgical procedures [30]. Based on the pathologic findings in this case, the presence of the omental graft within the prostate presented a potential pathway for the tumor to expand beyond the prostate throughout the abdomen; however, hematogenous and intraperitoneal spread was also a factor in metastasis of this neoplasm. Appreciating the possibility of omental involvement, the owners were presented with the option of surgical removal of the omental graft prior to definitive radiotherapy. They declined this option and selected palliative tomotherapy. Unfortunately, the prostatic tumor was refractory to the radiotherapy and chemotherapy, resulting in rapid dissemination of the cancer within the peritoneal cavity and a progression of the clinical signs.

In conclusion, prostatic omentalization, although useful for draining prostatic abscesses and cysts, may inadvertently serve to facilitate the spread of neoplastic lesions throughout the peritoneal cavity. To the author's knowledge, this case represents the first report of the dissemination of a canine prostatic carcinoma along the omentum after a prior prostatic omentalization procedure. Dogs undergoing prostatic omentalization may be at a higher risk for metastasis along this pathway if prostatic carcinoma develops at a future date, and surgeons should be aware of this potential complication when considering the procedure.

## Conflict of Interests

The authors declare that there is no conflict of interests with respect to their authorship or publication of this paper. There was no financial support provided.

## Acknowledgments

The authors would like to thank the Department of Medical Oncology and the Department of Radiation Oncology at the School of Veterinary Medicine, University of Wisconsin for their assistance with chemotherapy and tomotherapy.

## References

[1] R. A. White and J. M. Williams, "Intracapsular prostatic omentalization: a new technique for management of prostatic abscesses in dogs," *Veterinary Surgery*, vol. 24, no. 5, pp. 390–395, 1995.

[2] A. D. Weaver, "Fifteen cases of prostatic carcinoma in the dog," *Veterinary Record*, vol. 109, no. 4, pp. 71–75, 1981.

[3] A. M. Hargis and L. M. Miller, "Prostatic carcinoma in dogs," *Compendium on Continuing Education for the Practising Veterinarian,* vol. 5, pp. 647–653, 1983.

[4] F. W. Bell, J. S. Klausner, D. W. Hayden, D. A. Feeney, and S. D. Johnston, "Clinical and pathologic features of prostatic adenocarcinoma in sexually intact and castrated dogs: 31 cases (1970–1987)," *Journal of the American Veterinary Medical Association,* vol. 199, no. 11, pp. 1623–1630, 1991.

[5] B. E. LeRoy and N. Northrup, "Prostate cancer in dogs: comparative and clinical aspects," *Veterinary Journal,* vol. 180, no. 2, pp. 149–162, 2009.

[6] G. K. Ogilvie and A. S. Moore, *Managing the Canine Cancer Patient,* Veterinary Learning Systems, Yardley, Pa, USA, 2006.

[7] S. J. Withrow, D. M. Vail, and R. L. Page, *Small Animal Oncology,* WB Saunders, Philadelphia, Pa, USA, 5th edition, 2013.

[8] C. J. Henry and M. L. Higginbotham, *Cancer Management in Small Animal Practice,* Saunders Elsevier, 2010.

[9] T. Freitag, R. M. Jerram, A. M. Walker, and C. G. A. Warman, "Surgical management of common canine prostatic conditions," *Compendium: Continuing Education for Veterinarians,* vol. 29, no. 11, pp. 656–672, 2007.

[10] J. M. Turrel, "Intraoperative radiotherapy of carcinoma of the prostate gland in ten dogs," *Journal of the American Veterinary Medical Association,* vol. 190, no. 1, pp. 48–52, 1987.

[11] D. R. Proulx, D. M. Ruslander, M. L. Hauck et al., "Canine prostatic neoplasia. A retrospective analysis of 10 dogs treated with external beam radiation (1989–2001)," in *Proceedings of the 22nd Annual Conference of the Veterinary Cancer Society,* p. 40, 2002.

[12] C. R. Anderson, E. A. McNiel, E. L. Gillette, B. E. Powers, and S. M. LaRue, "Late complications of pelvic irradiation in 16 dogs," *Veterinary Radiology and Ultrasound,* vol. 43, no. 2, pp. 187–192, 2002.

[13] J. Obradovich, R. Walshaw, and E. Goullaud, "The influence of castration on the development of prostatic carcinoma in the dog. 43 cases (1978–1985)," *Journal of Veterinary Internal Medicine,* vol. 1, no. 4, pp. 183–187, 1987.

[14] K. U. Sorenmo, M. Goldschmidt, F. Shofer, C. Goldkamp, and J. Ferracone, "Immunohistochemical characterization of canine prostatic carcinoma and correlation with castration status and castration time," *Veterinary and Comparative Oncology,* vol. 1, no. 1, pp. 48–56, 2003.

[15] K. K. Cornell, D. G. Bostwick, D. M. Cooley et al., "Clinical and pathologic aspects of spontaneous canine prostate carcinoma: a retrospective analysis of 76 cases," *Prostate,* vol. 45, no. 2, pp. 173–183, 2000.

[16] B. E. LeRoy, M. V. P. Nadella, R. E. Toribio, I. Leav, and T. J. Rosol, "Canine prostate carcinomas express markers of urothelial and prostatic differentiation," *Veterinary Pathology,* vol. 41, no. 2, pp. 131–140, 2004.

[17] W. G. Nelson, A. M. de Marzo, T. L. DeWeese et al., "The role of inflammation in the pathogenesis of prostate cancer," *Journal of Urology,* vol. 172, no. 5, pp. S6–S12, 2004.

[18] C. A. Bradbury, J. L. Westropp, and R. E. Pollard, "Relationship between prostatomegaly, prostatic mineralization, and cytologic diagnosis," *Veterinary Radiology and Ultrasound,* vol. 50, no. 2, pp. 167–171, 2009.

[19] H. F. L'Eplattenier, S. A. van Nimwegen, F. J. van Sluijs, and J. Kirpensteijn, "Partial prostatectomy using Nd:YAG laser for management of canine prostate carcinoma," *Veterinary Surgery,* vol. 35, no. 4, pp. 406–411, 2006.

[20] J. M. Liptak, S. P. Brutscher, E. Monnet et al., "Transurethral resection in the management of urethral and prostatic neoplasia in 6 dogs," *Veterinary Surgery,* vol. 33, no. 5, pp. 505–516, 2004.

[21] C. Weisse, A. Berent, K. Todd, C. Clifford, and J. Solomon, "Evaluation of palliative stenting for management of malignant urethral obstructions in dogs," *Journal of the American Veterinary Medical Association,* vol. 229, no. 2, pp. 226–234, 2006.

[22] V. J. Poirier, L. J. Forrest, W. M. Adams, and D. M. Vail, "Piroxicam, mitoxantrone, and coarse fraction radiotherapy for the treatment of transitional cell carcinoma of the bladder in 10 dogs: a pilot study," *Journal of the American Animal Hospital Association,* vol. 40, no. 2, pp. 131–136, 2004.

[23] J. A. Lawrence and L. J. Forrest, "Intensity-modulated radiation therapy and helical tomotherapy: its origin, benefits, and potential applications in veterinary medicine," *Veterinary Clinics of North America—Small Animal Practice,* vol. 37, no. 6, pp. 1151–1165, 2007.

[24] C. J. Henry, D. L. McCaw, S. E. Turnquist et al., "Clinical evaluation of mitoxantrone and piroxicam in a canine model of human invasive urinary bladder carcinoma," *Clinical Cancer Research,* vol. 9, no. 2, pp. 906–911, 2003.

[25] K. U. Sorenmo, M. H. Goldschmidt, F. S. Shofer, C. Goldcamp, and J. Ferracone, "Evaluation of cydooxygenase-1 and cyclooxygenase-2 expression and the effect of cydooxygenase inhibitors in canine prostatic carcinoma," *Kleintierpraxis,* vol. 52, no. 1, p. 36, 2007.

[26] G. S. Palapattu, S. Sutcliffe, P. J. Bastian et al., "Prostate carcinogenesis and inflammation: emerging insights," *Carcinogenesis,* vol. 26, no. 7, pp. 1170–1181, 2005.

[27] A. M. de Marzo, E. A. Platz, S. Sutcliffe et al., "Inflammation in prostate carcinogenesis," *Nature Reviews Cancer,* vol. 7, no. 4, pp. 256–269, 2007.

[28] E. O. Kehinde, S. M. Abdeen, A. Al-Hunayan, and Y. Ali, "Prostate cancer metastatic to the omentum," *Scandinavian Journal of Urology and Nephrology,* vol. 36, no. 3, pp. 225–227, 2002.

[29] F. Zagouri, M. Papaefthimiou, A. N. Chalazonitis, N. Antoniou, M. A. Dimopoulos, and A. Bamias, "Prostate cancer with metastasis to the omentum and massive ascites: a rare manifestation of a common disease," *Onkologie,* vol. 32, no. 12, pp. 758–761, 2009.

[30] T. G. Nyland, S. T. Wallack, and E. R. Wisner, "Needle-tract implantation following US-guided fine-needle aspiration biopsy of transitional cell carcinoma of the bladder, urethra, and prostate," *Veterinary Radiology and Ultrasound,* vol. 43, no. 1, pp. 50–53, 2002.

# 12

# Regressing Multiple Viral Plaques and Skin Fragility Syndrome in a Cat Coinfected with FcaPV2 and FcaPV3

**Alberto Alberti,**[1] **Gessica Tore,**[1] **Alessandra Scagliarini,**[2] **Laura Gallina,**[2] **Federica Savini,**[2] **Chiara Caporali,**[3] **and Francesca Abramo**[4]

[1]*Department of Veterinary Medicine, University of Sassari, Via Vienna 2, 07100 Sassari, Italy*
[2]*Department of Veterinary Medical Sciences, University of Bologna, Via Zamboni 33, 40126 Bologna, Italy*
[3]*Private Practitioner, Via Giovanni da Verrazzano 19, 52100 Arezzo, Italy*
[4]*Department of Veterinary Sciences, University of Pisa, Viale delle Piagge 2, 56124 Pisa, Italy*

Correspondence should be addressed to Francesca Abramo; francesca.abramo@unipi.it

Academic Editor: Katerina K. Adamama-Moraitou

Feline viral plaques are uncommon skin lesions clinically characterized by multiple, often pigmented, and slightly raised lesions. Numerous reports suggest that *papillomaviruses* (PVs) are involved in their development. Immunosuppressed and immunocompetent cats are both affected, the biological behavior is variable, and the regression is possible but rarely documented. Here we report a case of a FIV-positive cat with skin fragility syndrome and regressing multiple viral plaques in which the contemporary presence of two PV types (FcaPV2 and FcaPV3) was demonstrated by combining a quantitative molecular approach to histopathology. The cat, under glucocorticoid therapy for stomatitis and pruritus, developed skin fragility and numerous grouped slightly raised nonulcerated pigmented macules and plaques with histological features of epidermal thickness, mild dysplasia, and presence of koilocytes. Absolute quantification of the viral DNA copies (4555 copies/microliter of FcaPV2 and 8655 copies/microliter of FcaPV3) was obtained. Eighteen months after discontinuation of glucocorticoid therapy skin fragility and viral plaques had resolved. The role of the two viruses cannot be established and it remains undetermined how each of the viruses has contributed to the onset of VP; the spontaneous remission of skin lesions might have been induced by FIV status change over time due to glucocorticoid withdraw and by glucocorticoids withdraw itself.

## 1. Introduction

Feline viral plaques (VPs) are well recognized uncommon skin lesions clinically appearing as solitary or multiple, raised, often pigmented, small plaques [1–4]. Cats are affected at any age [4] and they may be either immunocompromised [1, 2, 5] or immunocompetent [4]. Microscopically, a VP consists of well-demarcated foci of epidermal thickening, mild dysplasia, and presence of koilocytes. VPs are associated with the presence of *papillomavirus* (PV), predominantly with *Felis catus papillomavirus* type 2 (FcaPV2), but other PV types as well as multiple PVs in a single lesion have been less frequently reported [4–6]. The behavior of VPs is variable; progression to Bowenoid *in situ* carcinoma (BISC) and invasive squamous cell carcinoma (SCC) is a risk; the plaques can remain small for long time and regress; however,

very little information about follow-up is available from the published cases [7]. This paper reports a coinfection with 2 PV types, FcaPV2 and FcaPV3, in a FIV-positive cat with skin fragility syndrome (SFS) and spontaneous regressing multiple VPs. Papillomaviruses were molecularly characterized and relative viral loads were quantified.

## 2. Case Presentation

A short-haired adult neutered male cat was presented to a private veterinary clinic for bilateral pruritic alopecia and skin lesions on the trunk, noticed by the owners 5 months before, when the cat was found as a stray. The cat had been treated for a severe stomatitis and severe pruritus with two 20 mg/cat subcutaneous injections of

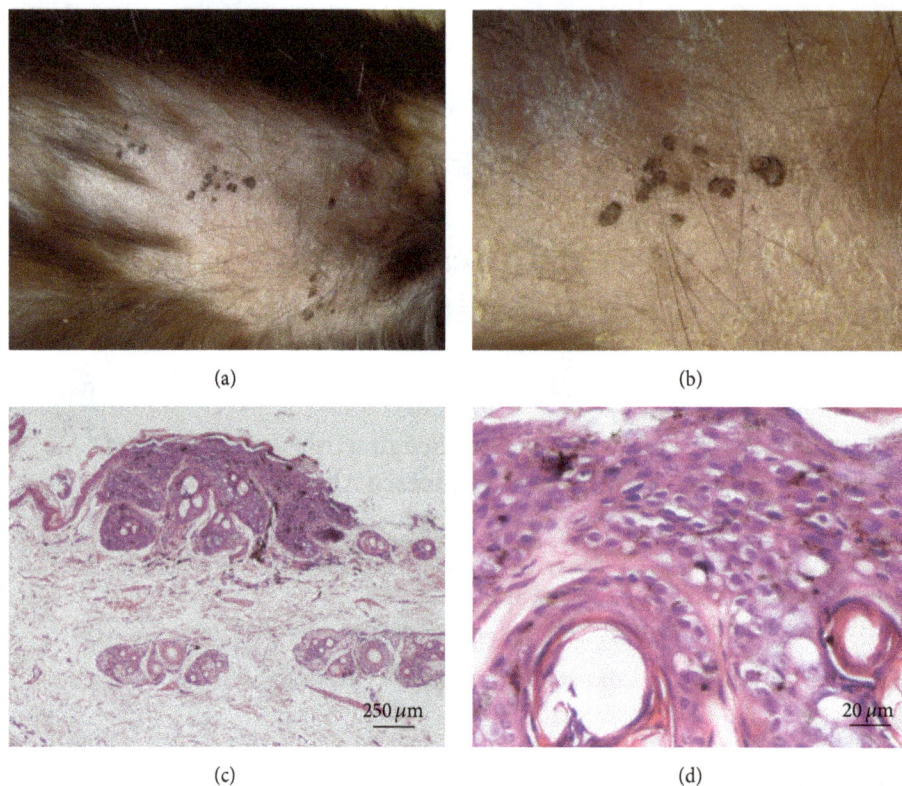

FIGURE 1: Macroscopic and microscopic features. Ill-defined alopecia in the cat trunk with multifocally grouped, 2 to 8 mm, pigmented, slightly raised, nonulcerated plaques (a). Detail of plaques arising from the alopecic and exfoliating skin (b): plaques have a rough surface and an irregular shape. Focal hyperplasia and dysplasia of the surface and follicular epidermis accompanied by mildly asynchronous keratinocyte maturation; note the loosely arranged and slightly fragmented collagen fibers in the dermis (c). Detail of (c): some keratinocytes have dark condensed nuclei and a clear cytoplasmic halo (koilocytes); others have a blue-grey cytoplasm (hematoxylin and eosin stain).

methylprednisolone acetate (Depo-Medrol Vet; Pfizer Italia S.r.l., Borgo San Michele, Italy) weekly and underwent full teeth extraction with the exception of the canines. Previously the cat had been administered undetermined courses of corticosteroids, without any detail about specific drug and dosages given by the owners. While general physical examination was unremarkable and mild stomatitis was seen at oral inspection, dermatological examination showed ill-defined alopecia on the trunk and flank with a very thin tissue paper skin, scaling, one wide laceration covered by necrotic material on the withers, and numerous small grouped slightly raised nonulcerated pigmented macules and plaques on the flank and posterior thorax (Figures 1(a) and 1(b)). Multiple skin scrapings and adhesive tape preparations showed no evidence of *Demodex* spp. mites, fungal culture was negative, and microscopic examination of hair shafts showed no abnormalities. A complete blood cell count and serum chemistry revealed mild leukocytosis (WBC 25,54 K/$\mu$L, reference values 5,50–19,50) with neutrophilia (18,77 K/$\mu$L, reference values 2,50–12,50) and increase of mononucleated cells (3,71 K/$\mu$L, reference values 0,15–1,70), hyperglycemia (385 mg/dL, reference values 71–159), and increased fructosamine levels (396 $\mu$mol/L, reference values 228–356). The cat was FeLV negative and FIV positive. CBC values, in particular persistent hyperglycemia, together with history of corticosteroid administration suggested iatrogenic hyperadrenocorticism. Liver lipidosis was considered unlikely for unchanged hepatic enzymes and for the good general condition of the cat. Clinical presentation indicated skin fragility and VP/BISC as main differential. Punch biopsies were taken from raised lesions, fixed in 10% buffered formalin, and routinely processed for histopathology. Histologically multiple sharply demarcated plaques of full-thickness epidermal and follicular dysplasia were seen, and groups of *in situ* proliferating keratinocytes showed loss of nuclear polarity (Figures 1(c) and 1(d)). A variable number of keratinocytes had cytoplasm enlarged by blue-greyish fibrillar material; some others had dark shrunken nucleus and clear cytoplasm (koilocytes). No invasion of the basal membrane into the dermis was detected. Epidermis adjacent to the neoplastic lesion was thin and keratotic, with collagen fibers of the underlying dermis markedly thin and loosely arranged. Collectively these features were indicative of SFS and concomitant multifocal VPs; despite the small dimension of the plaques, the possibility of progression to an early BISC was also indicated in the diagnostic report due to the follicular involvement and the dysplastic appearance of keratinocytes [8]. DNA was extracted from a fresh punch biopsy with the "DNeasy Blood and Tissue Kit" (Qiagen, Milan, Italy) according to vendor recommendations. To investigate the presence

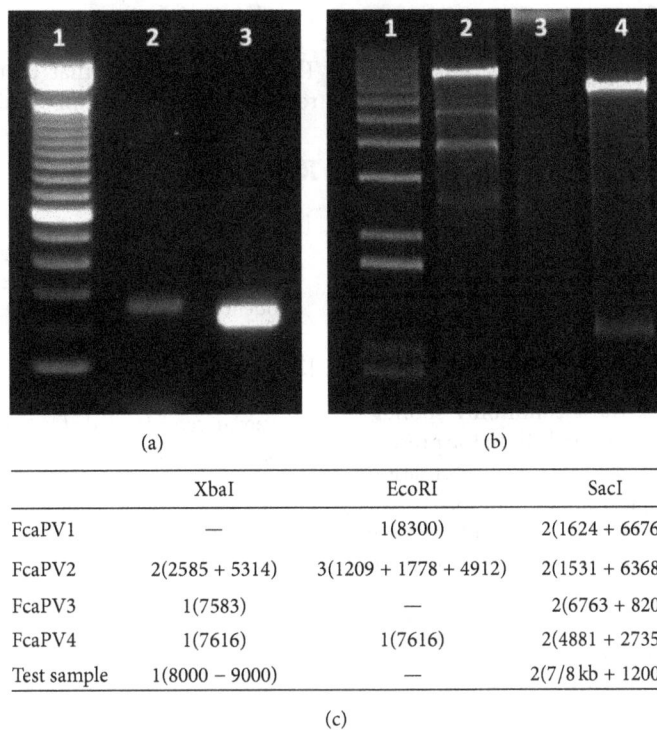

(a)                                    (b)

| | XbaI | EcoRI | SacI |
|---|---|---|---|
| FcaPV1 | — | 1(8300) | 2(1624 + 6676) |
| FcaPV2 | 2(2585 + 5314) | 3(1209 + 1778 + 4912) | 2(1531 + 6368) |
| FcaPV3 | 1(7583) | — | 2(6763 + 820) |
| FcaPV4 | 1(7616) | 1(7616) | 2(4881 + 2735) |
| Test sample | 1(8000 − 9000) | — | 2(7/8 kb + 1200) |

(c)

FIGURE 2: Molecular detection and typing of feline papillomavirus. In (a) PCR results demonstrating the presence of at least two PV types are shown (1, Life Technologies 100 bp DNA Ladder; 2, 3, positivity to primers FPV12F/R and FPV34F/R, resp.). Results obtained with rolling circle amplification (RCA) (b) and restriction enzyme digestions of the RCA products (c) indicating the presence of FcaPV3 in the lesion.

of feline PVs 2 sets of primers were used. Primers FPV12F/R (5′-TGCAAATAYCCTGACTACAT-3′/5′-CTATTRAAY-AATTGRGCCTC-3′) were designed to amplify 250 bp of the L1 of FcaPV1 and FcaPV2. Similarly primers FPV34F/R (5′-AGGACACTGAAAATCCCAAC-3′/5′-TCACACATT-TGACCATCCTC) targeted 230 bp of the L1 of FcaPV3 and FcaPV4. PCR profiles were set according to vendor recommendation for Taq polymerase (Qiagen, Milan, Italy). Notably, PCR was positive for both primer's pairs, indicating the presence of at least 2 distinct papillomavirus types (Figure 2(a)). Amplicons FPV12F/R and FPV34F/R were successfully cloned into pCR4-TOPO (Invitrogen, Milan, Italy). Three clones per amplicon were automatically sequenced. Upon submission to standard nucleotide blast, sequences obtained from amplicon FPV12F/R (GeneBank accession number KP868617) revealed 100% of nucleotide identity with the corresponding L1 region of FcaPV2 reference strain (EU796884) and sequences derived from amplicon FPV34F/R (GeneBank accession number KP868618) shared 99% of identity with FePV3 reference strain (JX972168). FcaPV2 and FcaPV3 viral loads were investigated by absolute quantification of DNA viral copies in the sample. Nucleic acid quantification was obtained by Real-Time PCR, performed with Rotor gene 3000 system (Corbett Research, Australia). With this aim, primers QFePV2F/R (5′-GCGGAG-GGAGCAACAATACACT-3′/5′-GGCCGCCTTCAAAAC-CAA-3′) and QFePV3F/R (5′-GCACAGGGGAGCATTGG-3′/5′-GGTGGACAGTCCCCCTTTTG-3′) were designed to amplify smaller fragments of the *Felis catus papillomaviruses* 2

(91 bp) and 3 (85 bp) L1, respectively. Absolute quantification of the viral DNA copies was obtained by plotting 10-fold dilutions (from $1.2 \times 10^1$ to $1.2 \times 10^4$ copies/$\mu$L) of 2 distinct pUC19 plasmids containing the cloned fragments. Based on Real-Time PCR, 4555 copies/microliter of FcaPV2 and 8655 copies/microliter of FcaPV3 were present in the sample. Rolling circle amplification and restriction enzyme digestions resulted in the detection of a patter compatible with FcaPV3 (Figure 2(b)).

Based on clinical and histopathologic features, wearing of a bodysuit was recommended to prevent further skin tearing from itching. Therapy was initiated with doxycycline of 10 mg/kg once daily for 2 months; this drug has been chosen for its dual antimicrobial and immunomodulatory action. No further treatment was administered for the VPs. The follow-up in the first three months showed improvement in skin lesions: ulcers progressively healed, hair started to regrow, VPs were still present but again no therapy was underwent, and mild stomatitis was present at oral examination. After 18 months from initial diagnosis, on demand from the referring veterinarian, the owner was allowed to revisit the cat and the raised pigmented multiple plaque as well as skin fragility had resolved while mild stomatitis was still present.

Since early reports of feline skin hyperplastic lesions related to papillomavirus [1, 2] numerous other cases and series of cases have been published so far, in which PVs are considered to have a causative role in different feline skin diseases [9, 10]. These include feline fibropapilloma or sarcoid

[11] and a wide spectrum of proliferative skin diseases ranging from nonneoplastic VPs to preneoplastic BISC and invasive SSC [12]. Viral plaques, BISC, and SCC may coexist in the same skin lesion or the first may progressively evolve to the others in a long period of time. In our case the clinical and histopathological resemblance between VP and BISC lead to the risk of overdiagnosing a preneoplastic lesion (BISC); however, regression of VP after discontinuation of glucocorticoid and general condition improvement is in line with a non-neoplastic nature of the plaques. Some histological features of VP are shared with BISC and a clear separation between the two entities may be difficult. SFS is an uncommon acquired disease of cats that has been reported in association with several concurrent diseases, most commonly spontaneous or iatrogenic hyperadrenocorticism [12]. In the present case, skin fragility was noted at the time of presentation together with multiple raised plaques, and both lesions might have been induced by the previous glucocorticoid therapy; moreover, the cat was FIV positive. VPs have already been documented in cats with underlying FIV or glucocorticoid immunosuppression [1, 2, 5]. Cat pruritus was diffuse when the cat was found and it was not possible to ascertain whether VPs on the flank and thorax might have developed by inoculation of virus in self-induced skin abrasions. The regression of skin lesions in the case reported suggests that glucocorticoid therapy and FIV status might have predisposed to VP.

Four PV types have been so far described in cats [6, 9, 13–15]. While association of FePV1 and FePV4 to disease remains to be clarified, an increasing number of reports indicate a correlation between the presence of FePV2 and FePV3 in VPs, BISCs, and SCCs [5, 13, 16]. FdPV-2 has been found in a high proportion of VPs and it has long been considered to be etiologically involved in the development of these skin lesions [4, 5]; however, more recently, Munday and Witham [17] have amplified FcaPV2 from 50% of swabs taken from the skin of clinically normal domestic cats, also suggesting a subclinical infection for this type of PV. A third PV, Feline Catus-PV3 (FcaPV3), has been also detected from a feline VP and BISC [4, 10]. Finally multiple PVs have been detected once in a single sample from a cat [5].

## 3. Conclusion

This paper reports a case of VP in which, by combining PCR test with sequencing and Real-Time PCR, coinfection with 2 PV types was recorded and their concentration was determined. Whether the role of the two viruses cannot be established in this case, FcaPV2 and FcaPV3 are present at comparable concentrations; it remains undetermined how each of the viruses might have contributed to the onset of lesions following immunosuppression. We hypothesize that one of the 2 viruses might have provided a more permissive environment for the other. Finally, spontaneous remission of skin lesions might have been induced by FIV status change over time due to glucocorticoid withdraw and by glucocorticoids withdraw itself.

## Conflict of Interests

The authors declare that there is no conflict of interests regarding the publication of this paper.

## References

[1] H. F. Egberink, A. Berrocal, H. A. D. Bax, T. S. G. A. M. van den Ingh, J. H. Walter, and M. C. Horzinek, "Papillomavirus associated skin lesions in a cat seropositive for feline immunodeficiency virus," Veterinary Microbiology, vol. 31, no. 2-3, pp. 117–125, 1992.

[2] H. C. Carney, J. J. England, E. C. Hodgin, H. E. Whiteley, D. L. Adkison, and J. P. Sundberg, "Papillomavirus infection of aged Persian cats," Journal of Veterinary Diagnostic Investigation, vol. 2, no. 4, pp. 294–299, 1990.

[3] J. L. Carpenter, J. W. Reider, J. Alroy, and G. M. Schmidt, "Cutaneous xanthogranuloma and viral papilloma on an eyelid of a cat," Veterinary Dermatology, vol. 3, no. 4-5, pp. 187–190, 1992.

[4] J. S. Munday and J. Peters-Kennedy, "Consistent detection of Felis domesticus papillomavirus 2 DNA sequences within feline viral plaques," Journal of Veterinary Diagnostic Investigation, vol. 22, no. 6, pp. 946–949, 2010.

[5] J. S. Munday, K. A. Willis, M. Kiupel, F. I. Hill, and M. Dunowska, "Amplification of three different papillomaviral DNA sequences from a cat with viral plaques," Veterinary Dermatology, vol. 19, no. 6, pp. 400–404, 2008.

[6] J. S. Munday, M. Kiupel, A. F. French, L. Howe, and R. A. Squires, "Detection of papillomaviral sequences in feline Bowenoid in situ carcinoma using consensus primers," Veterinary Dermatology, vol. 18, no. 4, pp. 241–245, 2007.

[7] H. Egberink, E. Thiry, K. Mostl et al., "Feline viral papillomatosis. ABC guidelines on prevention and management," Journal of Feline Medicine and Surgery, vol. 15, no. 7, pp. 560–562, 2013.

[8] T. L. Gross, P. J. Ihrke, and E. J. Walder, Skin Diseases of the Dog and Cat. Clinical and Histopathologic Diagnosis, Blackwell Science, Oxford, UK, 2nd edition, 2005.

[9] J. P. Sundberg, M. Van Ranst, R. Montali et al., "Feline papillomas and papillomaviruses," Veterinary Pathology, vol. 37, no. 1, pp. 1–10, 2000.

[10] J. S. Munday, M. Dunowska, S. F. Hills, and R. E. Laurie, "Genomic characterization of Felis catus papillomavirus-3: a novel papillomavirus detected in a feline Bowenoid in situ carcinoma," Veterinary Microbiology, vol. 165, no. 3-4, pp. 319–325, 2013.

[11] F. Y. Schulman, A. E. Krafft, and T. Janczewski, "Feline cutaneous fibropapillomas: clinicopathologic findings and association with papillomavirus infection," Veterinary Pathology, vol. 38, no. 3, pp. 291–296, 2001.

[12] W. H. Miller, C. E. Griffin, and K. Campbell, "Viral, rickettsial and protozoal skin diseases," in Muller and Kirk's Small Animal Dermatology, pp. 350–351, Elsevier Mosby, St. Louis, Mo, USA, 7th edition, 2013.

[13] R. Tachezy, G. Duson, A. Rector, A. B. Jenson, J. P. Sundberg, and M. Van Ranst, "Cloning and genomic characterization of Felis domesticus papillomavirus type 1," Virology, vol. 301, no. 2, pp. 313–321, 2002.

[14] M. Dunowska, J. S. Munday, R. E. Laurie, and S. F. K. Hills, "Genomic characterisation of Felis catus papillomavirus 4, a novel papillomavirus detected in the oral cavity of a domestic cat," Virus Genes, vol. 48, no. 1, pp. 111–119, 2014.

[15] M. Terai and R. D. Burk, "Felis domesticus papillomavirus, isolated from a skin lesion, is related to caine oral papillomavirus and contains a 1.3 kb non-coding region between the E2 and L2 open reading frames," *Journal of General Virology*, vol. 83, no. 9, pp. 2303–2307, 2002.

[16] J. S. Munday, "Papillomaviruses in felids," *Veterinary Journal*, vol. 199, no. 3, pp. 340–347, 2014.

[17] J. S. Munday and A. I. Witham, "Frequent detection of papillomavirus DNA in clinically normal skin of cats infected and noninfected with feline immunodeficiency virus," *Veterinary Dermatology*, vol. 21, no. 3, pp. 307–310, 2010.

# 13

# Hippocampal Necrosis in a Cat from Australia

## Carl Adagra[1] and Susan Amanda Piripi[2]

[1]Tropical Queensland Cat Clinic, Townsville City, QLD 4810, Australia
[2]University of Sydney, Sydney, NSW 2006, Australia

Correspondence should be addressed to Carl Adagra; cadagra@hotmail.com

Academic Editor: Paola Roccabianca

This paper reports findings from a feline case of hippocampal necrosis. A seven-year-old neutered female cat was seen with a history of behavioural change followed by complex focal seizures. The cat was severely pyrexic on presentation and anisocoria was present. It was treated with cooling, intravenous fluid, and phenobarbitone administration which was later changed to levetiracetam. An MRI was performed and revealed findings of a hypointense T1 and hyperintense T2 signal in the hippocampus and inferior temporal gyrus with mild gadolinium uptake, findings which were consistent with previous cases of hippocampal necrosis. The cat was witnessed to vomit and aspirate 24 hours after diagnosis leading to cardiac arrest and death. Postmortem examination revealed a subacute degenerative encephalopathy involving the hippocampus.

## 1. Introduction

Hippocampal necrosis is an infrequently reported MRI and postmortem finding in cats [1–6]. It has been predominantly associated with clinical signs of behavioral change and seizure activity and, to date, has been reported in cats from the UK, Switzerland, Italy, USA, and Austria [1–6]. Cats with this disease have been reported to show a myriad of symptoms including salivation, behavioural change, complex focal seizures, facial twitching, lip smacking, chewing, retching, vomiting, diarrhoea, circling, excessive swallowing, and postural deficits or weakness [1–6]. The reported prognosis for this disease is very poor with one case series reporting 4 survivors out of 17 cases (23%) over a four-month period [4].

The closest proposed analogues to hippocampal necrosis in the cat are hippocampal necrosis reported in rats [7], ischaemic hippocampal necrosis in humans [8], and mesial temporal lobe epilepsy with hippocampal sclerosis (MTLE-HS) in humans [9]. A study by Barbolt and Everett [7] in rats demonstrated that the majority of rats with hippocampal necrosis had a significant coexisting lesion likely to cause cerebral ischemia, with common lesions consisting of left sided atrial or valvular thrombosis, cerebral thrombosis,

large lymphocyte leukemia, or metastatic mesothelioma. Hippocampal necrosis in the rat was hypothesised to be frequently related to ischaemic injury.

In humans, the hippocampus is found to be the area of the brain most sensitive to ischemia and can be selectively damaged by this state [8]. MTLE-HS in humans is a disease with very similar clinical signs to hippocampal necrosis in cats. Similar MRI changes can be seen with the main difference being that MTLE-HS sufferers have less inflammatory change on histopathology than found in feline cases of hippocampal necrosis [9]. The aetiology of MTLE-HS is unknown, but many mechanisms are proposed including glutamate neurotoxicity and mitochondrial dysfunction leading to neuronal cell loss, immune factors leading to cell loss, a genetic predisposition to the disease, or a multifactorial disease process [9]. The accepted treatment of hippocampal necrosis is based on controlling the symptoms of the disease as there are no reports of resolution of lesions. Whilst a case of Hippocampal necrosis secondary to a pyriform lobe oligodendroglioma has been reported in a cat [1], the aetiology of the majority of feline hippocampal necrosis cases remains unknown and cases carry a guarded prognosis.

## 2. Case Presentation

A seven-year-old neutered female domestic short hair cat presented with a three-day history of behavioural change followed by salivation and a 40-second-complex focal seizure involving the head, neck, and forelimbs. The behavioural change consisted of excessive vocalization, facial territorial marking, and periuria. The cat lived an indoor only lifestyle and was fed with a mixture of commercial wet and dry cat food. There was no history of exposure to toxins.

On physical examination, the cat was agitated, hypersalivating, and severely pyrexic with a body temperature greater than 41 degrees centigrade (>105.8 F). Anisocoria was present with a miotic left pupil. The findings of behavioural change and seizures localised the neurologic lesion to the forebrain; a variety of possible differential diagnoses were considered including diseases of neoplastic, infectious, inflammatory, developmental, degenerative, idiopathic, metabolic, vascular, and toxic aetiology. The cat was immediately started on phenobarbitone (Phenobarbitone sodium 20 mg/0.5 mL; Mayne Pharma Ltd, Salisbury, South Australia) 3 mg/kg IV q12 h, body cooling, and intravenous fluids with Hartmann's solution at an initial rate of 5 mL/kg/hr. Diagnostic testing was initiated with a complete blood count, coagulation testing, and biochemistry panel. Abnormalities found were a mild elevation in albumin, hypernatraemia, and hyperchloraemia with mild eosinopaenia and neutrophilia.

With treatment, the cat's temperature reduced to 39.9 degrees centigrade (103.82 F) over a 4-hour period. Cooling was discontinued and the temperature continued to decrease to the normal range. The anisocoria and salivation also resolved; however, the cat became stuporous. This was considered to be partly related to sedative effects of phenobarbitone, but concurrent CNS disease seemed likely.

An ammonia tolerance test and toxoplasma IgM:IgG antibody and cryptococcus antigen test were performed. The cat was started on clindamycin (Dalacin; Pfizer Australia Pty Ltd, West Ryde, NSW.) 15 mg/kg IV q12 h pending toxoplasma titer results. Results returned within the reference ranges for all of these tests.

Prophylactic thiamine (Vitamin B1 injectable 125 mg/mL; Value Plus Animal Health Care Products Pty Ltd, Girraween, NSW.) supplementation was started at 25 $\mu$g/kg s/c q24 h for 3 days. Nutritional support was also started with supplemental syringe feeding as the cat's gag and swallowing reflexes remained intact. Treatment was started with prednisolone sodium succinate (Solu-Delta-Cortef; 1%. Pfizer Australia Pty Ltd, West Ryde, NSW.) 1 mg/kg IV q12 h prior to performing anesthesia for an MRI scan.

A follow-up blood profile was run 24 hours after presentation and prior to the MRI scan. This revealed a decrease in packed cell volume (PCV) to 17% with total protein remaining in the normal range. There was an increase in ALT to 330 $\mu$/L. Given the history of severe hyperthermia on presentation in combination with the initial blood test results, these changes were considered likely to be due to the secondary effects of hyperthermia with haemolysis and cellular breakdown in combination with the dilutional effect

of intravenous fluid administration. Therapy with phenobarbitone was discontinued due to its potential for hepatotoxicity and its sedative effects. Levetiracetam (Keppra, UCB Pharma, Malvern, Vic.) was started at a dose of 20 mg/kg PO q8 h. The decision was made to proceed with an MRI scan as the benefit of diagnosing the CNS lesion was considered to outweigh the risk of anesthetising the anemic patient. CSF collection was not performed at this time but planned for after MRI interpretation (to ensure that there were no changes associated with high intracranial pressure).

The cat proceeded to MRI, sagittal T1, transverse T2, and diffusion weighted images; dorsal STIR and gradient echo images were obtained through the brain, in addition to postgadolinium dorsal FLAIR and postgadolinium transverse and dorsal T1 weighted images. The ventricles were normal in size and position with no evidence of an intracranial mass lesion. Images through the inferior temporal lobes showed an increased T2 and decreased T1 signal in the hippocampus and inferior temporal gyrus on both sides. This change was associated with very mild enhancement after gadolinium but no definite mass lesion or abnormality was found on the diffusion weighted images. No abnormality was seen elsewhere in the brain. The findings of a hypointense T1 and hyperintense T2 signal in the hippocampus and inferior temporal gyrus with mild gadolinium uptake were consistent with changes reported in cats with hippocampal necrosis [6].

The cat started to exhibit improvement over the next 24 hours with an improved demeanor, return of appetite, and a normal neurologic examination without evidence of focal seizures, pyrexia, anisocoria, or salivation. The cat then suffered an episode of vomiting and aspiration of ingesta followed by the development of cyanosis and cardiorespiratory arrest. Initial resuscitation was performed with intubation, ventilation, and positive inotropes and was successful but was discontinued at the owners' request leading to death. Necropsy was performed.

All organs were grossly normal except for generalized pallor of the hepatic tissue. Histologic changes were present in the brain and most pronounced in the hippocampus with virtual sparing of the rest of the cerebrum. In all sections of the hippocampus, the majority of neurons were hypereosinophilic and shrunken, with nuclear karyorrhexis. Moderate background gliosis and patchy vacuolation of the neuropil were also noted. Capillaries were prominently lined by very plump endothelial cells and, in one section, several vessels within the hippocampus had moderate to marked lymphocytic cuffs which were limited to Virchow-Robbins space. In this section, there were also numerous plump gemistocytic astrocytes, with large nuclei and abundant brightly eosinophilic cytoplasm. No infectious agents or viral inclusion bodies were visible in the sections of brain examined. These findings were suggestive of a subacute degenerative encephalopathy involving the hippocampus and were consistent with previous reports of hippocampal necrosis. A photo micrograph from one section of brain is included in Figure 1.

Histologic changes were present within the liver but limited to the centrilobular area. Changes associated with acute necrosis were present. There was no evidence of

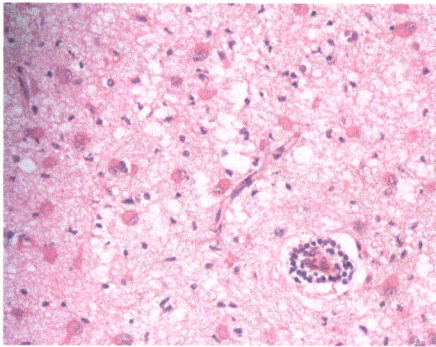

FIGURE 1

inflammation, haemorrhage, or toxic degeneration elsewhere in the liver.

## 3. Discussion

Hippocampal necrosis is a rare disease in the cat. This case was also complicated by the presence of severe hyperthermia at presentation. The hyperthermia was considered likely to be a secondary complication of the seizure activity and may suggest a longer seizure than was described by the owners or partial upper airway obstruction during the seizure. The aetiology of hippocampal necrosis is not fully understood in animals and may be due to hippocampal ischaemia due to underlying disease [7]. Whilst it is possible that hyperthermia was involved in the aetiopathogenesis of the hippocampal necrosis found in this case. This was considered less likely as behavioural change preceded seizure activity and hyperthermia.

Toxins were considered a possible cause of the original disease process in this cat but seemed unlikely based on history and postmortem findings. Whilst exposure to a cholinesterase-inhibiting compound causes similar presenting signs, in a previous case series cholinesterase activity was unremarkable in all cats with hippocampal necrosis in which the test was performed [5].

The lymphocyte cuffs found in a section of hippocampus may indicate that part of the blood-brain barrier in this region was damaged. It is possible that this is a primary lesion and these cuffs occurred due to an original event which was related to the hippocampal necrosis, but it is also possible that these are a change secondary to hyperthermia.

Elevations in ALT could have been related to hepatocellular injury or enzyme induction. This change was considered to be another effect of hyperthermia and most likely related to processes involving hepatocellular injury. The centrilobular necrosis found on histologic liver examination is typical of "shock necrosis"; this along with an ammonia tolerance test within the reference range suggests that the hepatic changes were secondary to other systemic disease rather than a primary cause of encephalopathy. The rapid elevation in ALT did raise concerns about phenobarbitone administration, as this drug has been identified as a potential hepatotoxin [10]. Phenobarbitone would be contraindicated with severe liver

disease of any aetiology and so the decision was made to change from anticonvulsant therapy with phenobarbitone to levetiracetam which is excreted predominantly in an unchanged form and considered a safer option for patients with hepatic disease [11]. Although unlikely, a thiamine deficiency was considered possible. Thiamine is essential for neuronal glucose metabolism and often deficient in times of increased metabolic demand [12]. Thiamine deficiency has been reported to cause symptoms of seizures, behavioural change, and ataxia in cats [13] so supplementation was considered appropriate in this case.

Hippocampal necrosis is reported to have a poor prognosis with high rates of death and euthanasia [1–6]. The outcome of this case is disappointing, but the management of this case was similar to the four reported surviving cases which were all managed with an anticonvulsant and supportive care [5]. The disease aetiology remains a mystery with many possible proposed mechanisms. Whilst neoplasia has been suggested as a possible cause of some cases of Hippocampal necrosis in cats [1], this was not found in this case at MRI or necropsy.

Hippocampal necrosis has not previously been reported in the southern hemisphere; finding this disease in Australia confirms that it is not limited geographically to Europe and the USA. This disease should be considered a differential diagnosis in cats presenting with seizure activity, behavioural change, or anisocoria.

## Conflict of Interests

The authors declare that there is no conflict of interests regarding the publication of this paper.

## References

[1] A. E. Vanhaesebrouck, B. Posch, S. Baker, I. N. Plessas, A. C. Palmer, and F. Constantino-Casas, "Temporal lobe epilepsy in a cat with a pyriform lobe oligodendroglioma and hippocampal necrosis," *Journal of Feline Medicine and Surgery*, vol. 14, no. 12, pp. 932–937, 2012.

[2] S. Schriefl, T. A. Steinberg, K. Matiasek, A. Ossig, N. Fenske, and A. Fischer, "Etiologic classification of seizures, signalment, clinical signs, and outcome in cats with seizure disorders: 91 cases (2000–2004)," *Journal of the American Veterinary Medical Association*, vol. 233, no. 10, pp. 1591–1597, 2008.

[3] R. Fatzer, G. Gandini, A. Jaggy, M. Doherr, and M. Vandevelde, "Necrosis of hippocampus and piriform lobe in 38 domestic cats with seizures: a retrospective study on clinical and pathologic findings," *Journal of Veterinary Internal Medicine*, vol. 14, no. 1, pp. 100–104, 2000.

[4] E. Brini, G. Gandini, I. Crescio, R. Fatzer, and C. Casalone, "Necrosis of hippocampus and piriform lobe: clinical and neuropathological findings in two Italian cats," *Journal of Feline Medicine and Surgery*, vol. 6, no. 6, pp. 377–381, 2004.

[5] A. Pakozdy, A. Gruber, S. Kneissl, M. Leschnik, P. Halasz, and J. G. Thalhammer, "Complex partial cluster seizures in cats with orofacial involvement," *Journal of Feline Medicine and Surgery*, vol. 13, no. 10, pp. 687–693, 2011.

[6] O. Schmied, G. Scharf, M. Hilbe, U. Michal, and K. T. F. Steffen, "Magnetic resonance imaging of feline hippocampal necrosis,"

*Veterinary Radiology and Ultrasound*, vol. 49, no. 4, pp. 343–349, 2008.

[7] T. A. Barbolt and R. M. Everett, "Hippocampal neuronal necorsis in control Fischer 344 rats," *Journal of Comparative Pathology*, vol. 103, no. 3, pp. 335–341, 1990.

[8] R. N. Auer and H. Benveniste, "Hypoxia and related conditions," in *Greenfield's Neuropathology*, D. I. Graham and P. L. Lantos, Eds., vol. 1, pp. 263–314, Arnold, London, UK, 6th edition, 1997.

[9] H.-G. Wieser, "Mesial temporal lobe epilepsy with hippocampal sclerosis," *Epilepsia*, vol. 45, no. 6, pp. 695–714, 2004.

[10] N. Kumar, "Neurologic presentations of nutritional deficiencies," *Neurologic Clinics*, vol. 28, no. 1, pp. 107–170, 2010.

[11] V. Palus, J. Penderis, S. Jakovljevic, and G. B. Cherubini, "Thiamine deficiency in a cat: resolution of MRI abnormalities following thiamine supplementation," *Journal of Feline Medicine and Surgery*, vol. 12, no. 10, pp. 807–810, 2010.

[12] K. A. Brown, "Factors modifying the migration of lymphocytes across the blood-brain barrier," *International Immunopharmacology*, vol. 1, no. 12, pp. 2043–2062, 2001.

[13] S. E. Bunch, "Hepatotoxicity associated with pharmacologic agents in dogs and cats," *Veterinary Clinics of North America: Small Animal Practice*, vol. 23, no. 3, pp. 659–670, 1993.

# 14

# Anesthetic and Airways Management of a Dog with Severe Tracheal Collapse during Intraluminal Stent Placement

**M. Argano,[1] K. Gendron,[2] U. Rytz,[3] and C. Adami[1]**

[1] Anesthesiology and Pain Therapy Division, Department of Veterinary Clinical Science, Vetsuisse Faculty, University of Berne, Switzerland
[2] Radiology Division, Department of Veterinary Clinical Science, Vetsuisse Faculty, University of Berne, Switzerland
[3] Surgery Division, Department of Veterinary Clinical Science, Vetsuisse Faculty, University of Berne, Switzerland

Correspondence should be addressed to M. Argano; martina.argano@gmail.com

Academic Editors: K. K. Adamama-Moraitou and J. S. Munday

This case report describes the anesthetic and airways management of a dog affected by 4th degree tracheal collapse and undergoing endoscope-guided intraluminal stent placement. After premedication with acepromazine and butorphanol, general anesthesia was induced with propofol and maintained with intravenous propofol and butorphanol in constant rate infusion. During intraluminal stent placement, oxygen was supplemented by means of a simple and inexpensive handmade device, namely, a ureteral catheter inserted into the trachea and connected to an oxygen source, which allowed for the maintenance of airways' patency and adequate patient's oxygenation, without decreasing visibility in the surgical field or interfering with the procedure. The use of the technique described in the present paper was the main determinant of the successful anesthetic management and may be proposed for similar critical cases in which surgical manipulation of the tracheal lumen, which may potentially result in hypoxia by compromising airways patency, is required.

## 1. Introduction

Tracheal collapse is a progressive condition which mainly affects small-breed dogs, characterized by degeneration of the hyaline cartilage rings and weakening of the dorsal trachealis muscle [1, 2]. Besides conservative medical management, which is reported to palliate clinical symptoms for several years in most cases [3], more invasive treatment options are either surgical application of extraluminal rings [4–8] or endoscope-guided intraluminal stent placement [9–14]. The latter, although considered minimally invasive [7], is the most challenging in terms of anesthetic management, owing to the difficulty of maintaining the airways patent throughout the entire procedure. In order to perform the surgery in a safely intubated patient, the endoscope's distal end may be inserted into the trachea through the endotracheal tube (ETT). However, this technique entails some drawbacks, such as limited visibility of the surgical field and, especially in toy breeds in which only small diameter ETT can be placed, obstruction of the ETT lumen. Thereby, it is generally preferred to have the trachea not to be intubated during intraluminal stents placement. On the other hand, even in case of nonintubated airways, the endoscope's tube itself may narrow the tracheal lumen enough to compromise oxygenation.

Oxygen supplementation may be provided by means of different methods, although none of them seem to be optimal for surgical procedures involving the tracheal lumen in terms of efficiency, simplicity, and practicability. Jet ventilation, either transtracheal, via percutaneous insertion of a hypodermic needle, or intratracheal via a semiflexible catheter, is regarded as a useful tool capable of providing efficient oxygenation even in case of nonpatent airways; nevertheless, not all facilities have such expensive and sophisticated equipment at their disposal. Flow by technique is simple and inexpensive and may be useful to provide oxygen supplementation in spontaneously breathing patients; however, because the mouth is the entry site of the tracheoscope tube, it may be difficult to position the oxygen source in a useful location without interfering with the surgical procedure.

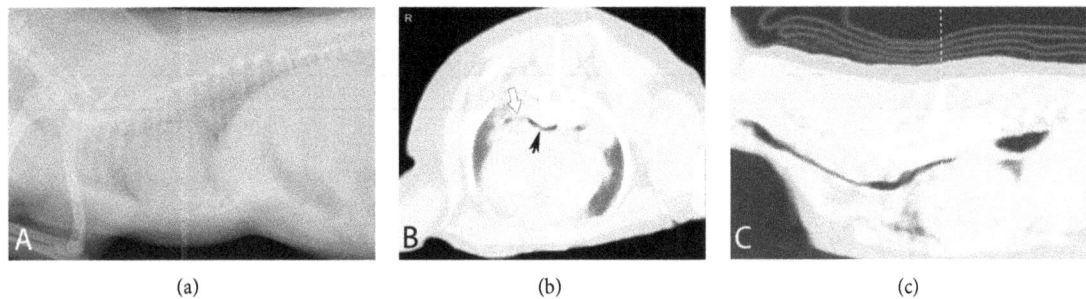

FIGURE 1: Preinterventional radiographic (a) overview of the thorax, left lateral projection. The thoracic volume is small and the caudoventral rib cartilages are pulled inwards. Pulmonary contrast is poor. The tracheal and mainstem bronchial lumen are partly reduced in width and opacified. Computed tomography (CT) was performed 12 h later, transverse view (b) at the level of the bifurcation (reference line) in the sagittal reconstruction (c). The scan performed without intubation is shown here. Severe dorsoventral tracheal flattening (black arrowhead) is present, and the right mainstem bronchus (solid white arrow) is also compressed.

We describe the use of a handmade, inexpensive, and simple device, composed of an oxygen source and a polyurethane ureteral catheter, to provide oxygen supplementation and ensure upper airways' patency in a dog undergoing endoscope-guided intratracheal stent placement. To the best of the authors' knowledge, such a technique has never been described in dogs.

## 2. Case Presentation

An 11-year-old, 2.8 kg female Yorkshire Terrier was referred to the Veterinary Teaching Hospital of the University of Berne with a history of stridor and respiratory distress no longer responsive to conservative medical treatment. On physical examination, physiological parameters were deemed normal, but stridor and louder inspiratory murmur were detected upon chest auscultation. Except for monocytosis (8%) and slightly elevated blood urea nitrogen (14 mmol/L) and creatine kinase (519 IU), blood biochemistry and hematology were within normal ranges for the species. Thoracic radiographic exam revealed smaller than normal lung volumes, a narrow effective cranial thoracic tracheal lumen, and hepatomegaly. Computed tomography showed a severe tracheal collapse of the cervical trachea, with practical closure from the fourth to seventh cervical vertebral bodies, and moderate-to-severe collapse of the remaining segments and mainstem bronchi (see Figure 1).

The dog was scheduled for tracheoscopy, followed by surgical correction of the tracheal collapse via endoscope-guided tracheal stent placement. After intramuscular premedication with acepromazine (Prequillan, Arovet AG, Dietikon, Switzerland, 0.01 mg/kg) and butorphanol (Morphasol, Dr. E. Graeud AG, Bern, Switzerland, 0.3 mg/kg), a 22 G intravenous catheter was placed aseptically in the left cephalic vein. The dog was subsequently preoxygenated for 5 minutes and general anesthesia was induced with intravenous propofol (Propofol 1% Fresenius, Fresenius Kabi AG, Oberdorf, Switzerland, 3 mg/kg) administered to effect to allow for endotracheal intubation. The 4.5 mm ETT was then connected to a circle breathing system to allow for 100% oxygen administration. Anesthesia was maintained with a constant rate infusion of propofol (0.3–1 mg/kg/min, IV) and butorphanol (0.2 mg/kg/h, IV). A balanced crystalloid solution (Plasmalyte A, Baxter AG, Volketswil, Switzerland) was administered at a rate of 5 mL/kg/h throughout the procedure. The dorsal metatarsal artery was catheterized with a 24 G indwelling catheter to allow for arterial blood sampling and blood gas analysis. Monitoring (Dräger Sulla 808V equipped with Datex-Ohmeda S3 Monitor) included lingual pulse oximetry, sidestream capnography, electrocardiography, and Doppler (Ultrasonic Doppler Flow Detector, Model 811-B, Parks Medical Electronics, INC. Aloha, Oregon, USA) for noninvasive blood pressure measurements. Cardiovascular and respiratory variables were manually recorded at 5-minute interval. The ETT tube was left in place until the beginning of the stent placement, to ensure airways' patency while performing tracheoscopy. In order to allow for the visualization of the entire trachea, the proximal end of the ETT was pulled rostrally so that its caudal tip was positioned just distal to the tracheal inlet. Thereafter, the trachea was extubated to improve endoscopic field visibility during tracheal stent placement. A portable oxygen flowmeter equipped with a humidifier was connected, through a 7 mm female adaptor, with a 1-meter long silicon tube, whose free end was joined together with the proximal end of a 16 Fr. silicon-coated polyvinylchloride ureteral catheter, with an external diameter of 1.5 mm and a straight atraumatic tip (ERU ureteral catheter, Teleflex Medical, Athlone, Ireland). In order to optimize the gas flow to the lungs, several handmade orifices had been previously made with a sterile 21 G percutaneous needle at the free end of the catheter, starting from approximately 6 cm from the distal tip (see Figure 2). The ureteral catheter was inserted into the tracheal lumen so that its tip and that of the endoscope's insertion tube were parallel and moved in a synchronous manner with the latter in order to optimize surgical field visibility and, at the same time, patient oxygenation (see Figure 3). The oxygen flowmeter was set to deliver 2-3 L/min oxygen throughout the procedure.

Immediately after stent placement, the operator temporarily required withdrawal of the catheter to achieve a greater field visibility and check the stent position. On this occasion, a rapid drop in $SpO_2$ to 78% occurred; a blood gas

TABLE 1: Cardiovascular and respiratory variables recorded from an 11-years-old female Yorkshire Terrier during and after an endotracheal stent placement.

| Variable | Reference range | Time point 1 | Time point 2 | Time point 3 |
| --- | --- | --- | --- | --- |
| Arterial blood pH | 7.37–7.43 | 7.146 | 7.054 | 7.205 |
| $FiO_2$ | 0.21–1 | 0.21 | ND | 0.50 |
| $PaO_2$ | 95–108 | 83.6 | 240.3 | 120.4 |
| $SaO_2$ | 97–100 | 93.1 | 99.1 | 97.6 |
| $PaCO_2$ | 34–40 | 38 | 73.4 | 43.1 |
| HR | 70–110 | 118 | 120 | ND |
| SAP | 100–130 | 110 | 102 | ND |

$FiO_2$: inspired fraction of oxygen; $PaO_2$: arterial partial pressure of oxygen as measured by the blood gas analyzer (mmHg); $SaO_2$: arterial oxygen saturation as calculated by the blood gas analyzer (%); $PaCO_2$: arterial partial pressure of carbon dioxide as measured by the blood gas analyzer (mmHg); HR: heart rate (beats per minute); SAP: systolic arterial pressure as measured by Doppler (mmHg); ND: not determined; time point 1: during intratracheal stent placement, some minutes after oxygen supplementation was discontinued; time point 2: still during intratracheal stent placement, some minutes after oxygen supplementation was reestablished; time point 3: during recovery phase, with the animal being extubated and kept awake in the oxygen cage.

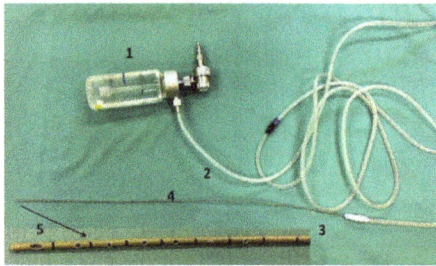

FIGURE 2: Handmade device developed to provide oxygen supplementation during tracheal stent. Placement: a portable oxygen flowmeter (1) is connected with a 1-meter long silicon tube (2). The free end of the silicon tube is joined together with the proximal end (3) of a 16 Fr. ureteral catheter (4), whose opposite end is modified with several handmade orifices (5) starting from approximately 6 cm from the distal tip.

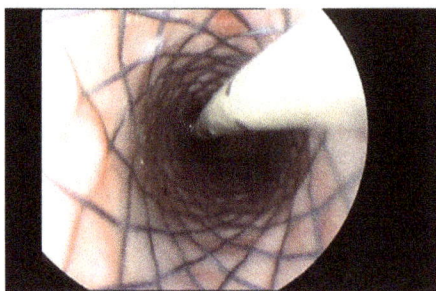

FIGURE 3: Endoscopic view of the tracheal lumen during the intraluminal stent placement. The white tube is the ureteral catheter used to provide oxygen supplementation.

analysis performed simultaneously confirmed the presence of hypoxemia ($PaO_2$: 84 mmHg; Table 1). The catheter was rapidly reinserted and oxygen supplementation was reestablished; this caused the $SpO_2$ to return to normal ranges. A new blood gas analysis confirmed an increase in a $PaO_2$ (240 mmHg), although at this time the dog was found to be moderately hypercapnic ($PaCO_2$: 73 mmHg; Table 1). At the end of the procedure, the dog was allowed to recover in

the intensive care unit of the hospital, in an oxygen cage set to deliver 50% oxygen. A blood gas analysis performed later with the dog staying awake revealed adequate oxygenation and ventilation (Table 1).

The day after, due to the occurrence of unexpected, sudden respiratory distress, further diagnostics were performed. Thoracic radiographs and tracheoscopy showed a complete tracheal collapse just distal to the stent's distal end and also a severe right bronchus collapse accompanied by right lung lobes atelectasis. Because of the poor prognosis, the dog was euthanized.

## 3. Discussion

To date, the literature pertaining to canine tracheal collapse has focused on various aspects of its pathogenesis and available treatment options [1, 3, 15, 16], but there is a lack of information regarding the anesthetic management when surgical correction of the tracheal narrowing is attempted. This case report describes the successful anesthetic and airways management of a dog affected by complete tracheal collapse during intraluminal stent placement by means of an innovative, practical, and inexpensive technique developed to maintain airway patency and, at the same time, provide effective oxygen supplementation.

Maintenance of airway patency and efficient oxygenation of the patient during intraluminal manipulation of a narrowed trachea may represent a real challenge for the anesthetist. Ideally, an airway access may be established by means of a catheter whose length, diameter, and physical properties would allow it to extend past the collapsed portion of the trachea, thus maintaining tracheal patency, while minimally interfering with the endoscopic field visibility during stent placement. Owing to its characteristics, the ureteral catheter we used fulfilled these requirements and allowed having safe, efficient, and practical airway management. The combination of silicon coating and atraumatic straight tip, together with the relative rigidity of a material such as polyvinylchloride, allowed for optimal remote control of the catheter's distal end position, without resulting in iatrogenic damages of the tracheal mucosa. In this way, the catheter could be guided to and fro into the tracheal lumen so that its distal tip would always parallel the endoscope's end; as a result, oxygen supplementation was optimized, while good endoscopic field visibility was maintained.

Owing to technical reasons, we were unable to measure the percentage of oxygen delivered to the patient by means of this novel method. In order to have a reliable measurement of the inspired fraction of oxygen, the distal end of the side stream sampling line for the gas analyzer should have paralleled the catheter's tip into the tracheal lumen. However, the presence of another device into an already narrowed trachea would have greatly decreased the field visibility and potentially increased the likelihood of tracheal damages. Furthermore, because gas sampling lines are usually manufactured with flexible materials, it would have been technically difficult to guide the aforementioned line to and fro in the trachea while avoiding bending and turning. Placing the sampling line at the proximal tip of the catheter, for instance by means of a hypodermic needle, may have been more practical; nonetheless, the measurement would have been unreliable as values obtained in this way more likely reflect the oxygen concentration as delivered by the gas source that was close to 100%, rather than the one really inspired by the patient. Although the real oxygen concentration delivered by means of this technique cannot be determined, we assume that this was adequate, as it resulted in normal $SaO_2$ and acceptable $PaO_2$ values (Table 1). The sudden, dramatic drop in $SpO_2$, $SaO_2$, and $PaO_2$ occurring immediately after oxygen supplementation that was discontinued confirms the clinical usefulness of the described technique in terms of maintenance of airways' patency and improvement of patient's oxygenation. During the aforementioned critical event, the blood gas results showed inconsistency between $SaO_2$ calculation and $SpO_2$ reading. This discrepancy could have been due to inaccurate pulse oximeter reading owing to manipulation of the tongue during the procedure; however, it should be noticed that while the value was recorded, the probe was properly positioned and a pulse waveform was correctly displayed. As an alternative explanation, the $SaO_2$ could have been overestimated by the blood gas analyzer. Indeed, such value is calculated based on the equation developed by Severinghaus, which only provides an estimate as it does not account for differences in temperature, pH, and concentrations of 2,3 DPG in red blood cells. As a result, an error of measurement cannot be excluded.

An effective teamwork, characterized by coordinated courses of action and excellent communication between surgeons and anesthetists, played a key role and was essential for the successful outcome. Indeed, when performing such a delicate procedure, poor planning and miscommunication between clinicians may increase the risk of complications, such as patient hypoxia and entrapment of the catheter between the tracheal mucosa and intraluminal stent, resulting in iatrogenic damage of the airways' mucous membranes.

In order to maintain a stable anesthetic level and avoid environmental pollution, which in the present case would have been unavoidable due to leakage of anesthetic gases through an unsealed connection between airways and fresh gas outlet, total intravenous anesthesia was selected as technique of choice. It was decided to administer propofol to maintain a stable anesthetic plane owing to its safety, short-context sensitive half time, and ease of use in constant rate infusion. Butorphanol was chosen as comaintenance agent due to its antitussive properties, which may improve the tolerance to the stent in the postanesthetic period and to the less pronounced respiratory effects in comparison to pure $\mu$-agonists. However, these intravenous agents are not devoid of side effects and both carry the potential for respiratory depression [17]. Hypoventilation and hypercapnia, as revealed by the blood gas analysis performed after oxygen supplementation was restored, did occur in this dog. Because propofol rate of infusion had been increased shortly before blood sampling in response to a superficialization of the anaesthetic depth, this hypercapnia was interpreted as the result of a transient respiratory depression, which resolved spontaneously within a few minutes without causing patient hypoxia. The impossibility to intubate the trachea with an appropriate size endotracheal tube without interfering with the surgical procedure prevented us from initiating intermittent positive pressure ventilation. However, should severe propofol-related respiratory depression occur, discontinuation of the procedure, followed by prompt intubation of the trachea and initiation of positive pressure ventilation, is strongly recommended.

## 4. Conclusion

Oxygen supplementation via a nondistensible, atraumatic ureteral catheter inserted into the tracheal lumen during intraluminal stent placement allowed for satisfactory airway management and patient oxygenation, without interfering with surgical field visibility or with completion of the procedure.

## Conflict of Interests

The authors do not have any potential conflict of interests to declare.

## References

[1] M. J. Dallman, R. C. McClure, and E. M. Brown, "Histochemical study of normal and collapsed tracheas in dogs," *American Journal of Veterinary Research*, vol. 49, no. 12, pp. 2117–2125, 1988.

[2] S. Ettinger, "Diseases of the trachea and upper airways," in *Textbook of Veterinary Internal Medicine*, S. J. Ettinger and E. C. Feldman, Eds., pp. 1073–1078, Elsevier Saunders, St. Louis, Mo, USA, 7th edition, 2010.

[3] R. White and J. Williams, "Tracheal collapse in the dog: is there really a role for surgery? A survey of 100 cases," *Journal of Small Animal Practice*, vol. 35, no. 4, pp. 191–196, 1994.

[4] R. Fingland, W. DeHoff, and S. Birchard, "Surgical management of cervical and thoracic tracheal collapse in dogs using extraluminal spiral prostheses: results in seven cases," *Journal of the American Animal Hospital Association*, vol. 23, pp. 173–181, 1987.

[5] R. Fingland, "Treatment of tracheal collapse: spiral ring technique," in *Current Techniques in Small Animal Surgery*, M. J. Bojrab, Ed., pp. 377–380, Lippincott Williams & Wilkins, Baltimore, Md, USA, 1998.

[6] S. A. Ayres and D. L. Holmberg, "Surgical treatment of tracheal collapse using pliable total ring prostheses: results in one experimental and 4 clinical cases," *Canadian Veterinary Journal*, vol. 40, no. 11, pp. 787–791, 1999.

[7] T. Glaus, J. Matos, P. Baloi, and M. Wenger, "Implantation intraluminaler Stents zur Behandlung des Trachealkollaps beim Hund," *Schweizer Archiv für Tierheilkunde*, vol. 153, no. 11, pp. 505–508, 2011.

[8] W. M. Becker, M. Beal, B. J. Stanley, and J. G. Hauptman, "Survival after surgery for tracheal collapse and the effect of intrahoracic collapse on survival," *Veterinary Surgery*, vol. 41, pp. 501–506, 2012.

[9] R. L. Eller, W. J. Livingston III, C. E. Morgan et al., "Expandable tracheal stenting for benign disease: worth the complications?" *Annals of Otology, Rhinology and Laryngology*, vol. 115, no. 4, pp. 247–252, 2006.

[10] S. A. Zakaluzny, J. D. Lane, and E. A. Mair, "Complications of tracheobronchial airway stents," *Otolaryngology—Head and Neck Surgery*, vol. 128, no. 4, pp. 478–488, 2003.

[11] M. J. Wallace, C. Charnsangavej, K. Ogawa et al., "Tracheobronchial tree: expandable metallic stents used in experimental and clinical applications. Work in progress," *Radiology*, vol. 158, no. 2, pp. 309–312, 1986.

[12] A. Moritz, M. Schneider, and N. Bauer, "Management of advanced tracheal collapse in dogs using intraluminal self-expanding biliary Wallstents," *Journal of Veterinary Internal Medicine*, vol. 18, pp. 31–42, 2004.

[13] W. T. N. Culp, C. Weisse, S. G. Cole, and J. A. Solomon, "Intraluminal tracheal stenting for treatment of tracheal narrowing in three cats," *Veterinary Surgery*, vol. 36, no. 2, pp. 107–113, 2007.

[14] A. R. Burningham, M. K. Wax, P. E. Andersen, E. C. Everts, and J. I. Cohen, "Metallic tracheal stents: complications associated with long-term use in the upper airway," *Annals of Otology, Rhinology and Laryngology*, vol. 111, no. 4, pp. 285–290, 2002.

[15] J. D. Payne, S. J. Mehler, and C. Weisse, "Tracheal collapse," *Compendium on Continuing Education for the Practicing Veterinarian*, vol. 28, no. 5, pp. 373–382, 2006.

[16] J. L. Buback, H. W. Boothe, and H. P. Hobson, "Surgical treatment of tracheal collapse in dogs: 90 cases (1983–1993)," *Journal of the American Veterinary Medical Association*, vol. 208, no. 3, pp. 380–384, 1996.

[17] C. E. Short and A. Bufalari, "Propofol anesthesia," *Veterinary Clinics of North America—Small Animal Practice*, vol. 29, no. 3, pp. 747–778, 1999.

# 15

# Cor Triatriatum Sinister in a French Bulldog

**Gustavo L. G. Almeida,**[1,2] **Marcelo B. Almeida,**[2] **Ana Carolina M. Santos,**[2] **Ângela V. Mattos,**[2] **Ludmila S. C. Oliveira,**[3] **and Rômulo C. Braga**[4]

[1] *Department of Internal Medicine, Faculty of Medicine, Gama Filho University, 20740-900 Rio de Janeiro, RJ, Brazil*
[2] *Cardiology Division, Centro Veterinário Colina, Rua Colina 60 Lj-09, Ilha do Governador, 21931-380 Rio de Janeiro, RJ, Brazil*
[3] *Clinical Division, Pet-Gávea, Marquês de São Vicente 07, Gávea, 22451-041 Rio de Janeiro, RJ, Brazil*
[4] *Radiology Department, CRV Imagem, Avenida das Américas 595, Barra da Tijuca, 22631-000 Rio de Janeiro, RJ, Brazil*

Correspondence should be addressed to Gustavo L. G. Almeida, glgouvea@cardiol.br

Academic Editors: C. Gutierrez and S. Stuen

A 3-year-old male French Bulldog was evaluated due to recent history of intolerance to exercise and coughing. The clinical, radiographic, and echocardiographic findings were consistent with cor triatriatum sinister (CTS), a congenital heart anomaly in which the left atrium is subdivided into two compartments by an abnormal fibromuscular membrane. This defect has been rarely recognized in humans and in domestic cats. To the best of our knowledge, this is the first report of the disorder in the canine species.

## 1. Introduction

Cor triatriatum (CT) literally means "heart with three atria." It is among the rarest developmental cardiac disorders reported in people [1, 2], dogs [3], and cats [4–6]. Cor triatriatum sinister (CTS) and dexter (CTD) consist of left or right atrium, respectively, divided into two chambers by a fibrous membrane. In CTS, the left auricle has two distinct compartments: one proximal that receives blood from pulmonary veins and one distal that communicates with the left ventricle through mitral valve. The embryogenesis of CTS is still subject of discussion, but the most accepted theory is that it results from lack of normal regression of the fetal pulmonary veins to form the roof of the left atrium [7, 8]. There are one or more small orifices in the separating membrane, allowing communication between both parts of the left auricle [4, 6]. CTS may be found as an isolated defect (classic) or may be associated with other cardiovascular anomalies—the atypical presentation [9]. The pathophysiological consequences of CTS are variable and strongly depend upon the size of the membrane's orifice. When associated with other cardiovascular defects, it usually represents a serious disorder [9, 10]. If the membrane's

foramen is large, the disease may show a benign course as seen eventually in adult humans with the classic type [8, 11, 12]. Since 1990s, the transthoracic echocardiography became the first choice imaging technique for the diagnosis of CT due to its high accuracy [1, 9, 10, 13]. This technique is essential not only to establish the diagnosis, but also to assess hemodynamic repercussions and to document eventual associated defects [8]. Other suitable methods for the diagnosis of CTS are cardiac computed tomography and magnetic resonance imaging [12], but they are expensive, rarely available in veterinary clinics, and also need general anesthesia to be performed. From the best of our knowledge, CTS in dogs was not reported before in the veterinary literature. The aim of this study was to describe this peculiar entity that was identified in an adult dog from Rio de Janeiro.

## 2. Case Presentation

In February 2012, a 3-year-old male French Bulldog was referred for cardiologic evaluation, due to coughing and dyspnea. The dog was on heartworm prophylaxis and had no relevant past medical history. A few days before our

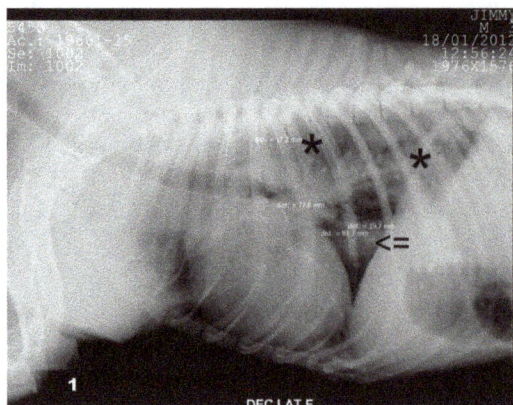

FIGURE 1: Lateral chest radiograph showing mild heart enlargement, signs of pulmonary congestion and oedema (*). The caudal vena cava (<=) is calibrous.

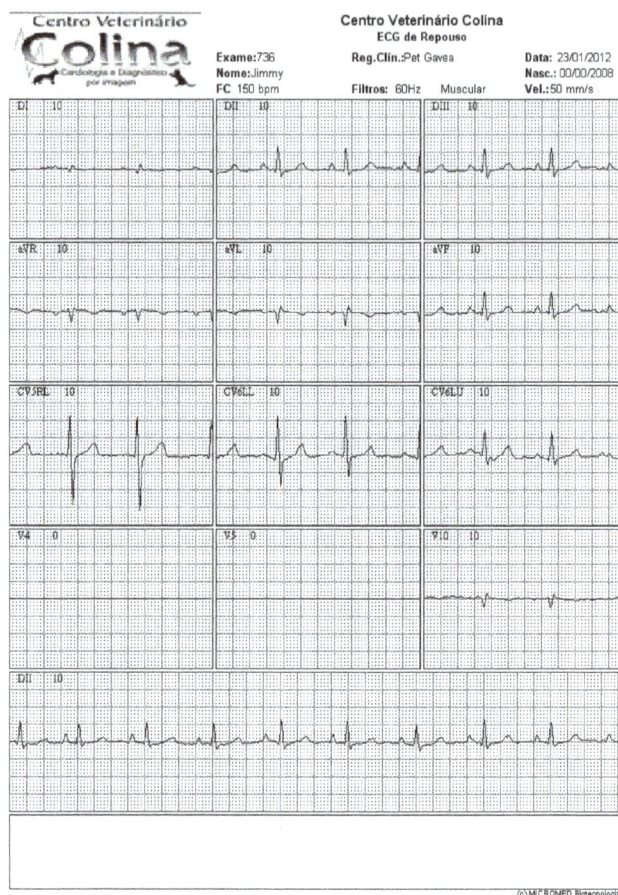

FIGURE 2: The ten-lead computed electrocardiographic tracing reveals sinus rhythm, main QRS axis falling between +80 and +90 degrees, heart rate of 150 beats per minute, and no criteria for chamber enlargement. Calibration: 1 cm = 1 mv and velocity of 50 mm per second.

evaluation, the patient began to be treated with benazepril and furosemide, showing significant clinical amelioration. The initial treatment has been maintained once the diagnosis of the malformation was made. The dog's owner refused to refer the patient for cardiac surgery, preferring clinical treatment. On physical examination, the dog was in good general physical condition, well active, and weighed 13,1 kg. He was too reactive during all examination but showed no dyspnea or coughing. The cardiac auscultation was normal, the heart rate was 144 beats per minute, the mucous membranes were not cyanotic, and the femoral pulse was regular, strong, and synchronous to the heart beats. The systolic arterial blood pressure measured by the Doppler method was 136 mm Hg. Blood test results (complete blood count, blood urea, creatinine, and fasting glucose) were within normal reference values. The chest radiograph showed a mildly augmented cardiac silhouette, signs of caudal vena cava engorgement, and arterial pulmonary congestion and edema (Figure 1). Also, hemivertebra affecting T3 and T5 to T8 was identified. The electrocardiogram (ECG) was normal (Figure 2). Transthoracic echocardiography revealed a left atrium subdivided by a transverse membrane into two distinct compartments, one proximal and one distal, the hallmark of CTS (Figures 3 and 4). The interatrial septum was seen intact. The left apical four-chamber view documented a continuous forward blood flow across the membrane's orifice (Figure 5). The mitral valve was morphologically normal, and the true left auricle was not enlarged. Mild pulmonary valve regurgitation was detected on the right paraesternal 4-chamber short-axis view at the level of the cardiac base. The patient has been showing good quality of life since four months ago when furosemide and benazepril were introduced.

## 3. Discussion

CTS was firstly described in human beings by Church in 1868 [1] and in the domestic cat by Gordon et al. more

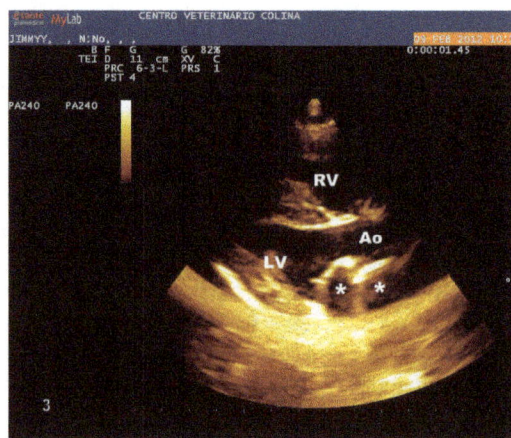

FIGURE 3: The transthoracic two-dimensional echocardiogram (parasternal long-axis view). Note a transverse membrane subdividing the left auricle into two distinct chambers (*), one proximal and one distal, the classical anatomic presentation of CTS. Right ventricle (RV), left ventricle (LV), and aorta (Ao).

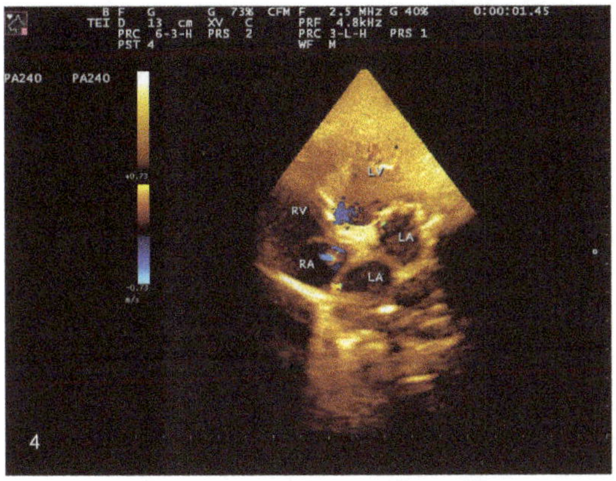

FIGURE 4: Left apical four-chamber view in systole, showing a transverse membrane and the two left atrial parts (*LA and **LA). Left ventricle (LV), right atrium (RA), and right ventricle (RV).

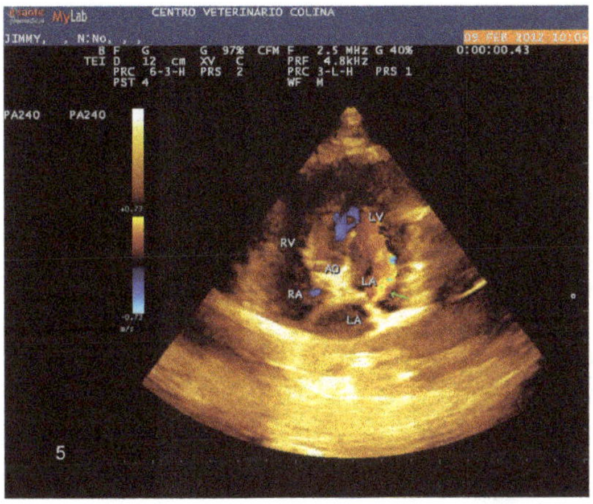

FIGURE 5: Transthoracic colour-Doppler echocardiogram (left apical four-chamber view) in diastole. Note a blood flow (green arrow) crossing a central orifice located in the intra-atrial membrane. Right atrium (RA), right ventricle (RV), left atrial chamber (LA), and aorta (AO).

than a century later [14]. Regarding canine species, only the dexter form has been reported [3, 4]. In CTS, the obstructive membrane causes increased pressure in pulmonary venous-capillary circulation, and, in consequence, pulmonary edema or pulmonary hypertension can develop secondarily to vasoconstriction [4]. This hemodynamic disorder may explain the clinical and radiographic changes observed in our case study. CTS may be very difficult to be distinguished from supravalvular mitral stenosis, another rare congenital defect in dogs that has similar physiology. The differentiation between both conditions is based on the level of the obstruction; in supravalvular stenosis the obstructive membrane is distal to left auricle and immediately above the mitral valvular plane, whereas in CTS it is proximal [6, 7, 15], as documented in this paper (Figures 3 and 4). Also, to help differentiation is that, in CTS, the flow crossing the orifice is continuous (Figure 5), while in supravalvular mitral stenosis is diastolic [16]. The peculiar anatomy of CTS can be well delineated by two-dimensional echocardiogram, while

the color-Doppler study permits identifying an increased flow velocity through the membrane's fenestration [12], as observed in our patient (Figures 3, 4, and 5). The electrocardiogram is nonspecific for this anomaly, and, in consequence, a normal ECG does not rule out the defect as reported in adult humans [8, 10–12]. In our patient, the ECG was within normal parameters. We believe that the cardiac condition was not severe enough to produce discernible changes on the ECG surface at the time of examination. In the dog, the pathological findings and natural history of the malformation are unknown but may be identical to that seen in cats [4, 6]. Given that the cardiac defect is obstructive by nature and if the membrane has a small hole, the hemodynamic changes tend to worsen with time. The disease progress may cause enlargement of left proximal atrial chamber, main pulmonary artery, right atrial dilatation, right ventricular dilatation, and eccentric hypertrophy [4, 6]. When heart failure develops, pharmacologic therapy with diuretics and angiotensin converting enzyme inhibitors (ACEIs) is beneficial [4, 17]. Furosemide is a drug of choice for heart failure because it is a potent diuretic that reduces preload and relieves congestion secondarily to cardiac dysfunction. In consequence, it reduces edema formation and dyspnea. However, because furosemide activates the rennin-angiotensin-aldosterone system, a concomitant use of an ACEI is advisable [6]. Benazepril hydrochloride is a long-acting ACEI that counterbalances the adverse effects caused by ACE activity, that is, exacerbated in heart failure. This drug produces significant prolongation of survival time of dogs with heart failure, improves the exercise capacity, and is well tolerated [17]. Although very rare, CTS should be included in the differential diagnosis of dogs with signs of heart failure and suspect congenital heart defect. This malformation is important to be early recognized because it is potentially correctable by surgery when clinically significant.

## References

[1] M. D. Rodefeld, J. W. Brown, D. A. Heimansohn et al., "Cor triatriatum: clinical presentation and surgical results in 12 patients," Annals of Thoracic Surgery, vol. 50, no. 4, pp. 562–568, 1990.

[2] R. Hamdan, N. Mirochnik, D. Celermajer, P. Nassar, and L. Iserin, "Cor Triatriatum Sinister diagnosed in adult life with three dimensional transesophageal echocardiography," BMC Cardiovascular Disorders, vol. 2010, article 54, 2010.

[3] P. Oliveira, O. Domenech, J. Silva, S. Vannini, R. Bussadori, and C. Bussadori, "Retrospective review of congenital heart disease in 976 dogs," Journal of Veterinary Internal Medicine, vol. 25, no. 3, pp. 477–483, 2011.

[4] M. D. Kittleson, "Other congenital cardiovascular abnormalities," in Small Animal Cardiovascular Medicine, M. D. Kittleson and R. D. Kienle, Eds., pp. 282–296, Mosby, St. Louis, Mo, USA, 1st edition, 1998.

[5] P. Menaut, V. L. Fuentes, and S. Dennis, "Cor Triatriatum Sinister in cats: 5 cases," in 15th FECAVA Eurocongress AFVAC—SAVAB—LAK, pp. 27–29, Lille, France, November 2009.

[6] E. Côté, K. A. MacDonald, K. M. Meurs, and M. M. Sleeper, "Congenital malformations," in *Feline Cardiology*, pp. 85–100, Wiley-Blackwell, West Sussex, UK, 1st edition, 2011.

[7] K. A. MacDonald, "Congenital heart diseases of puppies and kittens," *Veterinary Clinics of North America*, vol. 36, no. 3, pp. 503–531, 2006.

[8] R. P. Lima, C. Fonseca, F. Sampaio, J. Ribeiro, and V. G. Ribeiro, "Cor triatriatum sinistrum—description and review of four cases," *Revista Portuguesa de Cardiologia*, vol. 29, no. 5, pp. 827–836, 2010.

[9] M. Kelmendi, R. Bejiqi, G. Bajraktari, and R. Beqiraj, "Cor triatriatum sinister—three case reports," *Medicinski Arhiv*, vol. 63, no. 5, pp. 300–302, 2009.

[10] A. Thakrar, M. D. Shapiro, D. S. Jassal, T. G. Neilan, M. E. E. King, and S. Abbara, "Cor triatriatum: the utility of cardiovascular imaging," *Canadian Journal of Cardiology*, vol. 23, no. 2, pp. 143–145, 2007.

[11] R. Tasca, M. G. Tasca, P. A. Amorim, I. C. Do Nascimento, O. C. G. Veloso, and C. Scherr, "Clinical follow-up of a pregnant woman with Cor triatriatum," *Arquivos Brasileiros de Cardiologia*, vol. 88, no. 3, pp. e54–e56, 2007.

[12] P. N. Nassar and R. H. Hamdan, "Cor triatriatum sinistrum: classification and imaging modalities," *European Journal of Cardiovascular Mededicine*, vol. 1, no. 3, pp. 84–87, 2011.

[13] N. Alphonso, M. A. Nørgaard, A. Newcomb, Y. D'Udekem, C. P. Brizard, and A. Cochrane, "Cor triatriatum: presentation, diagnosis and long-term surgical results," *Annals of Thoracic Surgery*, vol. 80, no. 5, pp. 1666–1671, 2005.

[14] B. Gordon, E. Trautveter, and D. F. Patterson, "Pulmonary congestion associated with cor triatriatum in a cat," *Journal of the American Veterinary Medical Association*, vol. 180, no. 1, pp. 75–77, 1982.

[15] D. M. Fine, A. H. Tobias, and K. A. Jacob, "Supravalvular mitral stenosis in a cat," *Journal of the American Animal Hospital Association*, vol. 38, no. 5, pp. 403–406, 2002.

[16] D. Werner, A. Lienemann, S. Vogel et al., "Cor triatriatum sinister in an elderly patient-Findings in different imaging modalities and intraoperative correlation," *European Journal of Radiology Extra*, vol. 63, no. 1, pp. 25–28, 2007.

[17] The BENCH Study Group, "The effect of benazepril on survival times and clinical signs of dogs with congestive heart failure: results of a multicenter, prospective, randomized, double-blinded, placebo-controlled, long-term clinical trial," *Journal of Veterinary Cardiology*, vol. 1, no. 1, pp. 7–18, 1999.

# 16

# Elevated Testosterone and Progestin Concentrations in a Spayed Female Rabbit with an Adrenal Cortical Adenoma

**Katherine Baine,[1] Kim Newkirk,[2] Kellie A. Fecteau,[2] and Marcy J. Souza[2]**

[1]*Department of Small Animal Clinical Sciences, College of Veterinary Medicine, University of Tennessee, 2407 River Drive, Knoxville, TN 37996, USA*

[2]*Department of Biomedical and Diagnostic Sciences, College of Veterinary Medicine, University of Tennessee, 2407 River Drive, Knoxville, TN 37996, USA*

Correspondence should be addressed to Katherine Baine; tnexoticpetvet@gmail.com

Academic Editor: Maria Teresa Mandara

This case was described briefly in a recent book chapter (Lennox AM, Fecteau KA: 2014, Endocrine disease. In: BSAVA Manual of Rabbit Medicine, eds. Meredith A, Lord B, pp 274–276. British Small Animal Veterinary Association, Gloucester, UK). In the previous description, the tumor was described as a pheochromocytoma; however, further evaluation suggested that it more closely resembled an adrenal cortical adenoma. A 10-year-old, spayed female rabbit was presented for a behavior change of 8 months' duration. The rabbit was inappropriately urinating and defecating, as well as demonstrating aggressive behaviors such as chasing, biting, and mounting various objects. The rabbit had elevated progesterone, 17-hydroxyprogesterone, and testosterone concentrations, and ultrasound examination of the abdomen showed a round, homogenous nodule measuring $1.1 \times 0.8 \times 0.9$ cm in the region of the left adrenal gland. Necropsy revealed a unilateral adrenal cortical adenoma. To the authors' knowledge, this is the first complete description of a female rabbit with an adrenal cortical adenoma documented in the literature.

## 1. Case Presentation

A 10-year-old, spayed female rabbit was presented for a behavior change of 8 months' duration. The rabbit was inappropriately urinating and defecating, as well as demonstrating aggressive behaviors such as chasing, biting, and mounting various objects. The rabbit had been spayed in the first year of life.

On physical examination, the only significant finding was an enlarged clitoris (Figure 1). No significant abnormalities were present on either a complete blood count or biochemistry panel. However, the rabbit had elevated blood levels of progesterone (0.63 ng/mL; reference interval for a spayed female rabbit (RISF) 0.09–0.47 ng/mL), 17-OH progesterone (>25.0 ng/mL, extrapolated result 60.2 ng/mL; RISF 0.7–18.9 ng/mL), and testosterone (1.02 ng/mL; RISF 0.02–0.03 ng/mL) [1]. Cortisol (6.2 ng/mL; RISF 4.9–10.1 ng/mL) and androstenedione (1.2 ng/mL; RISF 0.96–4.0 ng/mL) levels were within normal limits [1]. Cortisol, progesterone, and testosterone assays (Coat-a-Count) were from Siemens Medical Solutions Diagnostics, Los Angeles, CA, and 17-OHP and androstenedione assays (ImmunChem Double Antibody) were from MP Biomedicals, Solon, OH.

Ultrasound examination of the abdomen showed a round, homogenous nodule measuring $1.1 \times 0.8$ cm in the region of the left adrenal gland (normal adrenal gland $0.72 \times 0.37$ cm) [2]; the nodule had an echogenicity approximately equal to the renal cortex. The right adrenal gland was not identified. The remainder of the examination was unremarkable. Due to the combination of clinical signs, elevated sex hormones, and a potential adrenal gland nodule, adrenal cortical disease was suspected. The owner declined exploratory surgery of the abdomen and adrenalectomy; therefore, medical management was recommended to potentially help alleviate clinical signs. Medical management was declined as well.

Six months following diagnosis, the patient was presented for progressive difficulty ambulating and rear limb ataxia; euthanasia was elected. On necropsy, the clitoris was markedly enlarged (measurements not obtained). The right adrenal gland measured 0.9 cm × 0.6 cm and had a 1:1:1

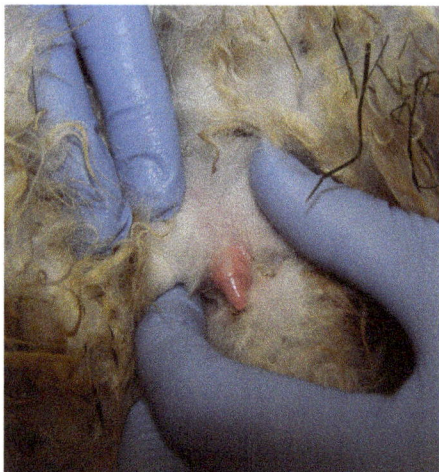

FIGURE 1: Clitoral enlargement in a 10-year-old, spayed female rabbit.

ratio of thickness of cortical layers and medulla. The left adrenal measured 1 cm × 1 cm. On cut section, the cortex was enlarged by a tan to red mass that compressed and replaced the medulla. The left adrenal gland was closely associated with the left renal vein. The kidneys were dark brown with many <1-mm depressions within the capsule; on cut section was white streaking within the right renal pelvis. Samples were collected and fixed in 10% neutral-buffered formalin and routinely processed for microscopic examination. Sections from each sample were stained with hematoxylin and eosin for further evaluation.

Histopathology revealed a neoplasm composed of cords and sheets of round to polygonal cells that expanded the left adrenal gland, compressed the cortex, and replaced the medulla (Figure 2(a)). The cells were frequently separated by vascular spaces and had distinct borders and moderate amounts of eosinophilic, often vacuolated cytoplasm. Nuclei were round and often had a single prominent nucleolus. There was minimal anisocytosis and anisokaryosis, and mitoses were rare to absent (Figure 2(a)). Only a small area of remaining medulla was present. A Churukian-Schenk stain, which highlights argyrophilic neurosecretory granules in the adrenal medulla, did not identify any granules in the neoplastic cells; however, a small piece of remaining adrenal medulla was positive (Figures 2(c) and 2(d)).

There was bilateral extracapsular adrenal cortical hyperplasia (Figure 2(a)). Both kidneys had multifocal linear areas where increased numbers of lymphocytes and plasma cells were present within the interstitium. The surrounding tubules were often atrophied and had a flattened epithelium (restitution) or hypertrophic cells (regeneration). Rare epithelial cells in these areas contained gram-positive organisms that were 2 μm in diameter (suspected Encephalitozoon cuniculi). In the brain were multifocal areas in the meninges where blood vessels were surrounded by small numbers of lymphocytes and plasma cells. These areas extended into the Virchow-Robin spaces of the underlying neuropil, with rare foci of

lymphocytes within the neuropil. Frequently, neurons contained lipofuscin; scattered vessels were also surrounded by lipofuscin-laden macrophages. Similar findings were present in multiple sections of the spinal cord. In addition, there were areas where scattered axons had dilated myelin sheaths, with rare macrophages within the myelin sheaths and occasional swollen axons. No infectious agents were identified within the brain and spinal cord with gram staining.

The final diagnoses included left adrenal cortical adenoma, widespread multifocal lymphocytic interstitial nephritis with intralesional protozoa (suspected E. cuniculi), multifocal mild lymphocytic meningoencephalitis, widespread multifocal mild lymphocytic neuritis, and myelitis with Wallerian degeneration (suspected E. cuniculi associated).

## 2. Discussion

Adrenocortical disease associated with elevated sex hormones has been diagnosed in many species, including canines, felines, ferrets, and humans [3–9]. In veterinary medicine, adrenocortical disease associated with elevated sex hormones has also been infrequently reported in rabbits: in 5 male and 1 additional female rabbit [5, 6, 9]. The pathogenesis of disease in rabbits is not well understood, but some hypothesize a similar mechanism to ferrets and mice in which gonadectomy contributes to adrenocortical hyperplasia and later tumorigenesis [3, 4, 10–12]. It is suspected that adrenocortical hyperplasia is secondary to the loss of feedback inhibition from the gonads to the hypothalamic-pituitary axis, which leads to chronic elevation in circulating luteinizing hormone, causing synthesis and secretion of sex steroids from the adrenal cortex [4, 12]. A previous study has suggested adrenal sex hormone production in normal ovariectomized rabbits, further supporting this hypothesis. Juvenile female rabbits after ovariectomy demonstrated continued sexual behaviors, which were then significantly reduced after adrenalectomy [13]. In contrast, ovariectomy eliminated all sexual behaviors in rats [14]. Given the increasing number of reported cases of adrenocortical disease in rabbits, additional research is needed to elucidate the pathophysiology of the disease in rabbits.

Based on other reported cases of adrenal cortical disease in rabbits, male rabbits are overrepresented 5 to 1 [5, 6, 9], and the average age of onset of clinical signs is reported to be 7.6 years old [5]. The age of onset of clinical signs in this case was 10 years. Except for the clitoral enlargement, the clinical signs in this case were similar to previous descriptions of rabbits with adrenal cortical disease, including urine and/or fecal marking, aggressive behaviors, and mounting various objects.

The diagnostic workup in this case was highly suggestive for adrenocortical disease; however, the right adrenal gland was not identified on ultrasound, and the left adrenal gland was not definitively identified and measured. Given the size, location, and appearance of the identified nodule, an association with the left adrenal gland was suspected.

Sex hormone reference ranges have been established for neutered rabbits of both sexes [1]. Unlike other described rabbit cases with adrenal cortical disease, including the other

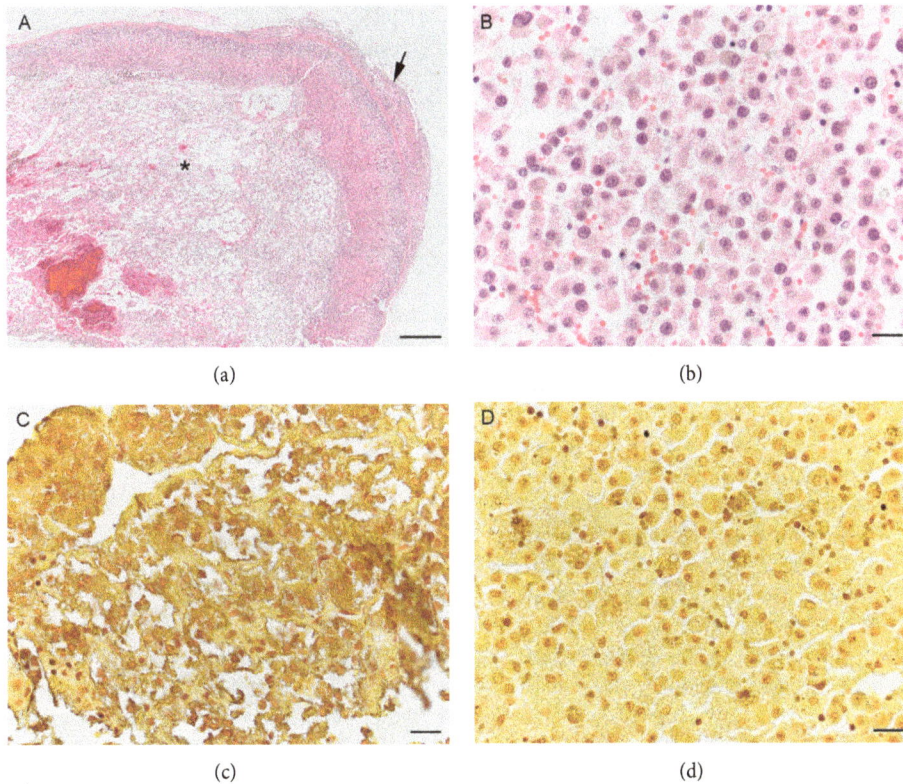

FIGURE 2: Adrenal gland from a rabbit. (a) The adrenal medulla is replaced by a well-demarcated mass of neoplastic cells (asterisk), which compresses the overlying adrenal cortex. There is also extracapsular adrenal cortical hyperplasia (arrow). Hematoxylin and eosin (H&E) stain. Bar = 200 $\mu$m. (b) The neoplastic cells are round to polygonal and occasionally form cords or nests, which are separated by vascular spaces. Occasionally the cytoplasm is vacuolated. H&E stain. Bar = 10 $\mu$m. (c) Compressed normal adrenal medulla with brown cytoplasmic granules. Churukian-Schenk stain. Bar = 10 $\mu$m. (d) The neoplastic cells do not contain brown cytoplasmic granules. Churukian-Schenk stain. Bar = 10 $\mu$m.

female rabbit mentioned briefly in a recent book chapter [5], progesterone and 17-hydroxyprogesterone concentrations were elevated in this case. Progesterone has been shown to induce a significant increase in aggression when administered to ovariectomized rabbits [15]. The increased levels in this case likely contributed to the aggression documented by the owner. Markedly elevated testosterone concentrations in this case likely also contributed to the clitoral enlargement and aggressive behaviors, which was similar to cases described with adrenal disease (aggressive behaviors) [5, 6, 9]. Testosterone levels were consistently increased in other cases of adrenocortical disease in rabbits, possibly due to the predominance of male rabbits previously described [5]. Additional possible causes for elevated sex hormones in a castrated animal include gonadal remnant, ectopic gonadal tissue, or other neoplasia. Human chorionic gonadotropin (hCG) stimulation testing has been used in rabbit patients to determine if an ovarian remnant or ectopic gonadal tissue is present [1, 15]; however, such testing was not pursued in this case.

Ultimately, the diagnosis of a unilateral adrenocortical adenoma was made on necropsy. Although extracapsular hyperplasia was identified bilaterally, it is an incidental finding in older horses, cats, and dogs [16]. Previous reports of

adrenal cortical disease in rabbits describe unilateral hyperplasia and carcinoma; adenomas have not been reported [5, 6, 9]. The adenoma was likely the cause for the elevated progesterone and testosterone in this case; however, since treatment was not pursued antemortem and immunohistochemical staining was not performed postmortem, there was no direct evidence that the adenoma caused increased hormone levels. A decreased testosterone level has been demonstrated in other cases of adrenal disease in rabbits after complete adrenalectomy [5].

The owner declined treatment for suspected adrenocortical disease in this case. The treatment of choice for unilateral disease is adrenalectomy [5], and although surgical removal may have been challenging due to the close association of the tumor to the left renal vein, complete surgical removal likely would have been curative. Medical management of adrenocortical disease using deslorelin, leuprolide acetate, finasteride, trilostane, or flutamide has been attempted in rabbits with variable success [5]. More research needs to be performed to evaluate the efficacy and safety of these therapies in rabbits.

Despite independent of the adrenal disease, ultimately, the clinical signs for which the patient was euthanized were secondary to *E. cuniculi* lesions within the central nervous system and kidneys. Encephalitozoonosis is a common disease of rabbits caused by obligate intracellular microsporidia. It can cause a nonsuppurative to granulomatous encephalitis and chronic interstitial nephritis [17]. Patients therefore can show a variety of neurologic signs and/or kidney failure. The rabbit in this case showed signs of neurologic disease prior to euthanasia (difficulty ambulating, ataxia); however, no clinical signs associated with renal disease were noted (polyuria/polydipsia) despite lesions found within the kidneys. Antemortem diagnostics were not performed to identify the underlying cause for the neurologic signs or determine if renal failure was present, although blood work performed 6 months previously was within normal limits. The lesions identified in the central nervous system and kidneys on histopathology were consistent with *E. cuniculi*; however, immunohistochemistry or polymerase chain reaction is required for a definitive diagnosis [17].

This case highlights the clinical signs, diagnostic workup, and necropsy findings associated with a unilateral adrenal cortical adenoma in an older, spayed female rabbit. Adrenal cortical disease should be considered in a spayed female rabbit demonstrating sexual behaviors (aggression, marking behaviors) and/or with an enlarged clitoris.

## Conflict of Interests

The authors declared no potential conflict of interests with respect to the research, authorship, and/or publication of this paper.

## Acknowledgment

The authors would like to thank Misty Bailey for editorial support.

## References

[1] K. A. Fecteau, B. J. Deeb, J. M. Rickel, W. J. Kelch, and J. W. Oliver, "Diagnostic endocrinology: blood steroid concentrations in neutered male and female rabbits," *Journal of Exotic Pet Medicine*, vol. 16, no. 4, pp. 256–259, 2007.

[2] S. Reese, "Abdomen," in *Diagnostic Imaging of Exotic Pets*, M. E. Krautwald-Junghanns, M. Pees, S. Reese, and T. Tully, Eds., p. 236, Schlütersche Verlagsgesellschaft mbH & Co. KG, Hannover, Germany, 2011.

[3] F. Beuschlein, S. Galac, and D. B. Wilson, "Animal models of adrenocortical tumorigenesis," *Molecular and Cellular Endocrinology*, vol. 351, no. 1, pp. 78–86, 2012.

[4] M. Bielinska, S. Kiiveri, H. Parviainen, S. Mannisto, M. Heikinheimo, and D. B. Wilson, "Gonadectomy-induced adrenocortical neoplasia in the domestic ferret (Mustela putorius furo) and laboratory mouse," *Veterinary Pathology*, vol. 43, no. 2, pp. 97–117, 2006.

[5] A. M. Lennox, "Surgical treatment of adrenocortical disease," in *BSAVA Manual of Rabbit Surgery, Dentistry, and Imaging*, F. Harcourt-Brown and J. Chitty, Eds., pp. 269–272, British Small Animal Veterinary Association, Gloucester, UK, 2014.

[6] A. M. Lennox and J. Chitty, "Adrenal neoplasia and hyperplasia as a cause of hypertestosteronism in two rabbits," *Journal of Exotic Pet Medicine*, vol. 15, no. 1, pp. 56–58, 2006.

[7] E. N. Meler, J. C. Scott-Moncrieff, A. T. Peter et al., "Cyclic estrous-like behavior in a spayed cat associated with excessive sex-hormone production by an adrenocortical carcinoma," *Journal of Feline Medicine and Surgery*, vol. 13, no. 6, pp. 473–478, 2011.

[8] H. M. Syme, J. C. Scott-Moncrieff, N. G. Treadwell et al., "Hyperadrenocorticism associated with excessive sex hormone production by an adrenocortical tumor in two dogs," *Journal of the American Veterinary Medical Association*, vol. 219, no. 12, pp. 1725–1728, 2001.

[9] M. Varga, "Hypersexuality in a castrated rabbit (*Oryctolagus cuniculus*)," *Companion Animal*, vol. 16, no. 1, pp. 48–51, 2011.

[10] M. K. de Jong, E. E. M. ten Asbroek, A. J. Sleiderink, A. J. Conley, J. A. Mol, and N. J. Schoemaker, "Gonadectomy-related adrenocortical tumors in ferrets demonstrate increased expression of androgen and estrogen synthesizing enzymes together with high inhibin expression," *Domestic Animal Endocrinology*, vol. 48, no. 1, pp. 42–47, 2014.

[11] N. J. Shoemaker, M. Schuurmans, H. Moorman, and J. T. Lumeij, "Correlation between age at neutering and age at onset of hyperadrenocorticism in ferrets," *Journal of the American Veterinary Medical Association*, vol. 216, no. 2, pp. 195–197, 2000.

[12] N. J. Schoemaker, K. J. Teerds, J. A. Mol, J. T. Lumeij, J. H. H. Thijssen, and A. Rijnberk, "The role of luteinizing hormone in the pathogenesis of hyperadrenocorticism in neutered ferrets," *Molecular and Cellular Endocrinology*, vol. 197, no. 1-2, pp. 117–125, 2002.

[13] C. Beyer, M. L. Cruz, and N. Rivaud, "Persistence of sexual behavior in ovariectomized-adrenalectomized rabbits treated with cortisol," *Endocrinology*, vol. 85, no. 4, pp. 790–793, 1969.

[14] C. Beyer, K. L. Hoffman, and O. González-Flores, "Neuroendocrine regulation of estrous behavior in the rabbit: similarities and differences with the rat," *Hormones and Behavior*, vol. 52, no. 1, pp. 2–11, 2007.

[15] K. L. Hoffman, E. Martínez-Alvarez, and R. I. Rueda-Morales, "The inhibition of female rabbit sexual behavior by progesterone: progesterone receptor-dependent and -independent effects," *Hormones and Behavior*, vol. 55, no. 1, pp. 84–92, 2009.

[16] C. C. Capen, "Endocrine system," in *Jubb, Kennedy and Palmers Pathology of Domestic Animals*, M. G. Maxie, Ed., pp. 325–482, Elsevier, Toronto, Canada, 5th edition, 2007.

[17] M. Leipig, K. Matiasek, H. Rinder et al., "Value of histopathology, immunohistochemistry, and real-time polymerase chain reaction in the confirmatory diagnosis of *Encephalitozoon cuniculi* infection in rabbits," *Journal of Veterinary Diagnostic Investigation*, vol. 25, no. 1, pp. 16–26, 2013.

# 17

# Algal Meningoencephalitis due to *Prototheca* spp. in a Dog

**Alexandre Le Roux,**[1] **Sanjeev Gumber,**[2] **Rudy W. Bauer,**[2] **Nathalie Rademacher,**[1] **and Lorrie Gaschen**[1]

[1] *Department of Veterinary Clinical Sciences, Section of Diagnostic Imaging, School of Veterinary Medicine, Louisiana State University, Skip Bertman Drive, Baton Rouge, LA 70803, USA*
[2] *Department of Pathobiological Sciences, School of Veterinary Medicine, Louisiana State University, Baton Rouge, LA 70803, USA*

Correspondence should be addressed to Alexandre Le Roux; aleroux@lsu.edu

Academic Editors: C. Hyun and I. Pires

A 6-year-old Boxer was examined because of progressive neurologic signs, with severe hindlimb ataxia and head tilt on presentation. There was no history of diarrhea or vomiting. MRI of the brain revealed multifocal ill-defined T1-enhancing lesions affecting the cerebrum, brainstem, and cervical meninges, without associated mass effect. Meningoencephalitis was considered the most likely diagnosis. Multiple algae were observed on the cytology of the CSF and were most consistent with *Prototheca* spp. Antiprotozoal treatment was denied by the owners, and 5 weeks after diagnosis, the dog was euthanized due to progression of the neurologic deficits, and a necropsy was performed. Histological changes in the brain were compatible with severe multifocal protothecal meningoencephalitis. The specific *Prototheca* species was not identified. The gastrointestinal tract was unremarkable on histology. According to this report, *Prototheca* spp. should be included in the differentials for neurological deficits even in the absence of gastrointestinal signs.

## 1. Introduction

Protothecosis is a rare disease described in many species, caused by a green alga, *Prototheca* spp. In the cases reported in dogs [1–3], the algae are usually disseminated within the organism, and the affected dogs commonly present large intestine diarrhea. Ocular and neurologic symptoms are also described with protothecosis, but these signs usually appear in a later stage of the disease. To the authors' knowledge, this is the first case report describing cerebral protothecosis without evidence of dissemination of the alga within the other organs, and more particularly within the gastrointestinal tract.

## 2. Case Presentation

A 6-year-old spayed female Boxer was referred for progressive ataxia of the hindlimbs of 3-week duration. The dog was previously diagnosed with bilateral cranial cruciate ligament rupture, treated surgically 4 months prior to presentation.

Physical examination was unremarkable. Neurologic examination revealed a severe hindlimb ataxia, worse on the left, and a left head tilt. Delayed hopping tests were noted in the forelimbs, and the dog fell when hopped in the rear. Crossing over and dragging of the hind feet were also observed. Cranial nerve examination was unremarkable, and there were no conscious proprioceptive deficits. Neurologic examination was consistent with brainstem and/or cerebellar localization. Based on the age, breed, and progressive neurological deficits, the following differentials were considered most likely causes of the clinical findings: neoplasia, such as meningioma or glioma, and an inflammatory lesion, such as an abscess or granuloma. Complete blood count was within normal reference range, and a mild hypercholesterolemia was noted on the chemistry panel.

Magnetic resonance imaging (MRI) of the brain was performed using a 1.5 T magnet (Echelon, Hitachi Medical Systems). Fast spin-echo T1-weighted, T2-weighted, fluid-attenuated inversion recovery (FLAIR), and gradient-echo (GRE) pulse sequences were acquired in a transverse plane. A T2-weighted pulse sequence was also acquired in a sagittal plane, and a T1-weighted pulse sequence was acquired in

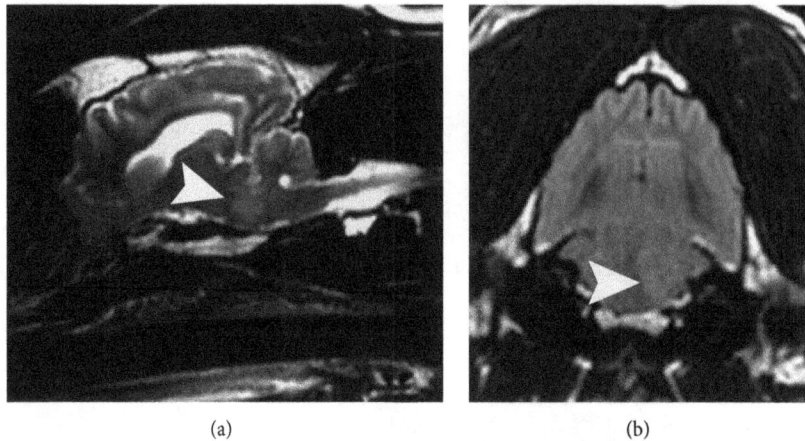

(a)                                                                        (b)

FIGURE 1: (a) T2-weighted sagittal and (b) FLAIR transverse pulse sequences of the brain, at the level of the pons. There is a broadbased ill-defined homogeneous hyperintense lesion (arrowhead) along the sphenoid bone, encompassing approximately fifty percent of the left side of the pons and extending dorsal to the fourth ventricle, which appears slightly displaced to the right.

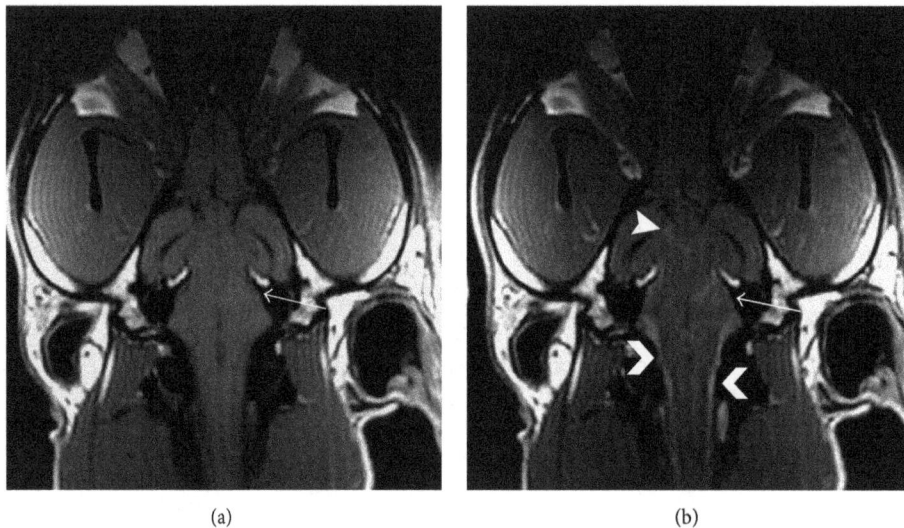

(a)                                                                        (b)

FIGURE 2: T1-weighted dorsal pulse sequences before (a) and after contrast (b), at the level of the brainstem. (a) On the T1-weighted precontrast images, a faint ill-defined hyperintense signal was visible in the left pons (long arrow). (b) On the T1-weighted postcontrast sequence, meningeal enhancement was observed around the pons, *medulla oblongata*, and cranial cervical spine (arrowheads). A broadbased enhancement was visible in the left aspect of the pons (long arrow). Faint ill-defined enhancing lesions were also observed in the right frontal lobe (solid arrowhead).

a dorsal plane. Postcontrast T1-weighted pulse sequences were acquired in dorsal and transverse planes, after intravenous administration of gadopentetate dimeglumine (Magnevist, Berlex Imaging; 0.1 mmol/kg intravenously).

A focal hyperintense lesion, 1 cm in diameter, was present on the T2-weighted, GRE, and FLAIR pulse sequences in the left pons and rostral medullary region (Figure 1), encompassing approximately 50% of the left side of the pons, extending dorsally to the fourth ventricle, mildly displacing it to the right. The lesion was broadbased along the sphenoid bone, in the region of the geniculate ganglion, and was faintly hyperintense on the T1-weighted sequences (Figure 2(a)). Additionally, faint ill-defined hyperintense lesions were also observed in the right frontal lobe and within the *corpus callosum* on

the FLAIR images. On the T1-weighted postcontrast pulse sequences, mild contrast enhancement of the pons lesion was present (Figure 2(b)). Meningeal enhancement was observed surrounding the pons, *medulla oblongata*, and cranial cervical spine (Figure 2(b)), and ill-defined areas of enhancement were visible within the thalamus, right frontal lobe, and *corpus callosum* and surrounding the lateral ventricles (Figure 3). Multifocal, contrast-enhancing disease affecting the cerebrum, brainstem, and cervical meninges was diagnosed. Meningoencephalitis was considered the most likely diagnosis, with differential diagnoses of metastatic neoplasia and lymphoma.

Following the MRI examination, cerebrospinal fluid was collected from the cerebellomedullary cistern, and it revealed

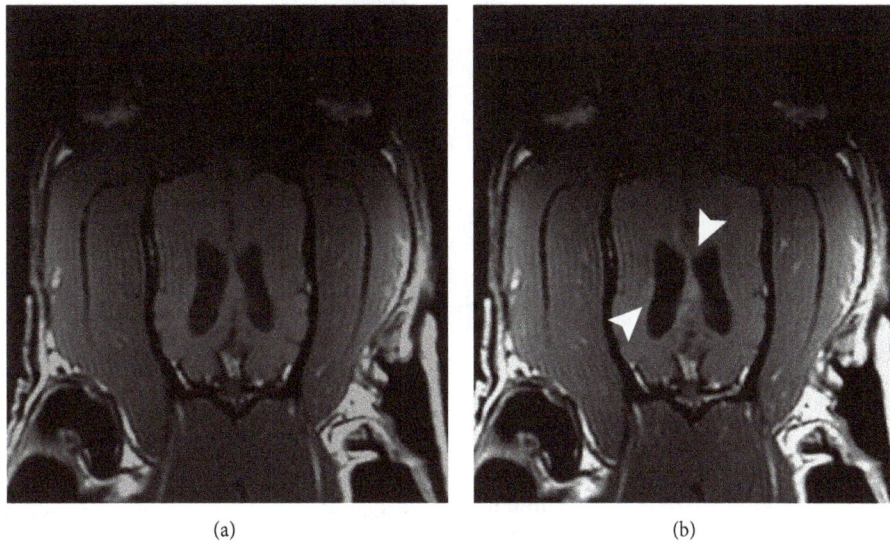

(a)                                                                                                (b)

FIGURE 3: T1-weighted dorsal pulse sequences before (a) and after contrast (b), at the level of the lateral ventricles. (a) The T1-weighted precontrast images were unremarkable. (b) On the T1-weighted postcontrast sequence, multiple ill-defined mildly enhancing lesions were visible within the right frontal lobe, temporal lobe, and *corpus callosum* and surrounding the lateral ventricles (solid arrowheads).

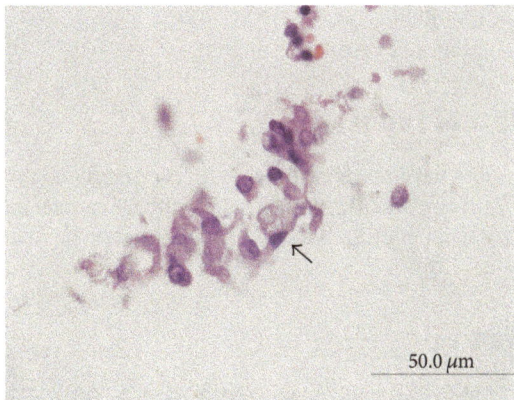

FIGURE 4: 1000x brain. A detached fragmented inflammatory focus of scattered histiocytes and few lymphocytes with extracellular, refractile, and round to oval thick-walled algal organism (arrow) which is 10–15 μm in diameter and composed of 2 to 3 wedge-shaped endospores is demonstrated. Hematoxylin and eosin stain: 1000x.

contained refractile, round to oval algae, 10–15 μm in diameter (Figure 4), with a 2-3 μm thick cell wall, confirmed by special stain (Gomori's methenamine silver). Rarely, these algal cells had 2-3 wedge-shaped endospores. The meninges were sporadically infiltrated with similar inflammatory cells. In the hepatic parenchyma, few scattered granulomas, composed of moderate numbers of histiocytes admixed with lymphocytes and eosinophils, were observed, as well as a high number of macrophages containing golden brown pigment (hemosiderin/bile), predominately in the portal areas. Special staining for algal organisms did not reveal any algal cells. Histological changes in the brain were compatible with severe multifocal prothecal meningoencephalitis. The hepatic changes were suggestive of a chronic infectious process, but no organisms could be identified in the histopathologic sections. No significant microscopic changes were present in the other organs, including the gastrointestinal tract. Culture of the brain for *Prototheca* spp. did not grow any organism after 7 days, and a specific *Prototheca* species could not be identified.

## 3. Discussion

Prothecosis is a rare disease that has been reported in many species including dogs [1–3], cats [4], cattle [5], and humans [6, 7]. It is caused by unicellular, achlorophyllous algae which exist in the environment as ubiquitous detritus inhabitants and contaminants of various substrates: raw and treated sewage, trees, soil, mud, and feces [7, 8] which may contaminate aquatic systems or food and subsequently be ingested by man and animals. Prothecosis can also occur secondary to traumatic inoculation [8]. Three species are currently recognized, with the most common two being *Prototheca wickerhamii* and *Prototheca zopfii*. They have a worldwide distribution and are both described to cause disease in

an eosinophilic pleocytosis with evidence of hemorrhage and intralesional yeast organisms, most consistent with *Prototheca* spp. Antiprotozoal treatment was denied by the owners, and 5 weeks after diagnosis, the dog was euthanized due to progression of the neurologic deficits. A postmortem examination was conducted. Macroscopically, the pons and *medulla oblongata* appeared slightly swollen with multifocal areas of dark brown to grey pinpoint foci in the hippocampus, thalamus, olfactory lobe, *medulla oblongata,* and pons. There was no other gross abnormality present.

Histopathologic examination of the brain revealed multiple random nodular aggregates of numerous lymphocytes, plasma cells, small numbers of histiocytes, and eosinophils centered on the blood vessels. Occasionally, few histiocytes dogs [2], while most human [6] and feline [4] cases are caused by *P. wickerhamii*.

The clinical signs of this disease are variable depending on the species affected. In humans and cats, it involves most commonly the skin, with vesiculobullous and granulomatous lesions observed, and it occurs more often in patients with underlying immunosuppression or concomitant disease [4, 7].

In dogs, there is currently no established breed, age, or sex predilections [9], but Collies [10–12] and Boxers [3] tend to be more frequently affected. The algae are usually widely disseminated throughout many organs including small intestines/colon, eyes, ears, skin, skeletal muscles, kidneys, liver, peritoneum, thyroid, heart, spinal cord, and brain [1–3]. The most common signs described are large bowel hemorrhagic diarrhea [1–3, 11–14] and ocular involvement [2, 10, 15–18] with retinal degeneration, chorioretinitis, or retinal detachment, potentially leading to blindness. Eventually, neurological signs can be observed in the form of lethargy, behavioral changes, paresis, head tilt, cervical pain, circling, ataxia, or seizures [2, 3, 19, 20]. In this case report, the neurological signs and histopathological results were similar to those of the previously published cases of canine central nervous system (CNS) prototothecosis [19, 20]. However, the dog in this report presented only neurologic symptoms. This atypical clinical presentation of prototothecosis has been previously described only in two instances [19, 21]. In our report, a few granulomas were observed in the liver during the necropsy, but no algal organisms were detected histopathologically. Microscopic examination of the eyes revealed only mild focal cataractous changes.

Only one report describing MR features of canine central prototothecosis has been reported in the literature [22]. In both, that case [22] and the case reported here, the MR lesions observed were suggestive of an inflammatory or infectious process. However, the lesion observed in the pons in our case was broadbased, which may be suggestive of an extra-axial neoplastic disease [23, 24], but it was also ill defined and poorly marginated, with only minimal displacement of the fourth ventricle to the right and only mild T1 post-gadolinium enhancement, without dural tail sign observed, which is more suggestive of an inflammatory lesion. Primary brain tumors are often contrast enhancing compared with inflammatory lesions [23, 24]. The combination of meningeal enhancement and multifocal parenchymal lesions favored an inflammatory or infectious disease process. In a study [25] of 25 dogs with inflammatory cerebrospinal fluid (24 infectious/inflammatory diseases and 1 choroid plexus tumor), MRI lesions observed in 19 dogs (76%) were described as T1-weighted or T2-weighted multifocal or diffuse intracranial lesions. Meningeal enhancement was identified in 28% of these dogs. According to this study, meningeal enhancement is suggestive of inflammatory cerebrospinal fluid, but it is a nonspecific sign. To better assess meningeal enhancement, the use of chemical fat suppression as well as delayed imaging following gadolinium may help in identifying its presence with an increased level of confidence [26]. Multifocal MR lesions such as in our patient are suggestive of inflammatory or metastatic disease, while a single lesion is usually observed more frequently in patients with primary brain tumors [23]. Multifocal primary brain tumors or combinations of primary and secondary tumors have been reported, however, in the same patient [27].

Cerebrospinal fluid analysis was important for the diagnosis in this dog. Other methods to diagnose *Prototheca* spp. infection include bacteriological culture, using blood agar and common mycologic media, from colonic scrapping, cerebrospinal fluid, or any other infected tissue [7, 14]. The reason for a negative culture in the dog in this report is unclear, but it could have been due to delayed tissue sampling, which was performed at the time of necropsy.

## 4. Conclusion

Although rare in dogs, *Prototheca* spp. infection should be considered when MR examination is suggestive of meningoencephalitis, even if there is no evidence of gastrointestinal disease.

## Abbreviations

CNS:   Central nervous system
FLAIR: Fluid-attenuated inversion recovery
GRE:   Gradient echo
MRI:   Magnetic resonance imaging.

## Conflict of Interests

The authors have no relevant affiliations or financial involvements with any organization or entity with a financial interest in or financial conflict with the subject matter or materials discussed in this paper.

## References

[1] G. Migaki, R. L. Font, R. M. Sauer, W. Kaplan, and R. L. Miller, "Canine prototothecosis: review of the literature and report of an additional case," *Journal of the American Veterinary Medical Association*, vol. 181, no. 8, pp. 794–797, 1982.

[2] S. R. Hollingsworth, "Canine prototothecosis," *Veterinary Clinics of North America—Small Animal Practice*, vol. 30, no. 5, pp. 1091–1101, 2000.

[3] V. J. Stenner, B. MacKay, T. King et al., "Prototothecosis in 17 Australian dogs and a review of the canine literature," *Medical Mycology*, vol. 45, no. 3, pp. 249–266, 2007.

[4] J. E. Dillberger, B. Homer, D. Daubert, and N. H. Altman, "Prototothecosis in two cats," *Journal of the American Veterinary Medical Association*, vol. 192, no. 11, pp. 1557–1559, 1988.

[5] L. G. Corbellini, D. Driemeier, C. Cruz, M. M. Dias, and L. Ferreiro, "Bovine mastitis due to Prototheca zopfii: clinical, epidemiological and pathological aspects in a Brazilian dairy herd," *Tropical Animal Health and Production*, vol. 33, no. 6, pp. 463–470, 2001.

[6] D. Thiele and A. Bergmann, "Prototothecosis in human medicine," *International Journal of Hygiene and Environmental Health*, vol. 204, no. 5-6, pp. 297–302, 2002.

[7] C. Lass-Flörl and A. Mayr, "Human prototothecosis," *Clinical Microbiology Reviews*, vol. 20, no. 2, pp. 230–242, 2007.

[8] R. S. Pore, E. A. Barnett, W. C. Barnes Jr., and J. D. Walker, "Prototheca ecology," *Mycopathologia*, vol. 81, no. 1, pp. 49–62, 1983.

[9] H. Tsuji, R. Kano, A. Hirai et al., "An isolate of Prototheca wickerhamii from systemic canine protothecosis," *Veterinary Microbiology*, vol. 118, no. 3-4, pp. 305–311, 2006.

[10] J. R. Cook Jr., D. E. Tyler, D. B. Coulter, and F. W. Chandler, "Disseminated protothecosis causing acute blindness and deafness in a dog," *Journal of the American Veterinary Medical Association*, vol. 184, no. 10, pp. 1266–1272, 1984.

[11] P. M. Rakich and K. S. Latimer, "Altered immune function in a dog with disseminated protothecosis," *Journal of the American Veterinary Medical Association*, vol. 185, no. 6, pp. 681–683, 1984.

[12] J. B. Thomas and N. Preston, "Generalised protothecosis in a collie dog," *Australian Veterinary Journal*, vol. 67, no. 1, pp. 25–27, 1990.

[13] T. S. Rallis, D. Tontis, K. K. Adamama-Moraitou, M. E. Mylonakis, and L. G. Papazoglou, "Protothecal colitis in a German Shepherd dog," *Australian Veterinary Journal*, vol. 80, no. 7, pp. 406–408, 2002.

[14] E. Strunck, L. Billups, and S. Avgeris, "Canine protothecosis," *Compendium on Continuing Education for the Practicing Veterinarian*, vol. 26, no. 2, pp. 96–103, 2004.

[15] J. R. Blogg and J. E. Sykes, "Sudden blindness associated with protothecosis in a dog," *Australian Veterinary Journal*, vol. 72, no. 4, pp. 147–149, 1995.

[16] W. W. Carlton and L. Austin, "Ocular protothecosis in a dog," *Veterinary Pathology*, vol. 10, no. 3, pp. 274–280, 1973.

[17] T. M. Donnelly, "Head tilt and sudden blindness in a dog," *Laboratory Animals*, vol. 33, pp. 25–29, 2004.

[18] T. E. Rizzi, R. L. Cowell, J. H. Meinkoth, and M. A. Gilmour, "More than meets the eye: subretinal aspirate from an acutely blind dog," *Veterinary Clinical Pathology*, vol. 35, no. 1, pp. 111–113, 2006.

[19] D. E. Tyler, M. D. Lorenz, J. L. Blue, J. F. Munnell, and F. W. Chandler, "Disseminated protothecosis with central nervous system involvement in a dog," *Journal of the American Veterinary Medical Association*, vol. 176, no. 10 I, pp. 987–993, 1980.

[20] C. Salvadori, G. Gandini, A. Ballarini, and C. Cantile, "Protothecal granulomatous meningoencephalitis in a dog," *Journal of Small Animal Practice*, vol. 49, no. 10, pp. 531–535, 2008.

[21] M. Marquez, S. Rodenas, J. Molin et al., "Protothecal pyogranulomatous meningoencephalitis in a dog without evidence of disseminated infection," *Veterinary Record*, vol. 171, article 100, 2012.

[22] M. Young, W. Bush, M. Sanchez, P. Gavin, and M. Williams, "Serial MRI and CSF analysis in a dog treated with intrathecal amphotericin B for protothecosis," *Journal of the American Animal Hospital Association*, vol. 48, no. 2, pp. 125–131, 2012.

[23] G. B. Cherubini, P. Mantis, T. A. Martinez, C. R. Lamb, and R. Cappello, "Utility of magnetic resonance imaging for distinguishing neoplastic from non-neoplastic brain lesions in dogs and cats," *Veterinary Radiology and Ultrasound*, vol. 46, no. 5, pp. 384–387, 2005.

[24] S. Hecht and W. H. Adams, "MRI of brain disease in veterinary patients part 2: acquired brain disorders," *Veterinary Clinics of North America—Small Animal Practice*, vol. 40, no. 1, pp. 39–63, 2010.

[25] C. R. Lamb, P. J. Croson, R. Cappello, and G. B. Cherubini, "Magnetic resonance imaging findings in 25 dogs with inflammatory cerebrospinal fluid," *Veterinary Radiology and Ultrasound*, vol. 46, no. 1, pp. 17–22, 2005.

[26] M. A. D'Anjou, E. M. Carmel, L. Blond, G. Beauchamp, and J. Parent, "MRI qualitative and quantitative characterization of meningeal enhancement in dogs and cats: effect of acquisition time and chemical fat suppression," in *Proceedings of the ACVR Annual Scientific Meeting*, Memphis, Tenn, USA, 2009.

[27] E. MacKillop, D. E. Thrall, R. S. Ranck, K. E. Linder, and K. R. Munana, "Imaging diagnosis—synchronous primary brain tumors in a dog," *Veterinary Radiology and Ultrasound*, vol. 48, no. 6, pp. 550–553, 2007.

# 18

# Successful Long-Term Use of Itraconazole for the Treatment of *Aspergillus* Diskospondylitis in a Dog

Emiko Van Wie,[1] Annie V. Chen,[2] Stephanie A. Thomovsky,[2] and Russell L. Tucker[2]

[1] *Texas A&M University College of Veterinary Medicine, 422 Raymond Stotzer Parkway, College Station, TX 77843, USA*
[2] *Washington State University College of Veterinary Medicine, P.O. Box 647010, Pullman, WA 99164, USA*

Correspondence should be addressed to Annie V. Chen; avchen@vetmed.wsu.edu

Academic Editors: F. Mutinelli, J. Orós, L. G. Papazoglou, and P. Roccabianca

A 5-year-old spayed female German shepherd dog was admitted with a history of generalized stiffness. Neurologic examination revealed mild paraparesis with multifocal spinal pain. Spinal radiographs and magnetic resonance imaging revealed diskospondylitis at L6-7 and multiple sites throughout the thoracolumbar spine. Biopsy of the intervertebral disk at L6-7 revealed a positive culture for *Aspergillus* species, and the dog was placed on itraconazole indefinitely. Clinical signs were significantly improved after two weeks of itraconazole. The dog was reevaluated 8 years later for unrelated reasons. No spinal pain was detected. Spinal radiographs revealed a fused L6-7 disk space and collapsed and sclerotic disk spaces at multiple sites. Itraconazole was tolerated by the dog with normal yearly liver enzyme values. To our knowledge, this is the first reported case of successful long-term use of itraconazole for the treatment of *Aspergillus* diskospondylitis in a dog.

## 1. Introduction

Diskospondylitis is an infection of the intervertebral disk with concurrent osteomyelitis in adjacent vertebral endplates. The most common cause of diskospondylitis is hematogenous spread of bacteria or fungi from urinary tract infections, dental infections, or endocarditis [1, 2]. Migrating foreign bodies, such as grass awns, have also been incriminated as a source of infection. *Staphylococcus aureus* is the most common cause of canine diskospondylitis.

*Aspergillus* is a fungus that is ubiquitous in the environment and an opportunistic pathogen. *Aspergillus terreus* is the most common species associated with disseminated aspergillosis [2]. Female German shepherd dogs are the most commonly affected breed with disseminated aspergillosis. It is speculated that German shepherd dogs have a hereditary immune defect that plays a significant role in the pathogenesis [1, 3]. In disseminated cases, it is not uncommon to find radiographic changes consistent with multiple sites of diskospondylitis [3, 4].

Aspergillosis can be localized to the spine only. There have been four published canine cases of *Aspergillus* diskospondylitis, without the presence of systemic involvement, in the veterinary literature [1, 5, 6]. All four cases were seen in German shepherd dogs; these dogs were euthanized due to poor prognosis or neurologic deterioration. The purpose of this report is to describe a case of nondisseminated *Aspergillus* diskospondylitis in a dog that was successfully treated with long-term itraconazole.

## 2. Case Presentation

A 5-year-old (41.2-kg) spayed female German shepherd dog was evaluated for a 3-month history of generalized stiffness that was refractory to pain medications. On admission, rectal temperature, heart rate, and respiration rate were within normal limits. Physical examination was unremarkable. Neurologic examination revealed kyphosis, paraparesis, and mild conscious proprioceptive deficits in the pelvic limbs. Spinal reflexes and cranial nerves were normal. Spinal palpation elicited pain in the midthoracic area and lower lumbar spine.

Complete blood count, serum biochemical analysis, and urinalysis were unremarkable. Spinal radiographs revealed

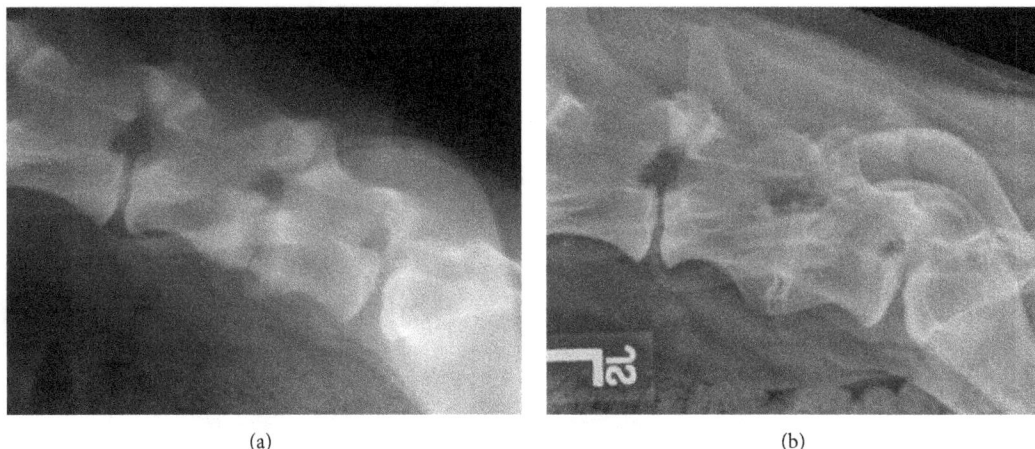

(a)                                             (b)

FIGURE 1: Lateral radiographs of the lower lumbar spine prior to (a) and after 8 years (b) of itraconazole treatment. (a) The L6-7 intervertebral disk space is collapsed and there is lysis of the endplates consistent with active diskospondylitis. (b) The L6-7 intervertebral disk space is collapsed and partially fused with smoothly marginated osseous proliferation between the ventral aspects of the vertebral bodies suggestive of healed diskospondylitis.

diskospondylitis at L6-7. Lumbar cerebrospinal fluid (CSF) revealed a mildly elevated protein count (55.5 mg/dL, reference <35 mg/dL) with mild blood contamination. Blood, urine, and CSF cultures for aerobic and anaerobic bacteria and fungal organisms were negative. Serum *Brucella* titer was negative via rapid slide agglutination test. Amoxicillin and clavulanic acid (Clavamox, Pzifer) was prescribed at 22 mg/kg orally every 8 hours. There was no improvement after three weeks; antibiotic therapy was changed to clindamycin and ciprofloxacin.

Six weeks later, the dog was re-evaluated for persistent spinal pain. Neurologic examination was unchanged from the initial visit. Spinal radiographs revealed further lysis of endplates and collapse of the disk space at L6-7 consistent with diskospondylitis (Figure 1(a)). Additionally, irregular endplates were found at T3-9 suspicious for diskospondylitis. Magnetic resonance (MR) imaging of the entire spine revealed multiple sites of diskospondylitis. On the T2-weighed images, irregular nucleus pulposus was seen at T2-10, T13-L1, and L6-7. On gadolinium dimeglumine (Magnvist, Bayer Health Care Pharmaceuticals) enhanced T1-weighted images, the intervertebral disk and endplates at L6-7 showed marked contrast enhancement along with moderate nerve root compression bilaterally (Figure 2).

A left-sided hemilaminectomy at L6-7 with a partial diskectomy was performed for nerve root decompression and intervertebral disk biopsy. Fungal hyphae were seen in the disk sample histologically and *Aspergillus* species were cultured. The specific species of *Aspergillus* was not available because fungal sequencing was not performed. Oral itraconazole (Sporanox, Janssen Pharmaceutica) was given at 5 mg/kg every 24 hours indefinitely. After 2 weeks of therapy, the dog was significantly improved clinically. By 6 weeks, the dog was 90% back to normal according to the owner.

The dog presented 8 years after the initiation of itraconazole therapy for unrelated reasons. The dog was on 5 mg/kg of itraconazole every 24 hours and tolerated treatment well

with normal yearly liver enzyme values. Physical exam was unremarkable. Neurologic exam revealed mild paraparesis, mild conscious proprioceptive deficits in the pelvic limbs, and no spinal pain.

Spinal radiographs showed collapse and partial fusion of the L6-7 intervertebral disk space with smoothly marginated osseous proliferation between the ventral aspects of the vertebral bodies (Figure 1(b)). Additionally, there were collapsed intervertebral disk spaces at T2-T11 and T13-L2. The endplates at T13-L1 and L1-L2 were also very irregular with sclerosis and potential lucency. Ventral bridging spondylosis was seen throughout the thoracic and thoracolumbar spine. Overall, the L6-7 diskospondylitis appeared to be healed; however, it could not be determined radiographically if the other sites were chronically healed or still active. Clinically, the patient had no spinal pain consistent with active diskospondylitis. However, due to the potential lucency noted at the T13-L2 endplates, continual therapy with itraconazole was recommended.

## 3. Discussion

In general, canine aspergillosis carries a poor prognosis [1, 4–8]. Most cases of disseminated aspergillosis with diskospondylitis are euthanized. A variety of treatments have been tried in several cases including itraconazole, ketoconazole, voriconazole, posaconazole, amphotericin B, and hamycin; however, euthanasia was elected within a year in most of the cases due to progression of disease [1, 4, 9–13]. There has been one reported survival of 4.3 years in a dog with disseminated aspergillosis and diskospondylitis treated with itraconazole alone for 2.7 years [9]. This dog was euthanized due to relapse of clinical signs after treatment was discontinued.

Nondisseminated *Aspergillus* diskospondylitis also carries a poor prognosis in dogs [1, 5, 6]. Of the 4 reported cases, all dogs were euthanized. Two of these dogs were

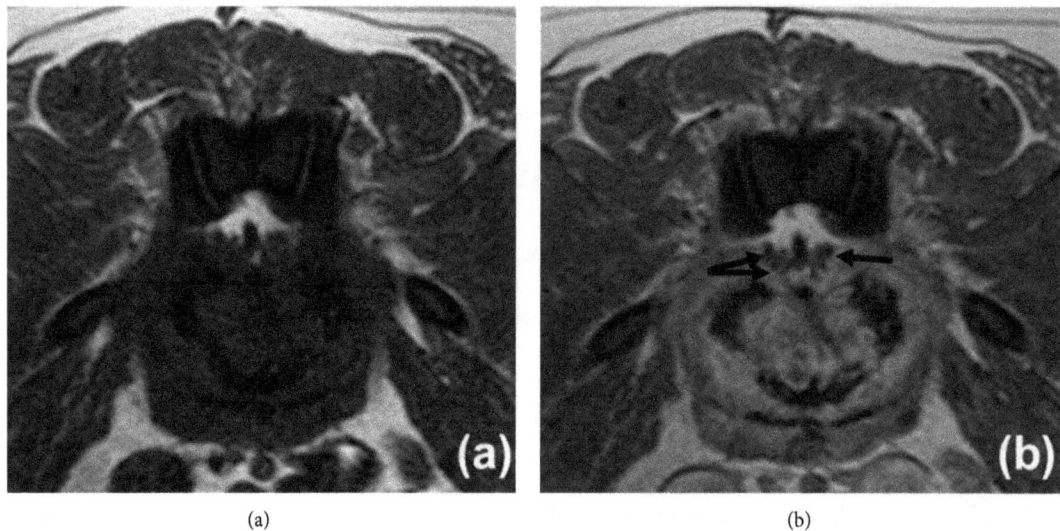

(a)                                                               (b)

FIGURE 2: Transverse T1-weighted before (a) and after (b) contrast MR imaging of the L6-7 intervertebral disk space. There is strong contrast enhancement of the intervertebral disk and endplates suggestive of active diskospondylitis. Nerve root compression (hypointense circles as indicated by arrows) from the inflamed disk is also noted bilaterally.

euthanized shortly after diagnosis. One dog was treated with ketaconazole for three weeks and was euthanized due to neurologic deterioration. The fourth dog was euthanized after lack of improvement on antibiotics and aspergillosis was diagnosed at necropsy.

In most current studies, azole antifungals were the choice of treatment for aspergillosis. Compared to amphotericin B and ketoconazole, itraconazole was more effective and had fewer side effects [2]. Itraconazole works by inhibiting fungal P450 enzyme necessary for ergosterol synthesis. Treatment with itraconazole alone has shown to extend survival time and improve clinical signs with aspergillosis diskospondylitis [9, 10]. However, long-term survival greater than 1 year has only been reported in one case [9]. Fluconazole has little activity against aspergillosis [2].

The dog in this case report had multiple sites of *Aspergillus* diskospondylitis without any signs of systemic dissemination. Initially, the dog was diagnosed with only one site of diskospondylitis even though multifocal spinal pain was noted. Six weeks later, radiographs and MR imaging revealed multifocal sites of diskospondylitis. It is not uncommon for radiographic evidence of diskospondylitis to lag behind the onset of clinical signs by as much as 2–6 weeks; thus, acutely affected patients can have equivocal or even normal radiographic findings [14, 15]. Follow-up radiographs 8 years later showed 2 additional sites of collapsed disk spaces and sclerotic endplates at T10-11 and L1-2 and potential lucency at the endplates of T13-L2. Because no follow-up radiographs were documented between these two time points, it is unknown when these additional sites became affected in the course of disease. Also, whether these sites were active or actually chronically healed sites could not be determined radiographically. One of the limitations of radiographs is the difficulty of differentiating chronic diskospondylitis from healing lesions or even degenerative changes of the spine [14, 15]. Advanced imaging techniques

such as MR imaging or computed tomography with contrast or nuclear scintigraphy may have been helpful to clarify this [16, 17].

This is the first reported case of nondisseminated *Aspergillus* diskospondylitis successfully treated with long-term itraconazole. The speculated reasons for success in this case may be related to an early surgical diagnosis which allowed for early treatment before dissemination of the disease and/or due to lifelong treatment with itraconazole, despite early resolution of clinical signs. This dog had no long-term side effects from itraconazole. Although the dog had no clinical signs consistent with diskospondylitis, radiographs suggest active aspergillosis may still be present. Indefinite, lifelong treatment with itraconazole should be considered in dogs with *Aspergillus* diskospondylitis, particularly German shepherd dogs with potential immune deficiency, in order to prevent progression of clinical signs or relapse. Treatment until resolution of clinical signs may not be sufficient.

## References

[1] W. L. Berry and A. L. Leisewitz, "Multifocal *Aspergillus terreus* discospondylitis in two German shepherd dogs," *Journal of the South African Veterinary Association*, vol. 67, no. 4, pp. 222–228, 1996.

[2] J. Lavely and D. Lipsitz, "Fungal infections of the central nervous system in the dog and cat," *Clinical Techniques in Small Animal Practice*, vol. 20, no. 4, pp. 212–219, 2005.

[3] M. J. Day, W. J. Penhale, C. E. Eger et al., "Disseminated aspergillosis in dogs," *Australian Veterinary Journal*, vol. 63, no. 2, pp. 55–59, 1986.

[4] R. M. Schultz, E. G. Johnson, E. R. Wisner, N. A. Brown, B. A. Byrne, and J. E. Sykes, "Clinicopathologic and diagnostic imaging characteristics of systemic Aspergillosis in 30 dogs," *Journal of Veterinary Internal Medicine*, vol. 22, no. 4, pp. 851–859, 2008.

[5] R. A. Weitkamp, "Aspergilloma in two dogs," *Journal of the American Animal Hospital Association*, vol. 18, no. 3, pp. 503–506, 1982.

[6] A. M. Wolf and G. C. Troy, "Deep mycotic disease," in *Textbook of Veterinary Internal Medicine; Diseases of the Dog and Cat*, S. Ettinger and E. C. Feldman, Eds., pp. 439–444, Saunders, Philadelphia, Pa, USA, 4th edition, 1995.

[7] S. S. Jang, T. E. Dorr, E. L. Biberstein, and A. Wong, "*Aspergillus deflectus* infection in four dogs," *Journal of Medical and Veterinary Mycology*, vol. 24, no. 2, pp. 95–104, 1986.

[8] J. Pastor, M. Pumarola, R. Cuenca, and S. Lavin, "Systemic aspergillosis in a dog," *Veterinary Record*, vol. 132, no. 16, pp. 412–413, 1993.

[9] S. E. Kelly, S. E. Shaw, and W. T. Clark, "Long-term survival of four dogs with disseminated *Aspergillus terreus* infection treated with itraconazole," *Australian Veterinary Journal*, vol. 72, no. 8, pp. 311–313, 1995.

[10] M. J. Dallman, T. L. Dew, L. Tobias, and R. Doss, "Disseminated aspergillosis in a dog with diskospondylitis and neurologic deficits," *Journal of the American Veterinary Medical Association*, vol. 200, no. 4, pp. 511–513, 1992.

[11] G. L. Wood, D. C. Hirsh, and R. R. Selcer, "Disseminated aspergillosis in a dog," *Journal of the American Veterinary Medical Association*, vol. 172, no. 6, pp. 704–707, 1978.

[12] S. J. Butterworth, F. J. Barr, G. R. Pearson, and M. J. Day, "Multiple discospondylitis associated with *Aspergillus* species infection in a dog," *Veterinary Record*, vol. 136, no. 2, pp. 38–41, 1995.

[13] A. C. Kaufman, C. E. Greene, B. A. Selcer, M. E. Styles, and E. A. Mahaffey, "Systemic aspergillosis in a dog and treatment with hamycin," *Journal of the American Animal Hospital Association*, vol. 30, no. 2, pp. 132–136, 1994.

[14] L. Hurov, G. Troy, and G. Turnwald, "Diskospondylitis in the dog: 27 cases," *Journal of the American Veterinary Medical Association*, vol. 173, no. 3, pp. 275–281, 1978.

[15] M. H. Shamir, N. Tavor, and T. Aizenberg, "Radiographic findings during recovery from discospondylitis," *Veterinary Radiology and Ultrasound*, vol. 42, no. 6, pp. 496–503, 2001.

[16] I. Carrera, M. Sullivan, F. Mcconnell, and R. Gonçalves, "Magnetic resonance imaging features of discospondylitis in dogs," *Veterinary Radiology and Ultrasound*, vol. 52, no. 2, pp. 125–131, 2011.

[17] L. Stern, R. McCarthy, R. King, and K. Hunt, "Imaging diagnosis—discospondylitis and septic arthritis in a dog," *Veterinary Radiology and Ultrasound*, vol. 48, no. 4, pp. 335–337, 2007.

**19**

# Aniridia in Two Related Tennessee Walking Horses

**Karen A. McCormick,**[1] **Daniel Ward,**[2] **and Kimberly M. Newkirk**[3]

[1] *Large Animal Clinical Sciences, University of Tennessee, College of Veterinary Medicine, 2407 River Drive, Knoxville, TN 37996, USA*

[2] *Small Animal Clinical Sciences, University of Tennessee, College of Veterinary Medicine, 2407 River Drive, Knoxville, TN 37996, USA*

[3] *Diagnostic and Biomedical Sciences, University of Tennessee, College of Veterinary Medicine, 2407 River Drive, Knoxville, TN 37996, USA*

Correspondence should be addressed to Karen A. McCormick; kkalck@utk.edu

Academic Editors: L. Espino López, S. Hecht, F. Mutinelli, and S. Stuen

Aniridia in horses is rare and has previously been reported to be genetically transmitted in Belgian horses and Quarter horses. This paper describes the defect in 2 related Tennessee Walking horses, with special reference to new findings regarding the molecular genetics of ocular development and how they might relate to equine aniridia. In addition to aniridia, these 2 horses possessed additional ocular abnormalities including cataracts and dermoid lesions. Euthanasia was elected, and the eyes were examined histologically. Iris hypoplasia, atypical dermoids, and cataracts were confirmed in both horses. Due to the heritability of aniridia in horses, breeding of affected animals is not recommended.

## 1. Introduction

Aniridia is a rare condition marked by partial or complete absence of the iris. This condition has been reported in horses [6–11], cattle [1], laboratory animals [2, 3], and humans [4, 5]. In Belgian horses [6] and Quarter horses [7], the defect has been reported to be genetically transmitted as an autosomal dominant trait, but at least one case in a Swedish Warmblood was not dominantly inherited [8]. In humans, the anomaly either presents as a familial condition with autosomal-dominant inheritance or is sporadic [4, 5]. Affected animals are usually photophobic with absent direct and indirect pupillary light responses bilaterally, and they often have additional ocular abnormalities including dermoid lesions and cataracts. Dermoid lesions, like many instances of aniridia, form during foetal development, and our understanding of the molecular genetics of ocular development has improved since the last case report of aniridia in horses [8]. Therefore, the purpose of this report is to describe the clinical and histologic features of aniridia in 2 related Tennessee Walking horses, especially considering "new" information about the genetics of ocular involvement.

## 2. Case Presentation

Two Tennessee Walking horses were presented to the University of Tennessee Equine Hospital for bilateral ocular abnormalities. Horse A was a 15-year-old mare, and horse B was her 12-month-old female offspring. Very limited history was available because both animals were rescued. Visual deficits had been recognized in both animals prior to presentation, and the new owners had noticed bilateral ocular opacities in both horses. On ophthalmic examination of horse A, both direct and indirect pupillary light responses were absent in both eyes. However, the horse did have positive menace responses bilaterally. The tips of the ciliary processes were visible in both eyes, and the iris could not be identified. The corneas showed evidence of chronic keratitis bilaterally with mild vascular infiltration of the cornea at the dorsal aspect. Fine cilia-like hairs were protruding from the superior corneoscleral limbus of the left eye, consistent with a limbal dermoid. There were also bilateral immature nuclear cataracts. Cataracts hid portions of the fundus, but those portions that were evaluable were normal.

(a)

(b)

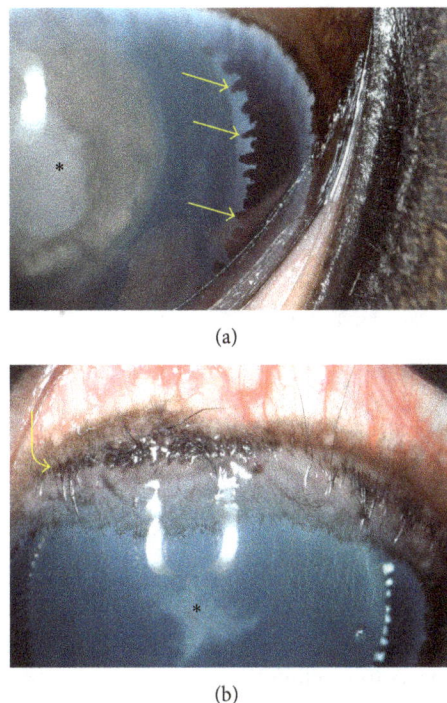

FIGURE 1: Horse B. (a) Left eye. Due to the absence of any grossly visible iris, the ciliary processes are easily seen (arrows). An immature nuclear cataract is also present (asterisk). (b) Right eye. Short hairs emanating from the corneoscleral limbus are considered variants of limbal dermoids (curved arrow). An incipient cataract is also present (asterisk).

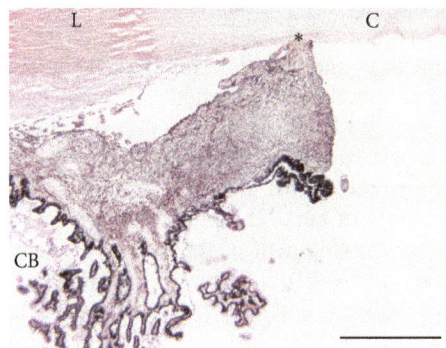

FIGURE 2: Horse A. The iris is markedly blunted and focally adhered to Descemet's membrane (peripheral anterior synechia) (asterisk). For orientation, C: cornea, L: limbus, and CB: ciliary body. Hematoxylin and eosin. Bar = 2 mm.

Ophthalmic examination of horse B, the yearling offspring of horse A, revealed similar findings. There was no evidence of an iris, and the ciliary processes were easily seen (Figure 1(a)). Chronic keratitis was present bilaterally, and limbal dermoid lesions were more pronounced than those in horse A (Figure 1(b)). Incipient to immature cataracts were present bilaterally.

Both horses were diagnosed with bilateral aniridia with chronic keratitis, limbal dermoids, and cataract formation. The rescue organization elected euthanasia for both animals due to the poor prognosis for improvement in long-term vision. Following euthanasia, the eyes of both animals were harvested and fixed in Davidson's solution.

## 3. Histopathology

In both eyes (one from each horse), the iris leaflets were present but markedly blunted (iris hypoplasia) (Figure 2). The blunted iris was frequently adhered to Descemet's membrane (peripheral anterior synechia) (Figure 2). The iris sphincter muscle was absent, and only poorly developed remnants of the dilator muscle were apparent with a Masson's trichrome stain (Figure 3). There were occasional nerve bundles within the iris leaflets. The iridocorneal angle was otherwise normal, but horse B had erythrocytes (haemorrhage) within the angle. On the posterior surface of the iris, the normally heavily pigmented, bilayered epithelium was disorganized and varied from poorly to heavily pigmented (Figure 3). The ciliary body and ciliary processes were within normal limits.

Horse A had mild, limbal, superficial corneal vascularization on one side of the eye; the clinically noted limbal dermoid was not present in the section. At the limbus of horse B, there was a single hair follicle with an associated sebaceous gland, consistent with a limbal dermoid. The surrounding collagen was haphazardly arranged and contained scattered blood vessels, lymphocytes, and plasma cells.

There was artifactual retinal detachment in both horses. Grossly, both horses had bilateral lens opacities; however, only the lens from the foal (horse B) was examined microscopically. There was splitting of the anterior lens capsule and lens epithelial cells metaplasia and hyperplasia. No other histopathologic lesions were present in the lens.

## 4. Discussion

Aniridia was first reported in horses in 1955 in a Belgian stallion and his offspring [6]. The defect identified in this group of related horses was heritable and passed via an autosomal dominant mode. Aniridia has also been described in a group of related Quarter horses, also with autosomal dominant inheritance [7, 9]. In single case reports in a Thoroughbred colt [10] and Welsh-Thoroughbred cross filly [11], hereditability was undetermined. Hereditability was undetermined for 5 in a series of 6 cases from Sweden, and dominant hereditability with complete penetrance was ruled out in one Swedish Warmblood. In humans, aniridia is inherited in about two-thirds of the cases and sporadic in the remainder [4]. In the inherited forms, the majority are autosomal dominant [4]. Although it is impossible to make a conclusion about inheritance in the 2 horses in this report, the presentation in a mare and its foal makes hereditability highly likely, and rarity of the syndrome makes dominant inheritance most likely.

The underlying pathophysiology of aniridia is not known with certainty. During ocular organogenesis, the epithelial layers of the normal iris are derived from the neuroectoderm of the anterior rim of the optic cup, while the stroma is derived from mesenchymal tissue of neural crest origin [12].

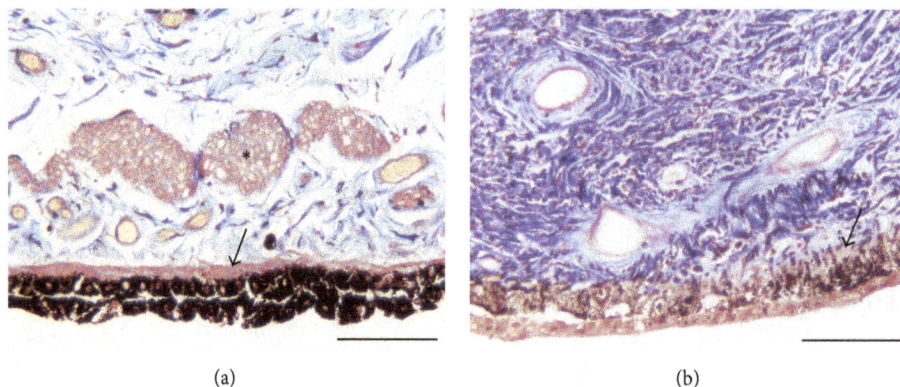

(a) (b)

FIGURE 3: (a) Control horse. Normal portion of the posterior surface of the pupillary margin of the iris with both the dilator muscle (arrow) and sphincter muscle present (asterisk). Masson's trichrome. Bar = 200 $\mu$m. (b) Horse B. Posterior surface of the iris with thin dilator muscle (arrow); the sphincter muscle was absent. Note also the poorly pigmented and disorganized epithelium on the posterior surface of the iris. Masson's trichrome. Bar = 200 $\mu$m.

Histologically, epithelium and stroma are both deficient in aniridia, so it is possible that defects in epithelial development prevent normal stromal maturation or that stromal maldevelopment causes failure of normal epithelial development [5]. A third theory suggests that aniridia is a result of excessive remodelling, with normal iris formation being followed by inappropriate iris tissue regression [13].

In humans, most cases are transmitted via autosomal dominant inheritance and are linked to defects in the *PAX6* gene, one of a family of transcriptional regulators that has a central role in controlling the development of the eye [4, 5]. Most mutations (nonsense mutations, splice mutations, frameshift deletions, etc.) cause premature translational termination on one of the alleles, resulting in haploinsufficiency with decreased expression of gene product [4, 5]. Because a critical dose of PAX6 protein is necessary to initiate transcription of target genes [14], the reduced amount could prove critical in preventing normal iris development. A high, continuous expression of *PAX6* in tissues of ectodermal origin (e.g., iridial epithelium) directly affects the regulation and structure of these tissues during organogenesis of the eye but is also necessary for the expression of signalling molecules that act on cells of mesenchymal origin (e.g., the iris stroma). In addition, a low and transient expression of *PAX6* is observed in cells of mesenchymal origin during development of the iris and other anterior segment tissues [15]. This favours a hypothesis that simultaneous defects in epithelial and mesenchymal development are involved in aniridia, with the former probably being more important. Missense mutations are relatively rare and result in a variety of phenotypes, including corneal dystrophy, Peter's anomaly, foveal hypoplasia, ectopia pupillae, congenital nystagmus, and presenile cataract [5]. Sporadic mutations also occur and may be associated with nephroblastoma (Wilms' tumour), genitourinary abnormalities, and mental retardation [4, 5]. While most of our knowledge about *PAX6* structure and function comes from humans and laboratory rodents, *PAX6* protein function is highly conserved across bilaterian species [4]. Therefore, it is easy to assume that most of the genetic features of aniridia described in humans would apply to

horses as well. Another equine ocular developmental disorder, multiple congenital ocular anomalies, also features maldevelopment and hypoplasia of the iris, but that syndrome appears to be clinically and genetically distinct from the equine aniridia syndrome [16, 17].

Clinically, aniridia in humans is usually found in association with other ocular defects such as cataracts, glaucoma, keratopathy, optic nerve hypoplasia, ectopia lentis, nystagmus, and photophobia [5]. The foregoing discussion of the importance of *PAX6* on ocular organogenesis focuses on the iris, but *PAX6* is equally important in the development of the cornea [18], lens [19], optic nerve/retina [20], and iridocorneal angle [15]. Multiple ocular defects are therefore not surprising. Both of the cases in this report had cataracts, corneal pathology, and limbal dermoids, and similar findings are common in previously published equine cases [7–10]. The dermoids were clinically atypical in that the aberrant hairs did not emanate from a skin-like mass of tissue but rather appeared in a regular row along the limbus and were very much like a row of cilia. The precise embryological errors leading to the development of the various presentations of dermoids are unclear, but it has been hypothesized that the pathogenesis of limbal dermoids may be related in part to aberrant development and fusion of the lids, with displacement of lid elements to the limbus [21], which would certainly correlate with the clinical appearance in our cases.

Aniridia is a complex heritable disorder of horses that has been reported in Belgians, Quarter Horses, and now in Tennessee Walking horses. The disorder most commonly follows an autosomal dominant mode of inheritance and results in impaired vision of affected animals due to chronic keratitis and cataract formation. There is no known treatment of the condition for horses; affected animals are managed based on clinical symptoms as they arise. Although horses have been reported to perform well with the condition [10], affected animals should not be used for breeding purposes.

## Acknowledgment

The authors would like to thank Misty R. Bailey, M. A., ELS, for his editorial assistance.

# References

[1] L. Z. Saunders and M. G. Fincher, "Hereditary multiple eye defects in grade Jersey calves," *The Cornell Veterinarian*, vol. 41, no. 4, pp. 351–366, 1951.

[2] T. Glaser, J. Lane, and D. Housman, "A mouse model of the aniridia-Wilms tumor deletion syndrome," *Science*, vol. 250, no. 4982, pp. 823–827, 1990.

[3] T. Glaser, D. S. Walton, and R. L. Maas, "Genomic structure, evolutionary conservation and aniridia mutations in the human PAX6 gene," *Nature Genetics*, vol. 2, no. 3, pp. 232–239, 1992.

[4] H. Kokotas and M. B. Petersen, "Clinical and molecular aspects of aniridia," *Clinical Genetics*, vol. 77, no. 5, pp. 409–420, 2010.

[5] H. Lee, R. Khan, and M. O'keefe, "Aniridia: current pathology and management," *Acta Ophthalmologica*, vol. 86, no. 7, pp. 708–715, 2008.

[6] K. Eriksson, "Hereditary aniridia with secondary cataract in horses," *Nordisk Veterinaermedicin*, vol. 7, pp. 773–779, 1955.

[7] J. R. Joyce, J. E. Martin, R. W. Storts, and L. Skow, "Iridial hypoplasia (aniridia) accompanied by limbic dermoids and cataracts in a group of related quarterhorses," *Equine Veterinary Journal*, vol. 22, no. 10, pp. 26–28, 1990.

[8] N. Håkanson, "Irishypoplasi hos häst," *Svensk Veterinärtidning*, vol. 45, pp. 99–103, 1993.

[9] J. Joyce, "Aniridia in a Quarter horse," *Equine Veterinary Journal*, vol. 15, no. 2, pp. 21–22, 1983.

[10] Y. Ueda, "Aniridia in a thoroughbred horse," *Equine Veterinary Journal*, vol. 22, no. 10, p. 29, 1990.

[11] N. L. Irby and G. D. Aguirre, "Congenital aniridia in a pony," *Journal of the American Veterinary Medical Association*, vol. 186, no. 3, pp. 281–283, 1985.

[12] C. S. Cook, "Ocular embryology and congenital malformations," in *Veterinary Ophthalmology*, K. N. Gelatt, Ed., pp. 3–36, Blackwell Publishing, Ames, Iowa, USA, 4th edition, 2007.

[13] G. R. Beauchamp and D. M. Meisler, "An alternative hypothesis for iris maldevelopment (aniridia)," *Journal of Pediatric Ophthalmology and Strabismus*, vol. 23, no. 6, pp. 281–283, 1986.

[14] A. Cvekl, C. M. Sax, E. H. Bresnick, and J. Piatigorsky, "A complex array of positive and negative elements regulates the chicken $\alpha$A-crystallin gene: Involvement of Pax-6, USF, CREB and/or CREM, and AP-1 proteins," *Molecular and Cellular Biology*, vol. 14, no. 11, pp. 7363–7376, 1994.

[15] D. C. Baulmann, A. Ohlmann, C. Flügel-Koch, S. Goswami, A. Cvekl, and E. R. Tamm, "Pax6 heterozygous eyes show defects in chamber angle differentiation that are associated with a wide spectrum of other anterior eye segment abnormalities," *Mechanisms of Development*, vol. 118, no. 1-2, pp. 3–17, 2002.

[16] D. T. Ramsey, S. L. Ewart, J. A. Render, C. S. Cook, and C. A. Latimer, "Congenital ocular abnormalities of Rocky Mountain Horses," *Veterinary Ophthalmology*, vol. 2, no. 1, pp. 47–59, 1999.

[17] S. L. Ewart, D. T. Ramsey, J. Xu, and D. Meyers, "The horse homolog of congenital aniridia conforms to codominant inheritance," *Journal of Heredity*, vol. 91, no. 2, pp. 93–98, 2000.

[18] J. Davis and J. Piatigorsky, "Overexpression of Pax6 in mouse cornea directly alters corneal epithelial cells: changes in immune function, vascularization, and differentiation," *Investigative Ophthalmology & Visual Science*, vol. 52, no. 7, pp. 4158–4168, 2011.

[19] A. Cvekl, Y. Yang, B. K. Chauhan, and K. Cveklova, "Regulation of gene expression by Pax6 in ocular cells: a case of tissue-preferred expression of crystallins in lens," *International Journal of Developmental Biology*, vol. 48, no. 8-9, pp. 829–844, 2004.

[20] F. Tremblay, S. K. Gupta, I. de Becker, D. L. Guernsey, and P. E. Neumann, "Effects of PAX6 mutations on retinal function: an electroretinographic study," *American Journal of Ophthalmology*, vol. 126, no. 2, pp. 211–218, 1998.

[21] W. H. Spencer and L. E. Zimmerman, "Conjunctiva," in *Ophthalmic Pathology: An Atlas and Textbook*, W. H. Spencer, Ed., vol. 1, pp. 109–228, WB Saunders, Philadelphia, Pa, USA, 3rd edition, 1985.

# 20

# Rattlesnake Envenomation in Three Dairy Goats

**Joseph Smith,**[1] **David Kovalik,**[2] **and Anita Varga**[3]

[1]*William R. Pritchard Veterinary Medical Teaching Hospital, University of California Davis, Davis, CA 95616, USA*
[2]*Union Veterinary Clinic, 609 2nd Street NE, Washington, DC 20002, USA*
[3]*Department of Medicine and Epidemiology, School of Veterinary Medicine, University of California, Davis, Tupper Hall, Davis, CA 95616, USA*

Correspondence should be addressed to Joseph Smith; joesmith@ucdavis.edu

Academic Editor: Luis Arroyo

Cases of rattlesnake envenomation in dairy goats are lacking. These cases present three dairy goats presented to a veterinary referral hospital for envenomation of Northern Pacific Rattlesnake (*Crotalus oreganus*). Treatments and clinical characteristics reported are similar to those for llamas, alpacas, and horses. These cases suggest that quick treatment in the event of a bite may have a more favorable clinical response. Existing rattlesnake bite scoring systems applicable to other species may be applicable to goats, and existing respiratory pathology may predispose goats to a less favorable outcome.

## 1. Introduction

To the author's knowledge this is the first reported case series of envenomation of dairy goats by the Northern Pacific Rattlesnake (*Crotalus oreganus*). Cases, treatment, and outcomes of rattlesnake envenomation have been reported for horses [1], llamas, and alpacas [2, 3] but veterinary literature is lacking in cases of rattlesnake envenomation in dairy goats. The following 3 cases, referred to the University of California-Davis William R. Pritchard Veterinary Medical Teaching Hospital (VMTH), between the years of 1994 and 2014, represent rattlesnake envenomation, where the rattlesnake was identified as the Northern Pacific Rattlesnake (*Crotalus oreganus*).

## 2. Case Selection

A retrospective search was done through the William R. Pritchard Veterinary Medical Teaching Hospital's record database (Veterinary Medical & Administrative Computer System, VMACs) for goat cases that were definitively diagnosed as rattlesnake envenomation. Search functions included a designation of caprine patients and then the term: "rattlesnake," "bite," "snakebite," "envenomation," and "snake." Records were then checked for the appearance of

a snakebite, and then either a witnessed bite or a witnessed account, by the owner, of a rattlesnake in close proximity to the snake near the time of envenomation. Cases that lacked a clear bite wound or some form of an eyewitness account of a rattlesnake were excluded.

## 3. Cases

Three cases fit the search criteria; all involved dairy goat breeds.

*3.1. Case 1.* A 3-year-old, female, open Toggenburg show doe presented to the VMTH after she was bitten on the left front leg shortly after the evening milking. This bite was witnessed by the owner and the snake was killed. The owner administered procaine penicillin (PPG) and flunixin meglumine. The affected limb was iced and the patient presented to the VMTH fewer than 2 hours after the bite occurred.

At presentation the doe was bright, alert, and responsive with a rectal temperature of 102.4 F (39.1°C), a slight tachycardia (96 beats/min; normal: 70–90) with a normal rhythm, and a mild tachypnea (56 breaths/min; normal: 15–30); mucus membranes were pink and moist. The left front leg was swollen from the distal aspect to the axillary region, with pitting edema observed. A bite was noted on the dorsal surface of fetlock. The owner noted the initial swelling had decreased after cooling the limb with ice. The remainder of the physical examination was within normal limits.

The doe was initially treated at the hospital with a maintenance rate of Lactated Ringer's Solution (2-3 mL/kg/hour), ampicillin (10 mg/kg IM, q 12 hours), methyl prednisolone (10 mg, IM, once), and flunixin meglumine (1.1 mg/kg SQ, q 12 hours). She was also treated with 10 mL of an equine origin antivenin IV (Crotalid). Hydrotherapy was utilized on the limb every 12 hours for 15 minutes.

On the second day of hospitalization the patient had normal temperature, pulse, and respiration values, and the leg was less swollen. Ampicillin, flunixin, LRS, and hydrotherapy were continued. The patient was walked several times during the day to improve lymphatic drainage with the hope of decreasing the swelling of the leg. Normal appetite, urinations, and defecation were noted, and the doe produced 50% as much milk as she did the day before the bite.

On the third day the patient showed continued improvement with reduced swelling on the proximal portion of the leg, but with edema still present on the fetlock. Milk production had also increased 0.45 kilograms from the previous day. Exercise and hydrotherapy were continued, and the patient was switched from ampicillin to ticarcillin and clavulanate due to limitations of pharmacy stock. Flunixin meglumine was discontinued at this time.

On the fourth day of hospitalization, the patient was discharged with instructions to administer sodium ceftiofur (2 mg/kg IM, q 12 hours) and PPG (22,000 IU/kg SQ, q 12 hours) for the next 8 days. Hydrotherapy was encouraged and the owner was instructed to observe the leg twice daily. The doe recovered uneventfully with no apparent complications after discharge. She went on to have a productive show career.

*3.2. Case 2.* A 10-month-old Alpine Doe was found recumbent by her owner with a swollen right front limb. Two puncture wounds were observed below the elbow, and severe swelling was noted on the right limb and ventral neck. She was administered procaine penicillin G (22,000 units/kg, IM), and flunixin meglumine (1.1 mg/kg, SC) by her owner and transported to the VMTH within two hours of discovery in the pasture.

On physical exam the doe was bright, alert, and responsive, with normal hydration and a weight of 50 kg. Her heart rate was within normal reference intervals, but she was tachypneic (50 breaths/minute), and her mucus membranes were pale with an increased capillary refill time (3 seconds). She was normothermic (102.7 F/39.3°C). Swelling was noted in the ventral neck area. The right forelimb was swollen, purple, and warm to the touch. Necrosis and sloughing of the skin were noted on the lateral aspect of the right forelimb. The swelling extended from carpus to shoulder and the patient was nonambulatory on the limb. Two puncture wounds were present below the elbow of this limb. The patient had normal pupillary light reflexes, menace responses, and no evidence of scleral injection. No stertor was observed, although frothing

saliva was noted. Normal rumen contractions and normal urinations were also noted during examination.

Upon arrival, a point-of-care chemistry analysis (iStat) revealed hyperglycemia (253 mg/dL; normal: 50–75), hypokalemia (2.7 mEq/L; normal: 3.5–6.7), increased bicarbonate (37 mEq/L: normal 24–28), hypocalcemia (0.81 mg/dL, ionized Ca; normal > 1.0), and hypoalbuminemia (2.4 g/dL; normal: 2.7–3.9). A urinalysis also revealed proteinuria (100–300; normal: negative to trace) and glucosuria (2000+; normal: negative). Packed cell volume was within normal ranges at 33% (normal 22–38) and total protein was decreased at 5.3 g/dL (normal 6.4–7.0). Radiographs revealed soft tissue swelling at the level of the radius and ulna with no evidence of fractures. A complete blood count (CBC) displayed a pronounced neutrophilia (13,341/$\mu$L; normal: 1,200–7,200) and thrombocytopenia (146,000/$\mu$L, normal: 300,000–600,000).

Treatment was initiated with the placement of an IV catheter and a 3 mL/kg bolus of polyionic fluids (Plasmalyte 148), followed by a maintenance rate of IV fluid therapy [2-3 mL/kg/hr; Plasmalyte 148 with 22 mL/L of calcium, phosphorous, magnesium, potassium solution (CMPK), and 40 mEq/L of potassium chloride (KCl) added]. The patient was also treated with a bolus of 2 liters of caprine plasma. Overnight the patient developed an acidosis (pH 7.172) and became obtunded. A repeat CBC showed a significant reduction in platelets (72,000/$\mu$L). The patient died the next day.

A necropsy was performed. The subcutaneous tissues and connective tissue planes between muscles along the ventral abdomen and left front leg were expanded by edema and hemorrhage. The muscles of the left front leg were dark red and edematous; these changes were more pronounced from the axillary to the carpal region. Aerobic and anaerobic cultures from the puncture wounds yielded no growth. Mild hemorrhage within the left ventricular free wall and diffuse petechiation of the omentum were noted. The lamina propria of the jejunum was infiltrated by inflammatory cells consisting mainly of lymphocytes, eosinophils, and lesser amounts of plasma cells. Tubular degeneration and glomerulonephritis were noted in the kidneys. Diffusely throughout the liver, hepatocytes were swollen and noted to contain one small, well-defined clear vacuole consistent with lipid accumulation. In sections of lymph node there was expansion of the cortex consistent with reactive follicular and parafollicular hyperplasia. The bone marrow was hyperplastic and was most likely a result of increased tissue demand for inflammatory cells.

The lungs were pink with multiple, dark red, ill-defined, atelectatic foci; all sections of lung floated in formalin. An infection with *Dictyocaulus filaria* was diagnosed based on the presence of inflammatory cell infiltrate within and around the bronchioles, profiles of parasites within the bronchiolar lumens, and thickening of the alveolar septa. The thickening of the alveolar septa and accumulation of blood and fibrin from the lungworm infection most likely led to impaired diffusion of oxygen and subsequent respiratory distress and contributed to the death of this animal along with envenomation.

*3.3. Case 3.* A 5-month-old La Mancha doe (18 kg) presented severe facial swelling of approximately 24-hour duration. The owners had noticed a rattlesnake in immediate proximity to the goat the day before presentation.

At presentation the doe was quiet, alert, and responsive with a rectal temperature of 103.5 F (39.7°C), and a heart rate of 150 beats/min (normal: 70–90), with a respiratory rate of 56 breaths/min (normal: 15–30). The doe's mucus membranes were not examined due to moderate to severe facial swelling and pain, but vulvar mucus membrane capillary refill time was noted to be 1-2 seconds (within normal limits). Two bites were observed, one on the right nostril and one on the nasal planum. Examination of the face was difficult due to severe bilateral swelling noted from the lips to the poll, and to the base of the neck. Some increased respiratory effort was noted on the initial examination. A moderate amount of edema was noted in the ventral neck region.

The doe was initially treated with dexamethasone sodium phosphate (1 mg/kg IV, once), flunixin meglumine (1 mg/kg IV, q 12 hours), sodium ceftiofur (1 mg/kg IM, q 12 hours), butorphanol (0.02 mg/kg IM, once), and given a subcutaneous (SC) bolus of 300 mL Normosol-R with KCl added (total K: 20 mEq/L). She was also vaccinated with a CDT toxoid (SC) and tetanus antitoxin (1500 units IM) was administered.

On the second day the doe's swelling had slightly reduced, and her activity continued to be reduced as she was observed in sternal recumbency for the majority of the day and observed standing only in the afternoon. She had a mild appetite when offered food. Therapy with sodium ceftiofur, flunixin meglumine, and 300 mL bolus fluids (q 4 hours, SC) was continued. PPG (22,000 IU/kg, IM q 12 hours) and morphine (0.25 mg/kg, IM, q 12 hours) were added to the therapeutic regimen.

On the third day more improvement was noted in behavior, although the swelling of the ventral neck persisted. A CBC and chemistry revealed normal CBC parameters in addition to hyperglycemia (98 mg/dL; normal: 50–75), hypoproteinemia (4.3 g/dL; normal: 6.4–7.0), hypokalemia (2.9 mEq/L; normal: 3.5–6.7), and hyponatremia (133 mEq/L; normal: 142–155 mEq/L). Furosemide (1 mg/kg, IV, once) was added to the treatment regimen and SC fluids were discontinued.

On the fourth day the doe was noted to be more physically active and playful. Her swelling had significantly decreased around the head and ventral neck. Her appetite appeared normal, but it was noted that in chewing she had a moderate amount of saliva oozing over her mandible. She had diminished facial nerve motor deficits on the left in the mandibular, auricular, and eyelid muscles. No strabismus or nystagmus was noted OU. The doe was discharged with instructions for continuing sodium ceftiofur (5 mg/kg, IM q 12 hours, for 3–5 additional days), and ophthalmic ointment (q 8 hours, until normal tear production was noted).

## 4. Discussion

While multiple studies outline the etiology and treatment of rattlesnake envenomation in llamas, alpacas [2, 3], horses [1], small animals, and humans [4], to the author's knowledge,

there are no studies or reports in current literature of this disease in dairy goats. Rattlesnakes are a common venomous snake species in North America and therefore represent a potential cause for veterinary emergencies. In the northern region of California, rattlesnake envenomation has been reported to have a 9% and 58% mortality rate in horses and new world camelids (NWC) [1, 2]. In this region of California the Northern Pacific Rattlesnake (*Crotalus oreganus*) is the most common rattlesnake species [1], and envenomation typically occurs seasonally, associated with the hibernation of rattlesnakes in the winter. All cases reported here occurred in June, within the rattlesnake season of May through August reported for NWC [2] and the rattlesnake season of March through October reported for horses [1] in the same region as these cases. Two bites occurred in lower limbs, and one occurred in the face. The most common sites of rattlesnake envenomation in NWC and horses have been reported as primarily the face and secondarily the legs [1–3]. Delays in treatment and increased mortality have been noted in horses [1], and it is noteworthy that the two goats in this case report that survived were promptly treated within hours, and the one that died experienced a several-day delay between the bite and treatment, which may be compounded by the concurrent lungworm infestation.

The clinical signs observed in horses and NWCs were noted in these goat cases. These patients displayed respiratory distress, fever, tachypnea, tachycardia [3], hyperthermia, and recumbency [2] as reported in NWC and horses [1]. Facial nerve paralysis has also been reported in horses with rattlesnake envenomation [1] and was noted in one of these cases. Cardiac arrhythmias have been reported in horses following envenomation, including atrial premature contractions, sinus pause, sinus tachycardia, sinus arrest, ventricular premature contractions, sinus arrhythmia, atrial fibrillation [10], as well as third-degree AV Block, among other arrhythmias [5]. No arrhythmias were noted in any of the goats, although no ECGs were performed.

In humans, the prophylactic treatment of rattlesnake bites with antibiotics is controversial with recommendations for [6] and against [7] this practice. A study of 15 rattlesnake venom cultures yielded 58 aerobic and 28 anaerobic bacteria, most commonly *Pseudomonas aeruginosa*, Proteus, coagulase negative staph, *Clostridium*, and *Bacteroides fragilis* [8]. Tissue edema and vascular compromise are common in rattlesnake envenomation and this environment predisposes a patient to infection. All 3 goats in this report were treated with antibiotics. However no uniform treatment was initiated due to different clinicians at time of admission. In 58 cases of rattlesnake envenomation of horses in California, almost all animals received antibiotics [1]. In a study of 12 NWC, all 10 that were alive on presentation were treated with procaine penicillin [2]. In the aforementioned Alpine doe case, culture of the wound at necropsy revealed no growth. This result could have been compromised by the antimicrobial therapy the doe received after envenomation, or could be because no bacteria was transmitted during the bite.

In all cases, anti-inflammatory therapy was used in the forms of flunixin meglumine, dexamethasone, dexamethasone sodium phosphate, or methyl prednisolone. Flunixin meglumine is a commonly used anti-inflammatory in both NWC [2, 3] and equine [1] envenomation. Corticosteroid treatment for snake envenomation has been linked to increased mortality in dogs [9], but in a recent NWC study, 10 of 27 rattlesnake envenomation cases were treated with corticosteroids (9 dexamethasone and 1 prednisolone) [3]. This study reported that treatment in NWC with either NSAIDS or corticosteroids was not associated with outcome. In a NWC study in the same geographical region as the 3 goat cases, 4 out of 5 animals that survived and 3 out of 7 that died were administered corticosteroids [2]. While controversial in its clinical application, dexamethasone may have a place in the treatment of rattlesnake envenomation as dexamethasone has been shown to inhibit Tumor Necrosis Factor- (TNF-) alpha synthesis [10]. Decreasing TNF-alpha could be beneficial in the management of systemic disease caused by rattlesnake envenomation in dairy goats.

All of these cases received some form of fluid therapy for medical management. Fluid therapies utilized were polyionic fluids and caprine plasma. Polyionic fluids utilized included Lactated Ringer's Solution, Normosol-R, and Plasmalyte 148. Potassium chloride and dextrose were utilized with fluid therapy. Two of the cases utilized furosemide in conjunction with fluid therapy.

Antivenin is another aspect of therapy for rattlesnake envenomation. Out of 58 snake-bitten horses, 9 received antivenin, and none of these animals died [1]. While that study was not designed to evaluate treatment regimens, the authors suggest that early administration of antivenin in the timeframe of envenomation could be beneficial for positive outcome in rattlesnake bites. Antivenin administration has also been associated with reduced morbidity in dogs and cats after snake envenomation [11]. This finding may be supported by the Toggenburg case (case 1). In the same area as the 3 cases in this study, as well as one NWC [2] and an equine [1] study, human snakebites were noted to have a 0% case fatality rate, but antivenin was much more heavily utilized, with some patients receiving as much as 12 vials [4].

In horses a rattlesnake-bite severity scoring (RBSS) system has been suggested [1]. This 12-point system scored patients in with 4 different variables (respiratory system, cardiovascular system, wound appearance, and hemostasis) with 0 being a normal presentation and 3 being a clinically severe presentation. It has been suggested that horses with a RBSS of 8 or higher should be watched especially carefully, as more aggressive treatment may be indicated for a patient with this score [1]. Enough clinical information is present to retrospectively apply this scoring system to the Alpine and the La Mancha cases. The Alpine case would have had a score of 8 with a score of 3 for the respiratory system (signs of respiratory distress), 0 for the cardiovascular system (no abnormalities), 3 for wound appearance (severe swelling spreading to the trunk), and a hemostasis score of 2 (platelets 72,000 $\mu$L on the second day). The La Mancha would have had a score of 6 with a score of 1 for the respiratory system (mild signs of respiratory distress evidenced by an increased respiratory effort), 2 for the cardiovascular system (a moderate tachycardia), 3 for wound appearance (severe swelling spreading to the neck), and a hemostasis score of

0 (no abnormalities). Using the previously recorded criteria, the Alpine case would have required more attention or more aggressive therapy. While more evaluations are needed, the outcome of the 2 cases (Case 2: score 8, mortality; Case 3: score 6, survival) suggests that the RBSS system may potentially be applicable to dairy goats.

Limitations of this report include its retrospective nature. Multiple clinicians and students were involved over an extended time frame. As such, cases were not worked up in an identical manner. While one of the bites was directly witnessed, 2 were not, and as such diagnosis of envenomation was based on proximity to a snake on discovery, recent observation of snakes on the premises, and appearance of bite wounds. The small sample size is also a limitation with this study. Long term follow-up (beyond 1 year) was only available for one goat in this study.

## 5. Conclusions

In conclusion, we report a case series of rattlesnake envenomation in dairy goats, which provides evidence of similar pathophysiology and treatment for rattlesnake envenomation in dairy goats as described for other large animal species. Faster implementation of treatment with respect to the timing of the bite may lead to a more positive treatment response. Similarly, the pathologic changes from coinfection with lungworms, such as Dictyocaulus filaria, may predispose a goat to a lesser prognosis in the case of rattlesnake envenomation. While this study was limited to three cases, more research is needed with respect to envenomation from different species of rattlesnake and therapy utilized to manage a snakebite, as well as the application of a bite scoring system to goats. These case descriptions provide basic information about rattlesnake envenomation that may be useful in managing cases of rattlesnake envenomation in dairy goats.

## Conflict of Interests

The authors declare that there is no conflict of interests regarding the publication of this paper.

## References

[1] C. Langdon Fielding, N. Pusterla, K. G. Magdesian, J. C. Higgins, and C. A. Meier, "Rattlesnake envenomation in horses: 58 cases (1992–2009)," Journal of the American Veterinary Medical Association, vol. 238, no. 5, pp. 631–635, 2011.

[2] S. Dykgraaf, N. Pusterla, and L. M. van Hoogmoed, "Rattlesnake envenomation in 12 New World camelids," Journal of Veterinary Internal Medicine, vol. 20, no. 4, pp. 998–1002, 2006.

[3] J. M. Sonis, E. S. Hackett, R. J. Callan, T. N. Holt, and T. B. Hackett, "Prairie rattlesnake envenomation in 27 new world camelids," Journal of Veterinary Internal Medicine, vol. 27, no. 5, pp. 1238–1241, 2013.

[4] A. N. Butner, "Rattlesnake bites in Northern California," The Western Journal of Medicine, vol. 139, no. 2, pp. 179–183, 1983.

[5] J. B. Lawler, M. A. Frye, M. M. Bera, E. J. Ehrhart, and J. M. Bright, "Third-degree atrioventricular block in a horse

secondary to rattlesnake envenomation," *Journal of Veterinary Internal Medicine*, vol. 22, no. 2, pp. 486–490, 2008.

[6] K. R. Kerrigan, "Bacteriology of snakebite abscess," *Tropical Doctor*, vol. 22, no. 4, pp. 158–160, 1992.

[7] R. S. Blaylock, "Antibiotic use and infection in snakebite victims," *South African Medical Journal*, vol. 89, no. 8, pp. 874–876, 1999.

[8] E. J. C. Goldstein, D. M. Citron, H. Gonzalez, F. E. Russell, and S. M. Finegold, "Bacteriology of rattlesnake venom and implications for therapy," *The Journal of Infectious Diseases*, vol. 140, no. 5, pp. 818–821, 1979.

[9] F. E. Russell and J. A. Emery, "Effects of corticosteroids on lethality of *Ancistrodon contortrix* venon," *The American Journal of the Medical Sciences*, vol. 241, pp. 507–511, 1961.

[10] L. L. Gilliam, T. C. Holbrook, C. L. Ownby et al., "Cardiotoxicity, Inflammation, and Immune Response after Rattlesnake Envenomation in the Horse," *Journal of Veterinary Internal Medicine*, vol. 26, no. 6, pp. 1457–1463, 2012.

[11] M. L. Pérez, K. Fox, and M. Schaer, "A retrospective evaluation of coral snake envenomation in dogs and cats: 20 cases (1996–2011)," *Journal of Veterinary Emergency and Critical Care*, vol. 22, no. 6, pp. 682–689, 2012.

# 21

# Peritoneal Effusion in a Dog due to *Babesia gibsoni* Infection

**Suresh Gonde,**[1] **Sushma Chhabra,**[1,2] **L. D. Singla,**[1] **and B. K. Bansal**[1]

[1]*College of Veterinary Science, Guru Angad Dev Veterinary and Animal Sciences University, Ludhiana, Punjab 141004, India*
[2]*Department of Veterinary Medicine, College of Veterinary Science, Guru Angad Dev Veterinary and Animal Sciences University, Ludhiana, Punjab 141004, India*

Correspondence should be addressed to Sushma Chhabra; chhabrasushma@rediffmail.com

Academic Editor: Paola Roccabianca

A five-year-old male Labrador was presented to Teaching Veterinary Clinics of GADVASU with a primary complaint of distended abdomen, fever, and anorexia. The dog was found to be dull with elevated rectal temperature (104°F), heart rate (148 per minute), and respiration rate (58 per minute). Blood smear examination and PCR assay revealed that dog was positive for *Babesia gibsoni*. Elevated bilirubin, alanine amino transferase (ALT), alkaline phosphatase (ALP), creatinine, blood urea nitrogen (BUN), total leucocyte count, hypoalbuminaemia, and hypoproteinaemia were haematobiochemical alterations. Radiography and ultrasonography showed ground glass appearance and anechoic area of abdomen, respectively.

## 1. Introduction

Canine babesiosis is one of the most important life-threatening tick borne haemoprotozoan diseases of dogs caused by intraerythrocytic protozoan parasites of the genus *Babesia* which are reported worldwide and in various parts of India including Punjab state [1, 2]. The variable prevalence of both *B. canis* and *B. gibsoni* has been observed in India (0.66 to 21.7%) and in Ludhiana the prevalence was recorded as 5.26 per cent [3]. The pathogenesis of canine babesiosis varies in different regions [4], possibly due to variation in the pathogenicity of different strains of *Babesia* species in various ecological conditions [5]. The severity of babesiosis is related to the extent of parasite replication in the host's red blood cells with subsequent cell lysis. A wide variety of clinical signs like anorexia, lethargy, icterus, vomition, and marked loss of body condition have been observed [6, 7] along with variable clinicopathologic abnormalities including haemoglobinuria, hypoglycemia, acid-base disturbances, azotemia, and elevations in the levels of liver enzymes [8]. Further, *B. gibsoni* causes regenerative hemolytic anemia and thrombocytopenia [9]. Spherocytosis and positive direct Coombs' test results suggest an immunomediate component. Thrombocytopenia is a frequent finding. In the present communication we describe the clinico-haematobiochemical, radiographic,

and ultrasonographic observations in a very rare case of peritoneal effusion due to the pathogenic effect of *Babesia gibsoni* infection.

## 2. Case Description

A five-year-old male Labrador dog was presented to the Veterinary Teaching Hospital of Guru Angad Dev Veterinary and Animal Sciences University, Ludhiana, July, 2013, with abdominal distension and persistent anorexia for the last two days. The dog had shown poor body condition. During the physical examination, the dog was pyretic (104°F), with heart rate of 148 beats per minute and a respiration rate of 58 breaths per minute. Mucous membranes were pale. Ticks were removed from the dog and were identified as *Rhipicephalus sanguineus*.

Blood samples were submitted for hematologic and serum biochemical analysis.

*2.1. Hematologic and Biochemical Analysis.* Hematologic and biochemical analysis revealed moderate to severe anaemia with elevated bilirubin, alanine amino transferase (ALT), alkaline phosphatase (ALP), creatinine, blood urea nitrogen (BUN), total leucocyte count, hypoalbuminaemia, and hypoproteinaemia were haematobiochemical alterations (Table 1).

TABLE 1: Haematobiochemical parameters in the dog infected with *Babesia gibsoni*.

| Parameters | Reference range[*] | Infected dog |
|---|---|---|
| Hb (g/dL) | 12–18 | 6 |
| TLC ($10^3/\mu L$) | 6–17 | 16 |
| TEC ($10^6/\mu L$) | 5.5–8.5 | 3.1 |
| PCV (%) | 35–55 | 18.4 |
| MCV (fL) | 60–70 | 59.4 |
| MCH (pg) | 19.5–24.5 | 19.4 |
| MCHC (g/dL) | 30–36 | 32.6 |
| Platelet ($10^5/\mu L$) | 2–9 | 1.58 |
| Neutrophils (%) | 60–70 | 72 |
| Lymphocytes (%) | 12–30 | 26 |
| Eosinophils (%) | 2–10 | 02 |
| Albumin (g/dL) | 2.6–4 | 1 |
| Total protein (g/dL) | 5.5–7.5 | 3.2 |
| Total bilirubin (mg/dL) | 0.1–0.6 | 1.8 |
| ALT (U/L) | 8.2–57 | 313 |
| ALKP (U/L) | 10.6–101 | 563 |
| BUN (mg/dL) | 8.8–26 | 30 |
| Creatinine (mg/dL) | 0.5–1.6 | 1.2 |
| Blood glucose (mg/dL) | 62–108 | 104 |

[*]Kahn et al. [15].

Chronic hepatic insufficiency in case of babesiosis could lead to hypoalbuminaemia [10]. Haematological parameters suggested that the dog might have blood parasites or other relevant infectious diseases. Pathogenesis of anemia appears to involve nonhemolytic and hemolytic mechanisms. Hemolysis may involve proteases produced by the invading parasite, an immune reaction to parasitized cells, and/or oxidative damage to erythrocytes. MCV, MCH, and MCHC values were just at borderline of the normal range (Table 1) indicating that anemia was not due to iron deficiency but MCV and MCHC frequently fail to correctly differentiate the various patterns of anemia [9]. The most common abnormality was thrombocytopenia. The reason for thrombocytopenia in babesiosis could be due to platelet sequestration in the spleen or immune mediated platelet destruction and development of disseminated intravascular coagulation [11].

*2.2. Parasitological Examination.* So to distinguish between these possibilities, the microscopic examination of Giemsa-stained thin blood smears prepared from the ear margin was carried out [12] under oil immersion (100x) lens. Examination revealed the presence of ring shaped, oval, parachute, and comma-like organisms, about 1–3 $\mu$m in diameter in the erythrocytes (Figure 1). On the basis of the size of the intracellular parasites in this case, the possibility that the dog has been infected with small *Babesia* spp., especially with *B. gibsoni*, was considered. The degree of parasitemia, calculated as the percentage of infected red blood cells by counting 1000 red blood cells, was 10.5%. Ticks present on

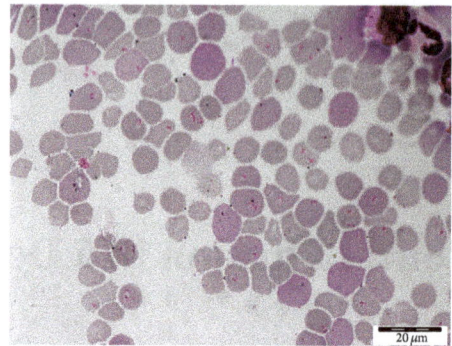

FIGURE 1: Photomicrograph of Giemsa-stained thin blood smear of the dog showing regenerative anemia and small circular shaped trophozoites of *Babesia gibsoni* in erythrocytes ×100.

the dog were identified as *Rhipicephalus sanguineus*. The fact that *B. gibsoni* cannot be distinguished from other canine small babesial isolates by microscopy prompted us to perform PCR for final diagnosis using *B. gibsoni* specific primer [13].

*2.3. DNA Extraction.* DNA from whole blood (300 $\mu$L) was extracted using the DNA purification kit (QIAGEN, GmbH, Germany) according to the manufacturer's instructions.

A primer set including forward primer (Gib599 F): 5′CTCGGCTACTTGCCTTGTC3′ and reverse primer (Gib1270R): 5′GCCGAAACTGAAATAACGGC3′ was used to amplify a 671 bp fragment of the 18 S rRNA gene region specific to *B. gibsoni* [13]. The PCR mix consisted of 1X molar concentration of 12.5 $\mu$L master mix (1X QIAGEN PCR buffer, 2.5 units of Taq DNA polymerase, 200 $\mu$M of each dNTP, and 1.5 mM $MgCl_2$), 1.5 $\mu$L of 10 pmol each of the respective primers, and 5 $\mu$L of template as DNA source.

After an initial denaturation at 95°C for 5 min, 30 cycles of denaturation (94°C for 45 sec), annealing (57°C for 1 min), and extension (72°C for 1 min) were conducted and the final extension was performed at 72°C for 8 min. A negative sample control (canine blood DNA only) and a negative DNA control (Milli-Q water in a substitute of DNA) were included in the PCR reaction. The PCR products were run on 1.5% agarose gel and stained with ethidium bromide. The size of the amplified PCR product was 671 bp (Figure 2).

*2.4. Peritoneal Fluid Analysis.* Based on abdominal distension ascites was suspected. A peritoneal tab was performed and 2 mL of clear peritoneal fluid was collected. Peritoneal fluid typically was examined for color, turbidity, total protein, and albumin concentration. The fluid was transparent and clear. Total protein and albumin were 0.4 g/dL and 0.2 g/dL, respectively, indicating hypoproteinaemia (0.4 g/dL) and hypoalbuminaemia (0.2 g/dL).

*2.5. Radiography and Ultrasonography.* Radiography and ultrasonography showed ground glass appearance and anechoic area of the abdomen, respectively (Figures 3 and 4). The

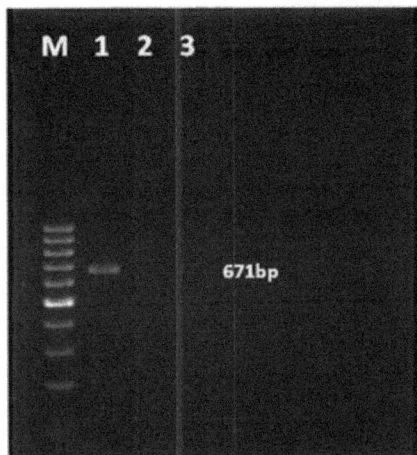

FIGURE 2: *Babesia gibsoni* species specific PCR assay. Lane M: GeneRuler 100 bp Ladder; lane 1: positive sample; lane 2: negative sample control; lane 3: negative DNA control.

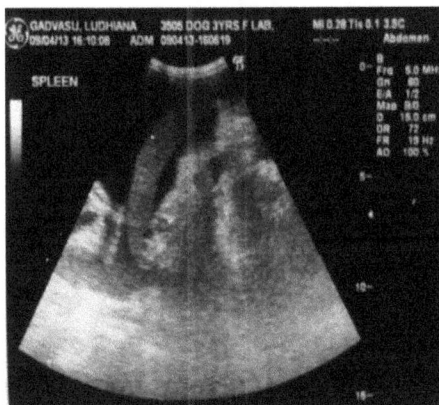

FIGURE 3: USG of abdomen showing anechoic area indicating free flowing fluid in abdomen.

case was thus confirmed as being ascites. Though most common clinical signs of babesiosis include anorexia, lethargy, recurrent fever, pale mucus membrane, and emesis [14], our findings revealed that it is important not to neglect babesiosis in differential diagnosis of ascites. Dogs with ascites should be subjected to classical parasitological or molecular diagnosis to rule out babesiosis. *Babesia* organisms infect the erythrocytes of dogs, leading to hemolytic anemia. Infection with *B. gibsoni* is known to cause more severe clinical signs than infection with large *Babesia* spp. and may result in multiple organ dysfunction syndromes [13]. As the dog was severely anaemic with other severe abnormalities in parameters related to vital organs it died within two days of treatment.

## 3. Conclusion

To the best of our knowledge, this is the first case report of peritoneal effusion in a dog associated with *B. gibsoni* infection diagnosed by microscopic examination and polymerase

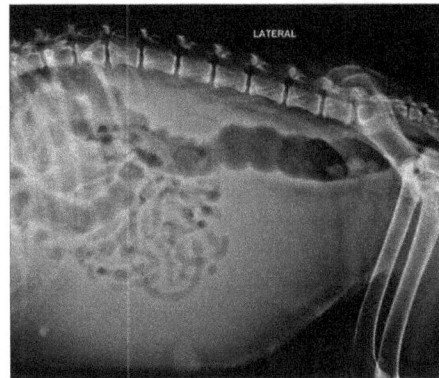

FIGURE 4: X-ray of abdomen showing ground glass appearance indicating free fluid in abdominal cavity.

chain reaction (PCR) in combination with peritoneal fluid analysis, radiography, and ultrasonography.

## Conflict of Interests

The authors declare that there is no conflict of interests regarding the publication of this paper.

## References

[1] S. M. E. Mohamed, L. D. Singla, A. A. M. Radya, and S. K. Uppal, "Morphometric variations in piroplasms of Babesia canis from naturally infected dogs from Punjab (India)," *Applied Biological Research*, vol. 14, pp. 207–210, 2012.

[2] N. Singla, L. D. Singla, and P. Kaur, "Babesiosis," in *Zoonosis: Parasitic and Mycotic Diseases*, S. R. Garg, Ed., pp. 207–223, Daya, New Delhi, India, 2014.

[3] S. M. E. Mohamed, *Clinico-diagnostic studies on vector transmitted haemoprotozoan diseases in dogs [M.S. thesis]*, Guru Angad Dev Veterinary and Animal Sciences University, Ludhiana, India, 2010.

[4] N. Saud and G. G. Hazarika, "Studies on the incidence and biochemical changes of Babesia infection in dogs," *Indian Veterinary Journal*, vol. 77, no. 11, pp. 944–947, 2000.

[5] R. E. Purnell, "Babesiosis in various hosts," in *Babesiosis*, M. Ristic and J. P. Kreier, Eds., pp. 25–63, Academic Press, New York, NY, USA, 1981.

[6] S. J. Ettinger and E. C. Feldman, *Text Book of Veterinary Internal Medicine*, pp. 643-644, W.B. Saunders Company, St. Louis, Mo, USA, 6th edition, 2005.

[7] H. J. Vial and A. Gorenflot, "Chemotherapy against babesiosis," *Veterinary Parasitology*, vol. 138, no. 1-2, pp. 147–160, 2006.

[8] P. J. Irwin, "Canine babesiosis," *Veterinary Clinics of North America: Small Animal Practice*, vol. 40, no. 6, pp. 1141–1156, 2010.

[9] D. J. Weiss and K. J. Wardrop, *Schalm's Veterinary Hematology*, Blackwell, Ames, Iowa , USA, 6th edition, 2010.

[10] L. M. Cornelius, "Abnormalities of the standard biochemical profile," in *Small Animal Medical Diadnosis*, M. D. Lorenza and L. M. Cornelius, Eds., pp. 539–591, 1987.

[11] A. L. Boozer and D. K. Macintire, "Canine babesiosis," *Veterinary Clinics of North America: Small Animal Practice*, vol. 33, no. 4, pp. 885–904, 2003.

[12] N. C. Jain, *Schalm's Veterinary Hematology*, Lea and Febiger, Philadelphia, Pa, USA, 4th edition, 1986.

[13] T. Miyama, Y. Sakata, Y. Shimada et al., "Epidemiological Survey of Babesia gibsoni infection in dogs in eastern Japan," *Journal of Veterinary Medical Science*, vol. 67, no. 5, pp. 467–471, 2005.

[14] D. R. Wadhwa, B. Pal, R. K. Mandial, A. Kumar, and R. K. Agnihotri, "Clinical, haemato-biochemical and therapeutic studies on canine babesiosis in Kangra Valley of Himachal Pradesh," *Journal of Veterinary Parasitology*, vol. 25, no. 1, pp. 39–41, 2011.

[15] C. M. Kahn, S. Line, and S. E. Aiello, *Reference Guide Table 6 and 7 in Merck Manual*, Merck & Co., White Housestation, NJ, USA, 9th edition, 2005.

# 22

# Fluoroscopic-Assisted Olecranon Fracture Repair in Three Dogs

**Stephen C. Jones,**[1,2] **Daniel D. Lewis,**[1] **and Matthew D. Winter**[1]

[1]*Department of Small Animal Clinical Sciences, College of Veterinary Medicine, University of Florida, Gainesville, FL 32610, USA*
[2]*Department of Veterinary Clinical Sciences, College of Veterinary Medicine, The Ohio State University, 601 Vernon L. Tharp Street, Columbus, OH 43210, USA*

Correspondence should be addressed to Stephen C. Jones; jones.5609@osu.edu

Academic Editor: Lysimachos G. Papazoglou

Olecranon fractures in dogs are often both comminuted and intra-articular. Anatomic reduction and stable internal fixation are thus paramount to achieving primary bone healing and mitigating the development of posttraumatic osteoarthritis. Intraoperative fluoroscopy can be useful to confirm accurate fracture reduction and facilitate precise implant placement, potentially reducing the surgical exposure required and additional trauma. Despite widespread use in human surgery, reports of fluoroscopic-assisted fracture repair in dogs are limited. Presented here are three dogs in which intraoperative fluoroscopy was used to facilitate accurate olecranon fracture reduction and implant positioning. The olecranon fractures appeared to heal by primary bone union, although the anconeal process failed to obtain osseous union in one dog. Despite the development of mild-to-moderate osteoarthritis in all three dogs, and the nonunion of the anconeal process in one dog, the clinical outcome was considered successful with all dogs subjectively free of lameness at long-term follow-up evaluation. Intraoperative fluoroscopy was found to be a useful modality during fracture reduction and implant placement in dogs with olecranon fractures.

## 1. Introduction

The olecranon is the most proximal segment of the ulna and is comprised of the olecranon tuber, the anconeal process, and the proximal portion of the trochlear notch [1]. The triceps brachii muscle group inserts on the olecranon which functions as a lever arm to mediate elbow extension and enable weight-bearing [1].

The majority of antebrachial fractures in dogs involve the radial and ulnar diaphyses [2] with surgical intervention often directed towards stabilization of the radius alone [3]. Isolated fractures of the olecranon are rare [2]. Olecranon fractures are often comminuted and commonly involve the articular surface of the trochlear notch [4]. Owing to the large tensile force exerted by the triceps brachii muscles and the frequent articular involvement, anatomic reduction and stable internal fixation of olecranon fractures are required to promote primary bone healing, mitigate the development of posttraumatic osteoarthritis, and optimize the probability of a return to prefracture limb function.

Intraoperative fluoroscopy is routinely used during human fracture repair [5–9] and is slowly being integrated in small animal orthopedics [10–14]. The use of fluoroscopy allows surgeons to accurately assess fracture reduction while facilitating and confirming proper implant placement. Intraoperative fluoroscopy helps to reduce additional surgical trauma, often allowing surgery to be done in a minimally invasive fashion [15]. This report describes the use of intraoperative fluoroscopy to facilitate the anatomic reduction and stabilization of intra-articular olecranon fractures in three dogs.

## 2. Case 1

A 1-year-old spayed female Bloodhound, weighing 29 kg, presented to the University of Florida Small Animal Hospital (UF SAH) in September 2008 for evaluation of a non-weight-bearing lameness of the left thoracic limb, which was sustained in a road traffic accident. Radiographic examination

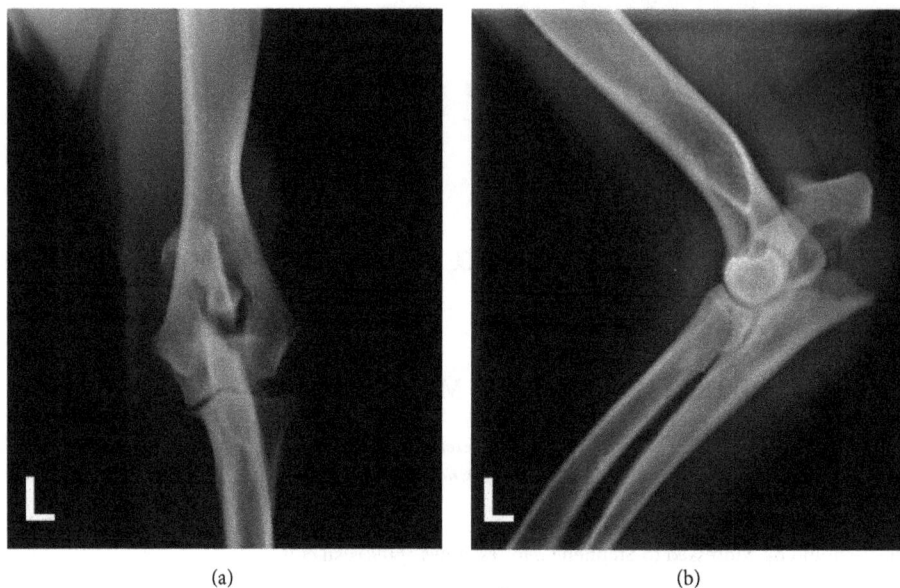

(a)                                                                                      (b)

FIGURE 1: Preoperative radiographs of dog 1. (a) Craniocaudal and (b) mediolateral radiographs showing a closed mildly comminuted short oblique fracture of the left olecranon. The fracture is seen extending into the articular margin of the ulnar trochlear notch, resulting in a proximally displaced olecranon tuber and anconeal process segment. There is a large osseous defect with adjacent mineral fragments in the lateral aspect of the humeral condyle. A linear, incomplete fissure is also seen in the proximal articular margin of the radial head.

revealed a closed, short oblique, mildly comminuted olecranon fracture extending in a caudoproximal-to-craniodistal orientation, terminating in the caudal articular margin of the ulnar trochlear notch. A linear, incomplete fissure was also detected in the proximal articular margin of the radial head. In the articular margin of the humeral capitulum, there was also a large lucent defect, with an associated displaced osteochondral fragment (Figure 1).

The dog was placed in dorsal recumbency, adjacent to the left edge of the table to facilitate fluoroscopic image acquisition. Fracture repair was accomplished via open reduction using a lateral approach [16]. The proximal olecranon fracture segment was visualized, directly reduced, and maintained in reduction with Vulsellum forceps (Schroeder Uterine Vulsellum Forceps, KNY-Scheerer Corporation of America, New York, NY). Intraoperative fluoroscopy (Siremobil Compact Fluoroscope, Siemens, Iselin, NJ) was used to assess the accuracy of reduction and implant placement. The fluoroscopic C-arm was covered with a disposable sterile plastic sleeve to prevent contamination of the surgical field. The C-arm was brought in from a caudal-to-cranial direction, positioning the elbow adjacent to the image intensifier; a member of the surgical team elevated the limb to prevent interference of the C-arm from the chest wall. Mediolaterally directed fluoroscopic images facilitated appropriate placement of an interfragmentary 1.1 mm Kirschner wire, which was placed perpendicular to the fracture line, in a caudodistal-to-cranioproximal direction. A 1.6 mm antirotational Kirschner wire was also placed in a similar orientation, under fluoroscopic guidance, immediately distal to the proximal wire. The proximal Kirschner wire functioned as a guide wire for the placement of a 3.5 mm lag screw. A 3.5 mm cannulated drill bit (Arthrex, Naples, FL, USA) was used to overdrill the cisfracture

segment; a drill sleeve was inserted into the hole over the Kirschner wire and a 2.5 mm cannulated drill bit (Arthrex, Naples, FL, USA) was used to drill through the transsegment. After tapping threads in the transsegment, a 3.5 mm cortical screw was placed in lag fashion. An eight-hole 2.7 mm String-of-Pearls locking plate (Orthomed, Vero Beach, FL, USA) was contoured and applied to the lateral surface of the ulna, with two bicortical screws engaging the proximal ulnar segment and four bicortical screws engaging the distal ulnar segment. The radial head fissure fracture was directly visualized via an approach between the lateral digital extensor and the extensor carpi ulnaris muscles; this fracture was stabilized using a 1.2/1.5 mm self-compressing pin (Orthofix Magic Pin, McKinney, TX, USA) and washer, and a 0.9 mm Kirschner wire, both inserted laterally to medially. Similarly, the humeral condylar fracture was stabilized with two diverging 0.9 mm Kirschner wires (Figure 2).

Recovery from surgery was uneventful. The dog was discharged from the hospital 36 hours after surgery; tramadol was administered (2 mg/kg PO every 8 hrs) for 14 days. A carpal flexion bandage was placed to discourage weight-bearing. This bandage was maintained for 4 weeks, with weekly evaluations and bandage changes. Passive range-of-motion exercises for the shoulder and elbow were conducted three times daily by the owner, for the first 6 weeks postoperatively. Radiographic examination of the fractures was conducted at 25, 53, and 80 days postoperatively. The fractures had obtained radiographic union by 80 days. There were no complications associated with the implants, but there was mild progression of periarticular new bone formation on the proximal aspect of the olecranon and the cranioproximal aspect of the radial head.

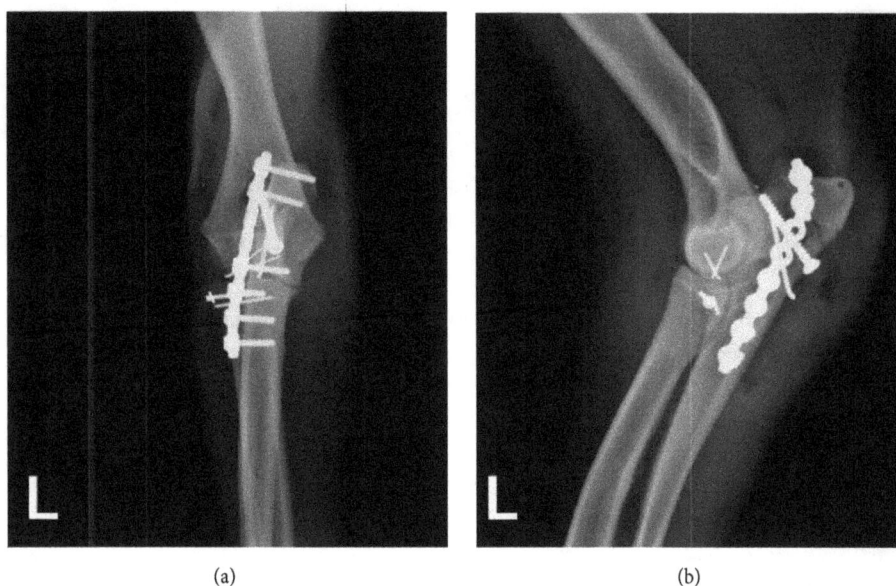

(a)                                                    (b)

FIGURE 2: Immediate postoperative craniocaudal (a) and lateral (b) radiographs of the left elbow of dog 1. A screw and a Kirschner wire have been placed across the olecranon fracture in a caudocranial direction. This fixation is supported by an eight-hole String-of-Pearls locking plate applied to the lateral olecranon and proximal ulnar diaphysis. Two divergent Kirschner wires are seen stabilizing the osseous fragment in the humeral capitulum. The self-compressing pin and Kirschner wire are seen stabilizing the fissure fracture of the proximal radius.

The owner was solicited to return the dog to the UF SAH for long-term evaluation, 5 years after surgery. There was no appreciable lameness or gait abnormality. The dog was comfortable on manipulation of the left elbow; small periarticular osteophytes were palpable, but the elbow was not effused. Range of motion of the left elbow (flexion = 25°, extension = 165°) was very similar to the right elbow (flexion = 20°, extension = 164°). Muscle atrophy was not evident with left brachial circumference (25.8 cm) being nearly identical to the right brachial circumference (25.9 cm). Gait was objectively evaluated by walking the dog on a force plate (Advanced Mechanical Technology Inc., Newton, MA, USA) and a pressure walkway (GAIT4Dog Walkway, Sparta, NJ, USA). Three successful trials were included for analysis. The mean peak vertical force (PVF) was slightly greater in the left (100.5 N/N) compared with the right (94.4 N/N) thoracic limb. The mean vertical impulse of the left (16.8 N-sec/N) and right (15.9 N-sec/N) thoracic limbs was also similar. The percentage of the gait cycle spent in the stance phase was again very similar between the left (59.8%) and right (61.3%) thoracic limbs. Radiographs obtained at this long-term evaluation revealed that the position of the implants was unchanged, with moderate osteophyte production and subchondral bone sclerosis of the ulnar trochlear notch, consistent with progression of elbow degenerative joint disease (Figure 3).

## 3. Case 2

A 7-year-old spayed female English Mastiff, weighing 71 kg, was examined at the UF SAH in July 2007 for left thoracic and left pelvic limb injuries, which were sustained in a road traffic accident. Radiographic examination of the left elbow revealed a closed, sagittally orientated, irregular olecranon fracture

that extended from the proximal margin of the olecranon distally through the caudal articular margin of the ulnar trochlear notch, resulting in a cranially displaced segment that included the anconeal process. There was a 1.5 cm fusiform osseous fragment located adjacent to the lateral humeral epicondyle, as well as moderate soft tissue swelling present surrounding the elbow, with displacement of the periarticular fat planes, suggestive of joint effusion (Figure 4). A concurrent left tarsometatarsal fracture-luxation was found when the left pes was radiographed.

The olecranon fracture was exposed using a lateral approach [16]. The fracture was reduced directly and reduction was maintained with point-to-point reduction forceps; reduction was assessed fluoroscopically and adjusted until there was anatomic apposition at the articular margins. Under fluoroscopic guidance (Siremobil Compact Fluoroscope, Siemens, Iselin, NJ) in a manner similar to that done in dog 1, a 1.1 mm interfragmentary Kirschner wire was placed across the fracture line, in a caudodistal-to-cranioproximal direction, purchasing the anconeal process proximally and cranially. An additional 1.1 mm Kirschner wire was then placed in the same orientation, approximately 13 mm proximally to the first wire. The distal Kirschner wire was used to guide accurate placement of a screw perpendicular to the fracture line. Using a 3.5 mm cannulated drill bit (Arthrex, Naples, FL, USA) placed over the guide wire, the cisfracture segment was overdrilled; a drill sleeve was placed in the hole over the wire, and the transsegment was drilled using a 2.5 mm cannulated drill bit (Arthrex, Naples, FL, USA). After tapping threads in the transsegment, a 3.5 mm cortical screw with an associated washer was placed in lag fashion. In similar fashion, a second 3.5 mm cortical screw and washer was placed in lag fashion using the proximally placed Kirschner

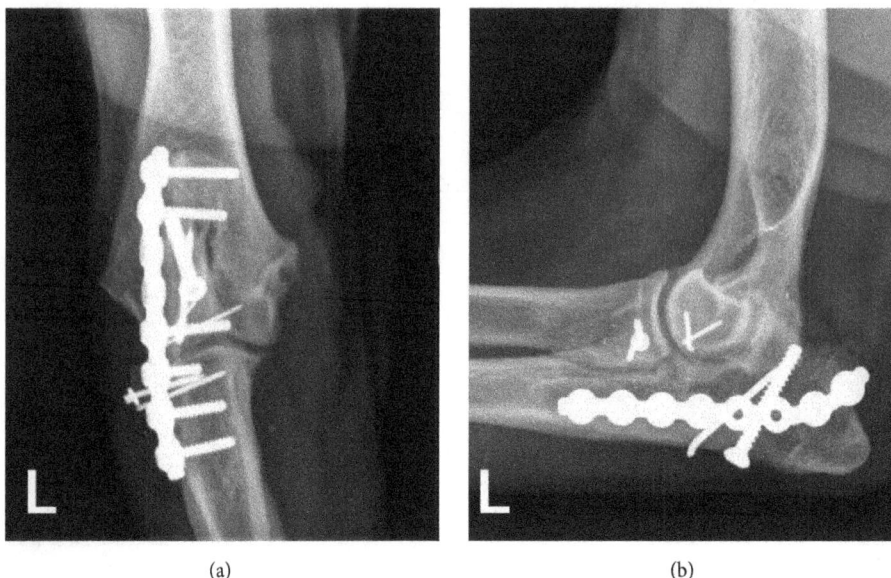

(a)                                              (b)

FIGURE 3: Radiographs of the left elbow of dog 1 obtained 5 years postoperatively. Craniocaudal (a) and mediolateral (b) radiographs show unchanged implants with modeling at the proximal margin of the String-of-Pearls plate. Moderate osteophyte production is present at the cranial margin of the humeroradial joint and the medial aspect of the humeroulnar joint and along the proximal margin of the anconeal process. Also note the mild sclerosis of the ulnar trochlear notch, with evidence of joint space narrowing. These findings are compatible with progressive degenerative joint disease.

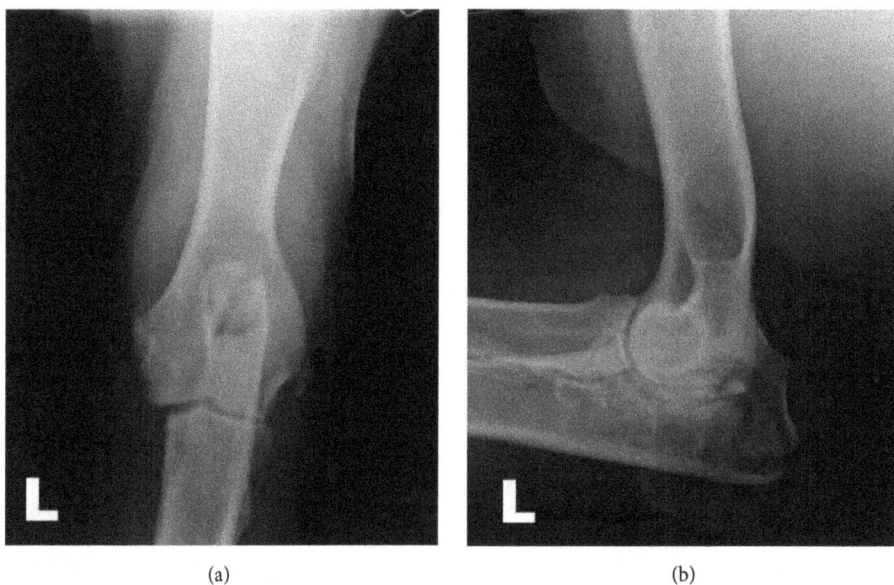

(a)                                              (b)

FIGURE 4: Craniocaudal (a) and mediolateral (b) radiographs of the left elbow of dog 2 obtained preoperatively. A sagittally oriented, irregular fracture was seen extending from the caudoproximal aspect of the olecranon cranially through the caudal articular margin of the ulnar trochlear notch. This resulted in displacement of a proximal ulnar segment that included the olecranon and anconeal process. Note the fusiform osseous fragment associated with the lateral humeral epicondyle, best seen on the craniocaudal view. There is a small osteophyte located on the medial coronoid process consistent with mild preexisting osteoarthritis.

wire to guide the process. Three 2.7 mm positional screws with washers were then placed through the fracture in a medial-to-lateral direction for additional fracture stabilization (Figure 5). A partial tarsal arthrodesis was performed using a laterally applied 13-hole 3.5 mm dynamic compression plate to stabilize the left pes.

The dog was reevaluated 45 days postoperatively. There was no appreciable lameness or gait abnormality. The dog was comfortable on manipulation of the left elbow; small periarticular osteophytes were palpable, but the elbow was not effused. A small hygroma had developed over the caudal aspect of the olecranon; no discomfort was elicited

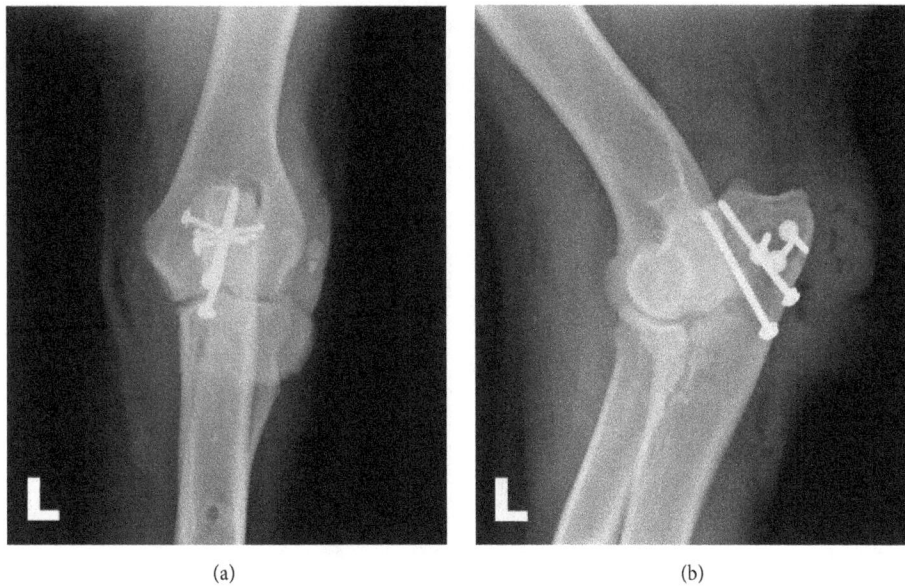

(a)　　　　　　　　　　　　(b)

FIGURE 5: Craniocaudal (a) and mediolateral (b) radiographs of the left elbow of dog 2 obtained immediately postoperatively. Two interfragmentary 3.5 mm screws with associated washers were placed in a caudodistal-to-cranioproximal orientation, purchasing the anconeal process proximally. Three additional interfragmentary 2.7 mm screws with associated washers were placed in a medial-to-lateral orientation.

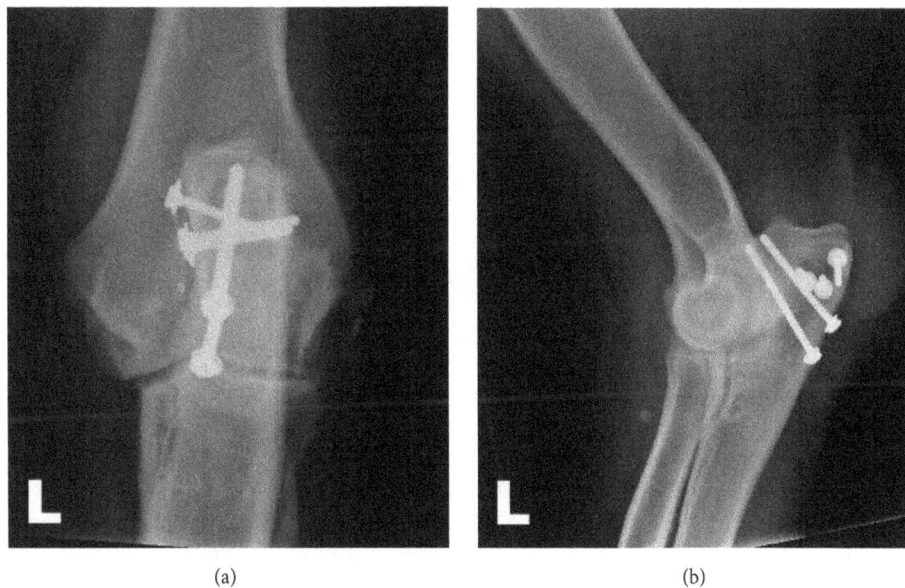

(a)　　　　　　　　　　　　(b)

FIGURE 6: Craniocaudal (a) and mediolateral (b) radiographs of the left elbow of dog 2 obtained 45 days postoperatively. The margins of the previously described sagittally orientated fracture line are now ill-defined, compatible with healing. Note the osteophyte production at the medial aspect of the humeroulnar joint and cranially at the level of the radial head. The hygroma is visible as soft tissue swelling, being caudal to the olecranon.

on palpation. Radiographically all implants remained stable (Figure 6). Only small regions of the initial fracture remained visible; however, the fracture had ill-defined margins and associated sclerosis, compatible with healing. Narrowing of the humeroulnar articulation was present, with associated sclerosis of the ulnar trochlear notch and early osteophyte formation at the medial aspect of the humeroulnar and the cranial aspect of the humeroradial articulations. The soft tissues surrounding the fracture as well as the elbow joint remained

thickened. The dog did not return to the UF SAH for 15 months, when it presented for evaluation of mild swelling over the previous tarsometatarsal arthrodesis site. The tarsal arthrodesis plate and screws were removed due to implant loosening secondary to an associated infection. At that time, there was no appreciable thoracic limb lameness and thus no radiographic examination was performed. The left elbow had a normal range of motion, with no discomfort elicited on manipulation and no palpable effusion. Three and half years

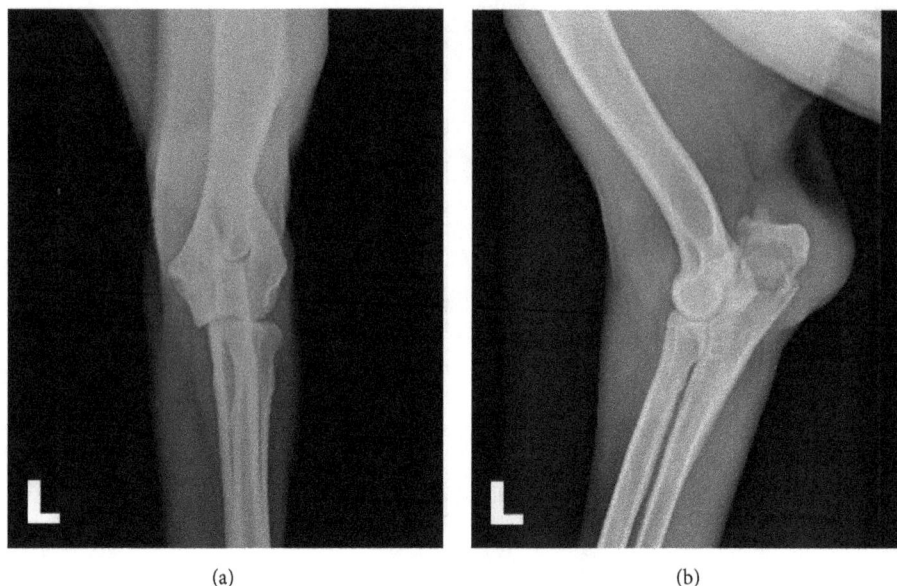

(a)                                                         (b)

FIGURE 7: Craniocaudal (a) and mediolateral (b) radiographs of the left elbow of dog 3 obtained preoperatively. A closed cranioproximal-to-caudodistally orientated olecranon fracture is seen extending into the ulnar trochlear notch. Comminution of the fracture resulted in cranial displacement of the anconeal process, seen best on the mediolateral radiograph.

after the initial fracture repair, the dog was examined by the UF Oncology Service and had a splenectomy to address splenic hemangiosarcoma. The dog was placed on a doxorubicin chemotherapeutic protocol and lived an additional 2 years before succumbing to the disease. No thoracic limb lameness or gait abnormalities were reported by the owner or observed by our Oncology Service up to the point of the dog's demise, 5.5 years following fracture repair.

## 4. Case 3

A 2-year-old intact male German shepherd, weighing 40 kg, presented to the UF SAH in April 2013 for evaluation of a non-weight-bearing lameness of the left thoracic limb, which was sustained in a road traffic accident. Preoperative radiographs and a computed tomographic (CT) scan showed a caudoproximal-to-craniodistally orientated, closed, comminuted olecranon fracture involving the articular margin of the ulnar trochlear notch, with cranioproximal displacement of the olecranon segment. The pattern of the fracture resulted in a comminution fragment that included the anconeal process, which was minimally, cranially displaced (Figure 7).

The fracture was exposed via a lateral approach [16], the proximal fracture segment, which included the olecranon tubercle, was directly reduced and reduction was maintained using point-to-point reduction forceps. Fluoroscopy (Ziehm Vision[2] FD, Ziehm Imaging, Nurnberg, Germany) was used, in the manner described in dog 1, to evaluate fracture reduction and to facilitate proper implant placement. Fracture fixation was accomplished by means of a laterally-to-medially directed 3.5 mm screw placed in lag fashion. The anconeal process was then anatomically reduced and held in reduction with point-to-point reduction forceps. Two 1.1 mm Kirschner wires were placed under fluoroscopic guidance, in

a caudal-to-cranial direction. The distal Kirschner wire was used as a guide wire for a cannulated drill bit to place a 2.7 mm screw, with a washer, in lag fashion. The tip of this screw was advanced to partially engage the transcortex of the anconeal process, ensuring the screw did not protrude through the cortex, avoiding potential impingement in the olecranon fossa. This primary repair was augmented with a caudally applied, eight-hole 2.7 mm locking compression plate (DePuy Synthes, West Chester, PA, USA) with one locking and two cortical screws engaging the proximal segment and two cortical and three locking screws engaging the distal ulnar segment. An additional 1.1 mm Kirschner wire was then placed into the anconeal process, from caudal-to-cranial, under fluoroscopic guidance (Figure 8) and postoperative radiographs were obtained (Figure 9).

Recovery from surgery was uneventful; the dog was discharged the following day. Postoperative therapy included administration of carprofen (1.9 mg/kg PO every 12 hrs for 5 days), tramadol (2.5 mg/kg PO every 12 hrs for 7 days), and cephalexin (25 mg/kg PO every 12 hrs for 14 days). The referring veterinarian performed 1- and 2-month postoperative follow-up examinations. The dog was reported to be using the limb well, with no loss of reduction or fixation and appropriate healing was documented radiographically.

The dog was evaluated at the UF SAH 6 months postoperatively. At that time, the dog had developed a hygroma over the caudal aspect of the left olecranon but ambulated without appreciable lameness. The left elbow had a very similar range of motion (flexion = 26°, extension = 152°) when compared with the right elbow (flexion = 27°, extension = 153°). Mild left elbow joint osteophytosis was palpable. Muscle atrophy was not detected, with the left and right brachial circumference being identical at 25 cm. Gait was objectively evaluated by walking the dog on a force plate (Advanced Mechanical

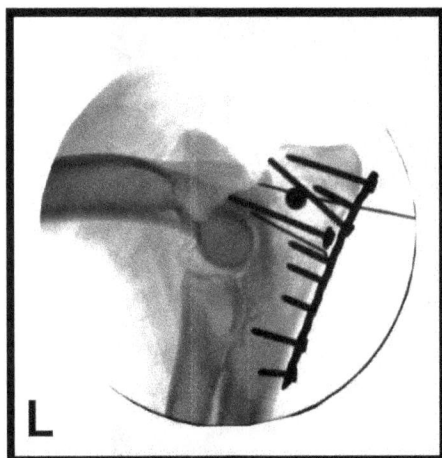

FIGURE 8: Mediolateral fluoroscopic image of the elbow of dog 3, acquired intraoperatively. This fluoroscopic image was used to assess proper placement of the proximal Kirschner wire in the anconeal process. Note the long protruding segment of the wire, which was subsequently cut adjacent to the caudal cortex of the ulna.

Technology Inc., Newton, MA, USA) and a pressure walkway (GAIT4Dog Walkway, Sparta, NJ, USA). Three successful trials were included for analysis. The mean PVF was found to be slightly decreased in left thoracic limb (123.3 N/N) compared with the right thoracic limb (134.3 N/N). The mean vertical impulse was also slightly decreased in the left (19.1 N-sec/N) compared to the right (21.1 N-sec/N) thoracic limb. The percentage of the gait cycle spent in the stance phase, however, was very similar between the left (60.7%) and right (60.0%) thoracic limbs. The mean pressure placed on the left thoracic limb (3.1 N/m$^2$) was also similar to the right thoracic limb (3.3 N/m$^2$).

Radiographic examination revealed osseous union of the olecranon tuber fracture (Figure 10). The anconeal component of the fracture, however, had not obtained union and had ill-defined, sclerotic margins. In addition, there was a fracture of the distal Kirschner wire and mild lucency surrounding the screw stabilizing the anconeal process, indicative of loosening. There was moderate sclerosis of the ulnar trochlear notch, with humeroulnar joint space narrowing. These changes were most severe at the level of the articular fracture and were compatible with healing and a component of degenerative joint disease. A large soft tissue mass was noted over the apex of the olecranon process, consistent with the clinically noted hygroma.

The dog was taken back to surgery and the previously placed plate and associated screws were removed. Under fluoroscopic guidance, the original 36 mm long, 3.5 mm screw in the anconeal process was replaced with a shorter (32 mm long) 3.5 mm screw. A shorter screw was used because there were concerns that the tip of the screw placed initially impinged on the cortical bone at the apex of the anconeal process, limiting the screw's ability to provide effective compression. The proximal and distal Kirschner wires in the anconeal process (apart from broken implanted segment) were removed. A 1.1 mm Kirschner wire was placed 11 mm

proximally to the screw. This wire served as a guide wire for drilling a hole to place a second 3.5 mm cortical screw in lag fashion (Figure 11).

Follow-up examination 2 months later (8 months after the initial surgery) revealed mild left thoracic limb lameness. Moderate left elbow effusion and mild fibrosis were palpable. On radiographic examination, the fracture involving the anconeal process persisted, with widening of the fracture gap and loosening of the distal screw (Figure 12). Both screws were removed under fluoroscopic guidance.

The dog was reevaluated 14 months after the initial surgery and was not appreciably lame. Pain was not elucidated on manipulation of the left elbow and there was no palpable effusion. Range of motion in the left elbow (flexion = 27°, extension = 155°) was again very similar to the right elbow (flexion = 21°, extension = 157°). No appreciable muscle atrophy was palpable with right (23.6 cm) and left (23.9 cm) brachial circumference measurements being similar. Gait was again objectively evaluated by walking the dog on a force plate (Advanced Mechanical Technology Inc., Newton, MA, USA) and a pressure walkway (GAIT4Dog Walkway, Sparta, NJ, USA), with three successful trials included for analysis. The mean PVF was found to be slightly decreased in left thoracic limb (103.5 N/N) compared with the right thoracic limb (107.9 N/N). The mean vertical impulse was also slightly decreased in the left (14.5 N-sec/N) compared to the right (16.2 N-sec/N) thoracic limb. The percentage of the gait cycle spent in the stance phase, however, was very similar between the left (64.6%) and right (64.9%) thoracic limbs. The mean pressure placed on the left thoracic limb (3.9 N/m$^2$) was also similar to the right thoracic limb (3.7 N/m$^2$).

## 5. Discussion

Despite widespread application in human orthopedic surgery [5–9], and an apparent increased usage in small animal surgery [15], reports detailing the results associated with fluoroscopic-assisted fracture stabilization in dogs are limited. Intraoperative fluoroscopy has been shown to be advantageous for assessing fracture reduction and facilitating accurate implant placement in human patients [6]. Previous work has described the use of fluoroscopy to aid in closed reduction and lag screw fixation of humeral condylar fractures in dogs [10], to assist in the placement of transilial rods or lag screws in dogs with sacroiliac luxation [11, 12], and for the application of external skeletal fixation in dogs with vertebral column [13] and appendicular long bone trauma [17, 18].

One major challenge associated with open reduction and internal fixation of olecranon fractures, utilizing a standard lateral approach [16], is the ability to fully visualize the articular margins of the fracture. Despite adequate soft tissue dissection and retraction, the capitulum and lateral epicondylar crest of the humerus overlies the trochlear notch, often restricting visualization of the fracture margins. We found that fluoroscopy was useful for assessing our initial fracture reduction, prompting improvement if necessary. Recognizing and correcting inaccuracies in reduction at the articular surface help mitigate abnormal cartilage wear and the development of posttraumatic osteoarthritis [19].

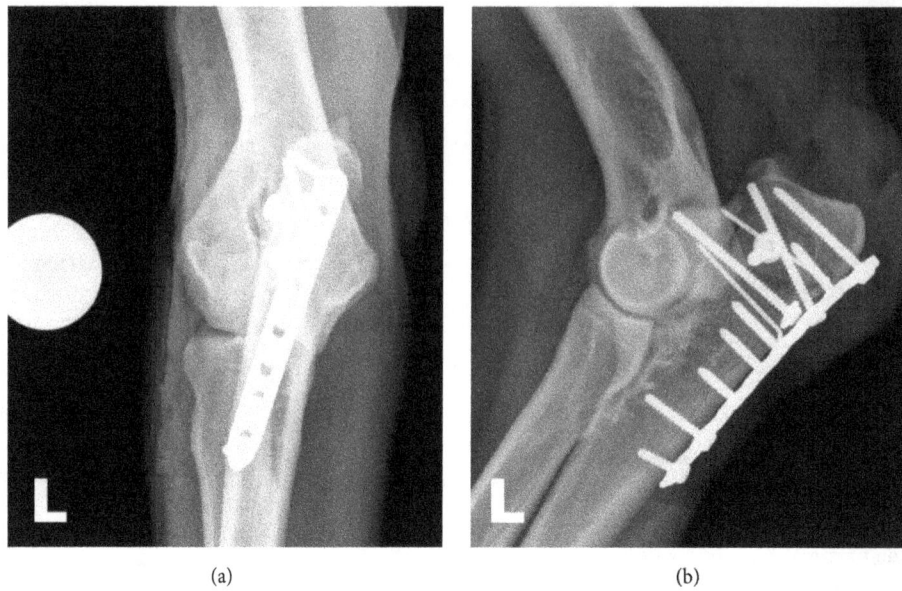

(a)                                                                           (b)

FIGURE 9: Craniocaudal (a) and mediolateral (b) radiographs of the left elbow of dog 3 obtained immediately postoperatively. The olecranon fracture was repaired with a laterally-to-medially directed screw, inserted in lag fashion. The anconeal process is stabilized with one screw inserted in lag fashion and two Kirschner wires, inserted in a caudal-to-cranial orientation. This repair was augmented with a caudally applied eight-hole 2.7 mm locking compression plate, with three screws engaging the proximal olecranon segment and five screws engaging the distal segment.

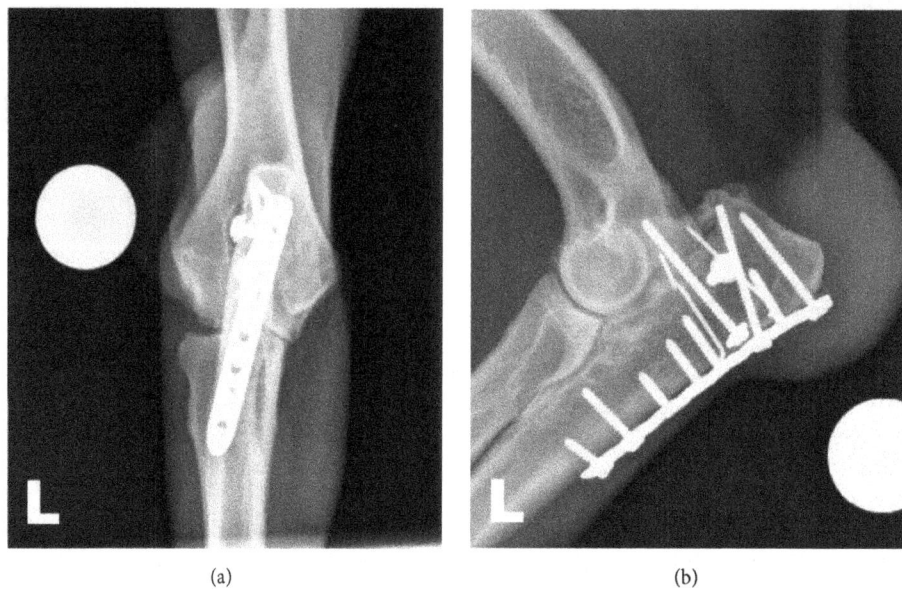

(a)                                                                           (b)

FIGURE 10: Craniocaudal (a) and mediolateral (b) radiographs of the left elbow of dog 3 obtained 6 months postoperatively. The fracture associated with the olecranon tuber is fully healed. The fracture margin associated with the anconeal process, however, remains visible, with ill-defined, sclerotic margins, indicating a nonunion. Note the lucency around the lag screw in the anconeal process and the fractured Kirschner wire seated distally in the anconeal process.

In agreement with previous findings [4], all three olecranon fractures in this report had articular involvement. In addition to assisting with accurate fracture reduction, intraoperative fluoroscopy was useful in facilitating appropriate implant placement. Accurate positioning of the Kirschner wires and the use of cannulated drill bits facilitated accurate

screw placement in the small juxta-articular and articular fracture segments [20]. Given that all three fractures in this report had articular components, placing the interfragmentary lag screws perpendicular to the fracture line was considered optimal to prevent a loss of reduction as the screws were tightened. Apart from the nonunion of the anconeal process

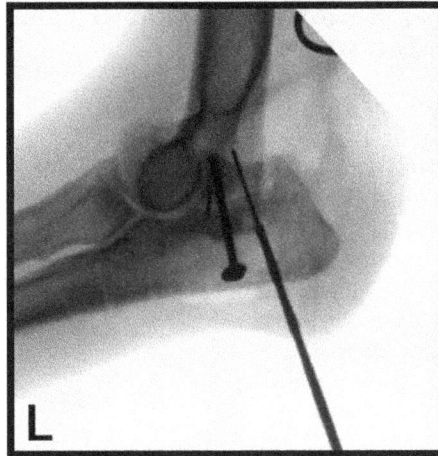

FIGURE 11: Mediolateral intraoperative fluoroscopic image of the elbow of dog 3. The previously placed caudal ulnar plate and associated screws have been removed. A new Kirschner wire has been placed to function as a guide wire to assist placement of an additional screw. Note the cannulated drill bit inserted over the guide wire, ensuring that the drill-tract and subsequently the screw are appropriately positioned.

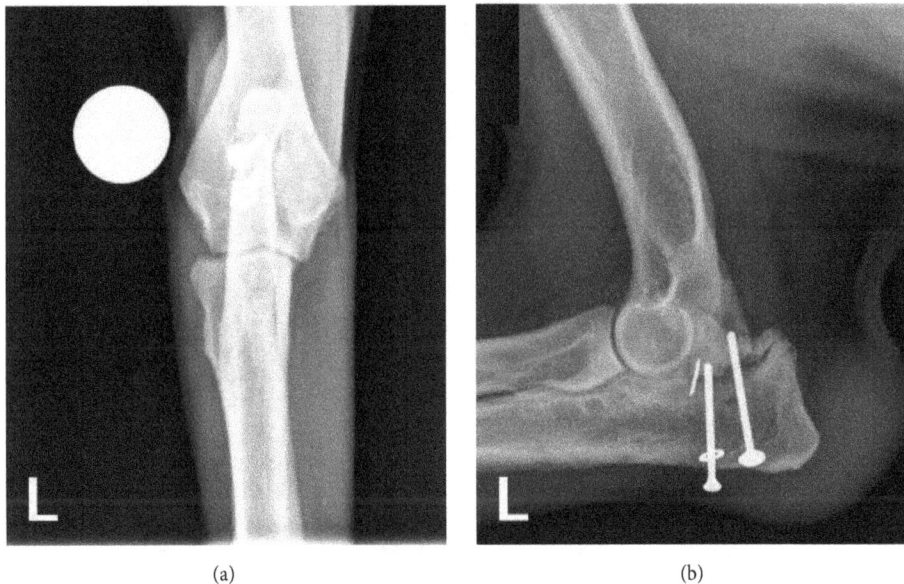

(a)                                                                 (b)

FIGURE 12: Craniocaudal (a) and mediolateral (b) radiographs of the left elbow of dog 3 obtained 8 months postoperatively. The fracture margin associated with the anconeal process is widened when compared with previous radiographs, with ill-defined, sclerotic margins. The distal screw has loosened.

in the third dog, the fractures appeared to undergo primary bone healing with limited callus formation.

There are biomechanical advantages to both caudal and lateral plate placement when stabilizing the proximal ulna [21]. In further agreement with the findings of Muir and Johnson we found that the use of a caudally or laterally applied ulnar plate was not associated with any implant failure or fracture-healing complications [4]. The proximal fracture fragment in dog 2 was prohibitively small to permit application of a plate. Placement of multiple interfragmentary screws, however, provided sufficient stability to allow this fracture to achieve union.

In the third dog, the olecranon tubercle fracture healed, but the anconeal process did not obtain radiographic union.

Recent reports suggest that optimal treatment for younger dogs with an ununited anconeal process (UAP) involves lag screw fixation in conjunction with proximal ulnar osteotomy [22, 23]. This method of treatment theoretically reduces excessive contact pressure on the anconeal process and addresses contributing elbow incongruity, while simultaneously permitting reduction and compression of the UAP [23]. The anconeal process is considered to be the primary stabilizer of the dog's elbow when the joint is subjected to pronation and is considered a secondary stabilizer when the joint is subjected to supination [24]. These findings suggest that the anconeal process is subjected to large torque moments during ambulation, and our fixation of the anconeal process was likely inadequate in dog 3. Neither the lag screw nor the interfragmentary Kirschner wires fully engaged the transcortex of the anconeal process, as we did not want these implants to penetrate the articular surface. This may have reduced fracture stability and contributed to the development of the nonunion. Similarly, a previous study found that stabilization of an UAP by placement of a lag screw alone resulted in failure of apophyseal fusion in 8 out of 9 joints [25]. Although UAP is a developmental disease and thus has a different etiology than the traumatic anconeal fracture presented in dog 3, the poor fusion rate [25] highlights the need for rigid fixation to neutralize the large forces exerted on the anconeal process during daily activities. In retrospect, we may have achieved a better outcome if we had initially placed two screws in the anconeal process, with both screws fully engaging the transcortex.

Development of mild to moderate posttraumatic osteoarthritis was documented in all dogs in this report, corroborating findings of previous reports [4, 19]. Varitimidis et al. reported that concomitant arthroscopic and fluoroscopically assisted articular radial fracture repair in human patients helped guide fracture reduction and was associated with improved clinical outcomes, when compared with fluoroscopic assistance only [8]. Patients in that study treated with arthroscopic and fluoroscopic assistance were found to have improved supination, flexion, and extension at all time points, compared with those patients in which only fluoroscopy was used [8]. The feasibility of incorporating closed arthroscopic reduction in dogs thus warrants investigation. The clinical outcome of the three dogs in this report was considered successful, despite the progression of osteoarthritis, even in the third dog in which the anconeal process fracture did not obtain union. All dogs were subjectively free of lameness at the time of the last documented follow-up examination. Our observations in all three dogs were supported by objective assessments of limb function in the first and third dogs.

This report is limited by its retrospective nature, which restricted our ability to obtain standardized outcomes over defined time points for each dog. In addition, we do not have a control group of dogs with similar fractures, managed without fluoroscopic-assisted surgery, for comparison. A further limitation of this report is the small number of dogs, precluding valid statistical comparison of fixation methods and clinical outcomes.

The use of intraoperative fluoroscopy allowed us to confirm anatomic fracture reduction intraoperatively and facilitated accurate implant placement. Anatomic reduction and stable fixation of these articular fractures permitted a successful return to function without appreciable lameness at the time of long-term follow-up evaluation in all three dogs.

## Abbreviations

UAP:      Ununited anconeal process
UF SAH: University of Florida Small Animal Hospital.

## Conflict of Interests

The authors declare that there is no conflict of interests regarding the publication of the paper.

## Acknowledgment

The authors would like to acknowledge the assistance of Ms. Debby Sundstrom in the collection of objective gait data and in the preparation of the figures.

## References

[1] H. E. Evans and A. de Lahunta, "The skeleton," in *Miller's Anatomy of the Dog*, H. E. Evans and A. de Lahunta, Eds., pp. 134–136, Elsevier Saunders, St. Louis, Mo, USA, 4th edition, 1996.

[2] I. R. Phillips, "A survey of bone fractures in the dog and cat," *Journal of Small Animal Practice*, vol. 20, no. 11, pp. 661–674, 1979.

[3] P. Muir and P. A. Manley, "Stabilisation of fractures of the proximal radius and ulna in a dog by application of a single plate to the ulna," *Veterinary Record*, vol. 134, no. 23, pp. 599–601, 1994.

[4] P. Muir and K. A. Johnson, "Fractures of the proximal ulna in dogs," *Veterinary and Comparative Orthopaedics and Traumatology*, vol. 9, no. 2, pp. 88–94, 1996.

[5] M. S. H. Beerekamp, G. S. I. Sulkers, D. T. Ubbink, M. Maas, N. W. L. Schep, and J. C. Goslings, "Accuracy and consequences of 3D-fluoroscopy in upper and lower extremity fracture treatment: a systematic review," *European Journal of Radiology*, vol. 81, no. 12, pp. 4019–4028, 2012.

[6] B. L. Norris, D. H. Hahn, M. J. Bosse, J. F. Kellam, and S. H. Sims, "Intraoperative fluoroscopy to evaluate fracture reduction and hardware placement during acetabular surgery," *Journal of Orthopaedic Trauma*, vol. 13, no. 6, pp. 414–417, 1999.

[7] B. Carelsen, R. Haverlag, D. T. Ubbink, J. S. K. Luitse, and J. C. Goslings, "Does intraoperative fluoroscopic 3D imaging provide extra information for fracture surgery?" *Archives of Orthopaedic and Trauma Surgery*, vol. 128, no. 12, pp. 1419–1424, 2008.

[8] S. E. Varitimidis, G. K. Basdekis, Z. H. Dailiana, M. E. Hantes, K. Bargiotas, and K. Malizos, "Treatment of intra-articular fractures of the distal radius," *The Journal of Bone & Joint Surgery—British Volume*, vol. 90, no. 6, pp. 778–785, 2008.

[9] M. Kraus, S. von dem Berge, H. Schöll, G. Krischak, and F. Gebhard, "Integration of fluoroscopy-based guidance in orthopaedic trauma surgery—a prospective cohort study," *Injury*, vol. 44, no. 11, pp. 1486–1492, 2013.

[10] J. L. Cook, J. L. Tomlinson, and A. L. Reed, "Fluoroscopically guided closed reduction and internal fixation of fractures of the lateral portion of the humeral condyle: prospective clinical study of the technique and results in ten dogs," *Veterinary Surgery*, vol. 28, no. 5, pp. 315–321, 1999.

[11] J. L. Tomlinson, J. L. Cook, J. T. Payne, C. C. Anderson, and J. C. Johnson, "Closed reduction and lag screw fixation of sacroiliac luxations and fractures," *Veterinary Surgery*, vol. 28, no. 3, pp. 188–193, 1999.

[12] C. S. Leasure, D. D. Lewis, C. W. Sereda, K. L. Mattern, C. T. Jehn, and J. L. Wheeler, "Limited open reduction and stabilization of sacroiliac fracture-luxations using fluoroscopically assisted placement of a trans-iliosacral rod in five dogs," *Veterinary Surgery*, vol. 36, no. 7, pp. 633–643, 2007.

[13] J. L. Wheeler, D. D. Lewis, A. R. Cross, and C. W. Sereda, "Closed fluoroscopic-assisted spinal arch external skeletal fixation for the stabilization of vertebral column injuries in five dogs," *Veterinary Surgery*, vol. 36, no. 5, pp. 442–448, 2007.

[14] C. A. Tonks, J. L. Tomlinson, and J. L. Cook, "Evaluation of closed reduction and screw fixation in lag fashion of sacroiliac fracture-luxations," *Veterinary Surgery*, vol. 37, no. 7, pp. 603–607, 2008.

[15] B. S. Beale and A. Pozzi, "Minimally invasive fracture repair," *Veterinary Clinics of North America—Small Animal Practice*, vol. 42, no. 5, pp. 963–1096, 2012.

[16] D. L. Piermattei and K. A. Johnson, "The forelimb," in *An Atlas of Surgical Approaches to the Bones and Joints of the Dog and Cat*, D. L. Piermattei and K. A. Johnson, Eds., pp. 186–189, Saunders, Philadelphia, Pa, USA, 4th edition, 2012.

[17] J. P. Farese, D. D. Lewis, A. R. Cross, K. E. Collins, G. M. Anderson, and K. B. Halling, "Use of IMEX SK-circular external fixator hybrid constructs for fracture stabilization in dogs and cats," *Journal of the American Animal Hospital Association*, vol. 38, no. 3, pp. 279–289, 2002.

[18] K. A. Kirby, D. D. Lewis, M. P. Lafuente et al., "Management of humeral and femoral fractures in dogs and cats with linear-circular hybrid external skeletal fixators," *Journal of the American Animal Hospital Association*, vol. 44, no. 4, pp. 180–197, 2008.

[19] W. J. Gordon, M. F. Besancon, M. G. Conzemius, K. G. Miles, A. S. Kapatkin, and W. T. N. Culp, "Frequency of post-traumatic osteoarthritis in dogs after repair of a humeral condylar fracture," *Veterinary and Comparative Orthopaedics and Traumatology*, vol. 16, no. 1, pp. 1–5, 2003.

[20] D. D. Lewis, "Femoral neck fracture repair," in *Small Animal Orthopedics, Rheumatology and Musculoskeletal Disorders*, D. D. Lewis and S. J. Langley-Hobbs, Eds., pp. 113–114, CRC Press, Boca Raton, Fla, USA, 2nd edition, 2014.

[21] D. D. Lewis and S. J. Langley-Hobbs, "Olecranon fracture repair," in *Small Animal Orthopedics, Rheumatology and Musculoskeletal Disorders*, D. D. Lewis and S. J. Langley-Hobbs, Eds., pp. 55–56, CRC Press, Boca Raton, Fla, USA, 2nd edition, 2014.

[22] U. Krotscheck, D. A. Hulse, A. Bahr, and R. M. Jerram, "Ununited anconeal process: lag-screw fixation with proximal ulnar osteotomy," *Veterinary and Comparative Orthopaedics and Traumatology*, vol. 13, no. 4, pp. 212–216, 2000.

[23] R. A. Pettitt, J. Tattersall, T. Gemmill et al., "Effect of surgical technique on radiographic fusion of the anconeus in the treatment of ununited anconeal process," *Journal of Small Animal Practice*, vol. 50, no. 10, pp. 545–548, 2009.

[24] K. W. Talcott, K. S. Schulz, P. H. Kass, D. R. Mason, and S. M. Stover, "In vitro biomechanical study of rotational stabilizers of the canine elbow joint," *American Journal of Veterinary Research*, vol. 63, no. 11, pp. 1520–1526, 2002.

[25] A. Meyer-Lindenberg, I. Nolte, and M. Fehr, "The ununited anconeal process: retro- and prospective investigations on surgical treatment," *Tierärztliche Praxis Ausgabe K: Kleintiere Heimtiere*, vol. 27, no. 5, pp. 309–320, 1999.

# 23

# Bilateral Telencephalic Gliomatosis Cerebri in a Dog

**Mario Ricciardi,**[1] **Antonio De Simone,**[1] **Pasquale Giannuzzi,**[1] **Maria Teresa Mandara,**[2] **Alice Reginato,**[2] **and Floriana Gernone**[1]

[1] "Pingry" Veterinary Hospital, Via Medaglie d'Oro 5, 70126 Bari, Italy
[2] Department of Biopathological Science and Hygiene of Food and Animal Productions, Faculty of Veterinary Medicine, University of Perugia, 06126 Perugia, Italy

Correspondence should be addressed to Mario Ricciardi; ricciardi.mario@alice.it

Academic Editor: Paola Roccabianca

An 8-year-old intact male Lagotto Romagnolo was presented with forebrain signs. Neuroanatomic localization was diffuse prosencephalon. MRI revealed diffuse, bilateral, and symmetric T2 and FLAIR hyperintensities in the parieto-occipital white matter and corpus callosum. No mass effect or contrast enhancement was noted. Analysis of cerebrospinal fluid revealed normal protein content and mild mononuclear pleocytosis. Atypical cells were not identified. 15 days later because of the worsening of clinical condition the patient was euthanized upon owner's request. Neuropathological investigations were consistent with gliomatosis cerebri (GC). Such an unusual imaging pattern appeared similar to some cases of human GC and to a previous reported case in a dog, suggesting a possible repeatable imaging findings for this rare brain neoplasm. GC should be included in the MRI differentials for diffuse bilateral white matter signal changes and specific MRI findings described in this report may help in reaching a presumptive diagnosis of this tumor.

## 1. Case Presentation

An 8-year-old intact male Lagotto Romagnolo was evaluated for a 1-month history of abnormal mental status. Clinical and neurological examination findings included depression, decreased postural reactions in all four limbs, especially on the right side, and decreased menace response in both eyes. During clinical examination the dog had seizures. The medical case was considered to be consistent with a diffuse forebrain lesion. Because of the age of the patient and the absence of hyperthermia neoplasm was considered the most probable cause of neurological signs while inflammation was considered to be less likely. Complete blood count, serum chemistry, and urinalysis results were within normal limits.

MRI of the brain was performed under general anesthesia using a 0.25 Tesla permanent magnet (ESAOTE VET-MR GRANDE, Esaote, Genoa, Italy). MRI sequences protocol included Fast Spin Echo T2-weighted images acquired in sagittal and transverse plane, a FLAIR acquired in the transverse plane, and Spin Echo T1-weighted images acquired in the transverse plane before and after intravenous

administration of paramagnetic contrast medium (Magnegita—gadopentatedimeglumine 500 mmol/mL—insight agents; 0.15 mmol/kg BW). MRI showed extensive, bilateral, and symmetric T2 and FLAIR hyperintensity of the parieto-occipital periventricular and subcortical white matter. The occipital lobes appeared severely involved. The lesions were isointense on T1-weighted images and did not enhance after contrast medium administration (Figures 1 and 2). On sagittal T2-weighted images the aboral part of the corpus callosum lacked homogeneous signal intensity and had ill-defined margins (Figure 3). Mass effect or loss of anatomical architecture was not present. Based on the imaging findings toxic-metabolic or degenerative disorders involving white matter (leukoencephalopathy) were considered the main differential diagnoses, while an inflammatory process, either immunomediated or infectious, and a diffuse infiltrative neoplasm were believed less likely.

Analysis of CSF collected from cerebellomedullary cistern revealed normal protein content (20 mg/dL; range, <25 mg/dL) and mild mononuclear pleocytosis (30 cells/$\mu$L; range, <5 cells/$\mu$L). Atypical cells were not identified. The dog

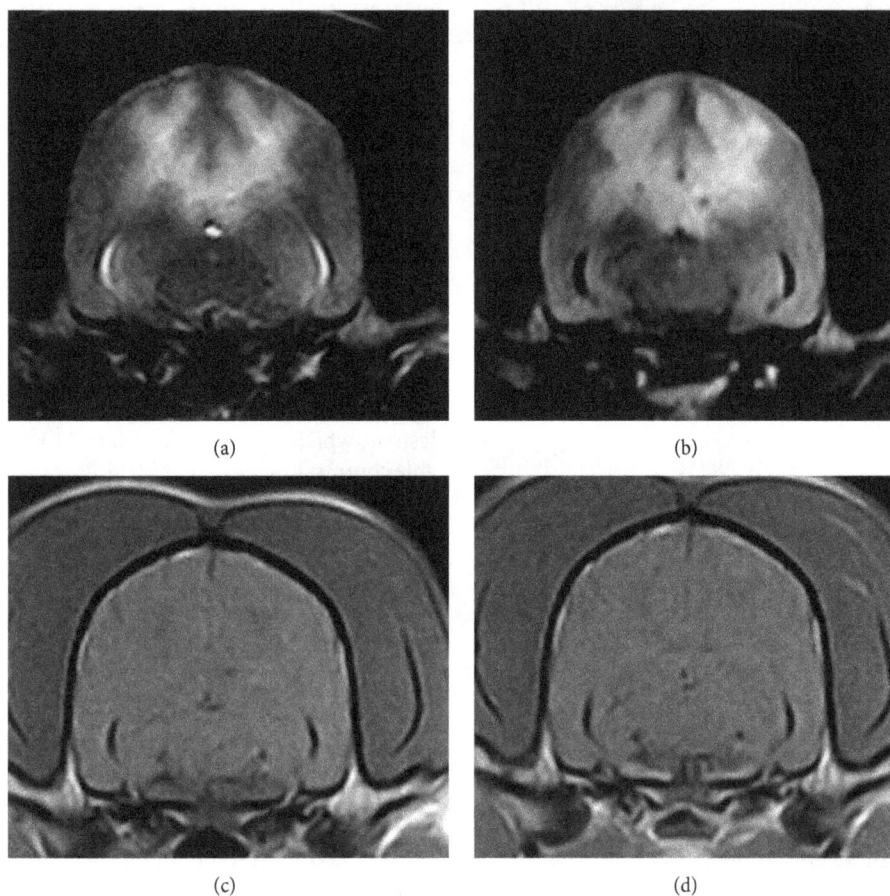

FIGURE 1: (a) T2-weighted (TR = 3720 ms, TE = 90 ms, slice thickness = 3,5 mm), (b) FLAIR (TR = 4000 ms, TE = 100 ms, TI = 1000 slice thickness = 3,5 mm), and (c) T1-weighted (TR = 600 ms, TE = 18 ms, slice thickness = 3,5 mm) pre- and (d) postcontrast transverse images at the level of the caudal mesencephalic aqueduct. There is bilateral and symmetric T2 and FLAIR hyperintensity within the parieto-occipital periventricular and subcortical white matter. The lesions are isointense on T1-weighted images and did not enhance after contrast medium administration. No mass effect is present.

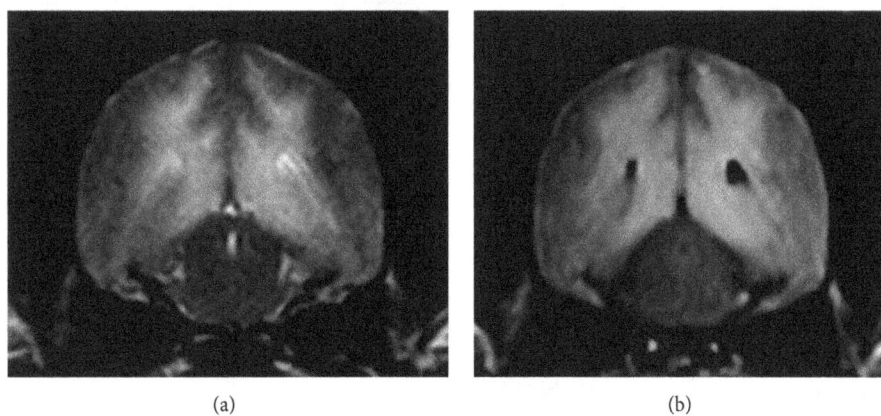

FIGURE 2: (a) T2-weighted (TR = 3720 ms, TE = 90 ms, slice thickness = 3,5 mm), (b) FLAIR (TR = 4000 ms, TE = 100 ms, TI = 1000 slice thickness = 3,5 mm) at the level of the rostral mesencephalon. There is bilateral and symmetric T2 and FLAIR hyperintensity of the parietal periventricular white matter and corona radiata. No mass effect is present.

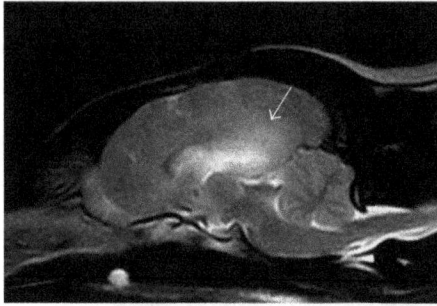

FIGURE 3: Sagittal T2-weighted image (TR = 3720 ms, TE = 90 ms, slice thickness = 3,5 mm). There is ill-defined T2 hyperintensity of the splenium of corpus callosum. No mass effect is evident.

was treated with phenobarbital (5 mg/kg *q* 12 hr). Pending on the PCR tests on the CSF sample for canine distemper virus, *Toxoplasma gondii*, *Neospora caninum*, *Ehrlichia canis*, and *Rickettsia* spp., clindamycin (15 mg/kg *q* 12 hr) was added on. All the required PCR investigations turned out to be negative. After 15 days the dog was reevaluated. Because of the worsening of clinical condition the dog was euthanized upon owner's request.

Soon after death the dog was submitted to necropsy that did not reveal significant gross visceral lesions. At neuropathological examination performed on formalin-fixed coronal brain sections, cortical white matter of centrum semiovale was markedly expanded to the detriment of cortical gray matter. No more gross brain lesions were observed.

At histologic examination a severe diffuse infiltration of neoplastic cells was observed affecting centrum semiovale, periventricular white matter, corpus callosum, septum pellucidum, fimbria fornix, and parahippocampal gyrus. The neoplastic cells had round to elongated nuclei with coarsely stippled chromatin and indistinct cytoplasm borders. They were haphazardly arranged in a finely fibrillary neuropile (Figure 4(a)). Focally the neoplastic invasion was associated with a diffuse vacuolization of white matter and a coexisting foam cell infiltration. A mild neoplastic infiltration of the fourth ventricle floor was also observed associated with necrosis of the medial vestibular nucleus. Immunolabeling on selected paraffin-embedded brain sections was performed with avidin-biotin peroxidase complex staining for GFAP (GFAP, rabbit polyclonal antibody, 1 : 500, Dako, Carpenteria, CA, USA). It showed a diffuse marked GFAP-immunoreaction of the neoplastic cells (Figure 4(b)). The histological findings were consistent with GC of astrocytic type.

## 2. Discussion

GC is a primary wide and diffuse infiltration of the CNS by neoplastic glial cells [1]. It has been reported in humans, with approximately 300 described cases [2–6], and very rarely in dogs, cats, and goats [7–15]. In humans two general forms of GC are recognized. Type I GC is characterized by neoplastic infiltration with good architecture preservation and without a grossly visible mass. Type II GC consists in

a neoplastic infiltration accompanied by a mass lesion with ill-defined margins [1, 2, 4, 5, 7, 16]. Affected patients show clinical signs reflecting tumor localization. In humans GC is primarily localized in the telencephalon with mono- or bilateral involvement of different brain lobes. However, more areas may also be affected such as basal nuclei, thalamus, hypothalamus, corpus callosum, cranial nerves, cerebellum, brainstem, and spinal cord [17, 18]. Infiltration of the brain parenchyma typically occurs along the myelinated fibres producing extensive demyelination of the affected areas [19]. This condition gives a histological pattern, which strictly correlates with the hemispheric white matter signal changes seen on MRI [18–20]. In human medicine, MRI features of histologically confirmed GC include extensive, symmetrical, or asymmetrical and often poorly delineated T2-hyperintense lesions, which tend to be T1-iso to T1-hypointense with variable contrast enhancement [2, 16, 21, 22]. However, these findings are considered nonspecific for GC so that the differential diagnosis includes immunomediated or virus induced white matter diseases, leukodystrophy, and other brain tumors such as primary brain lymphoma or glioblastoma multiforme [18]. In people, the involvement of commissural structures such as the corpus callosum has been unequivocally related to GC allowing differentiating this neoplasm by a demyelinating disease [20, 21].

To date 12 cases of GC have been reported in dogs with multiple distributions of the lesions throughout the brain and spinal cord, while MRI patterns have been described in five cases [7, 9, 11, 12, 22–24]. Three dogs had telencephalic involvement [9, 11, 13] but only one of them showed bilateral and symmetric white matter T2 and FLAIR hyperintensities without any apparent mass effect or anatomical distortion [11]. Based on the MRI features in that case the lesions were misdiagnosed as a leukoencephalopathy of unknown origin. However information about the involvement of the corpus callosum was not available in the referred study [11].

In this report we describe a similar imaging pattern with bilateral and symmetric involvement of dorsal parieto-occipital white matter and corpus callosum, that showed inhomogeneous T2-hyperintensity at level of the splenium. Interestingly in people the involvement of corpus callosum has been reported in 8 out of 9 cases of cerebrum GC [17]. This is why this finding is nowadays considered very suggestive for GC [20, 21, 25].

Generally, bilateral and symmetric involvement of specific anatomic areas of CNS, without relevant mass effect and with anatomic preservation, is typical of metabolic-toxic and degenerative diseases [26–28]. On the contrary, primary CNS tumors usually appear as space-occupying lesions with mass effect and peritumoral edema of variable grade [26–28]. This peculiar distribution pattern of GC clearly subverts these rules and makes the MRI-based ante mortem diagnosis difficult.

Similar and sometimes overlapping imaging findings have been described in dogs with different brain diseases [13, 28–30]. In NLE, MRI findings are characterized by bilateral but not symmetric T2 and FLAIR hyperintensities in the telencephalic white matter [13, 29]. Moreover anatomical distortion may be present. Also in necrotizing leukoencephalitis

(a)

(b)

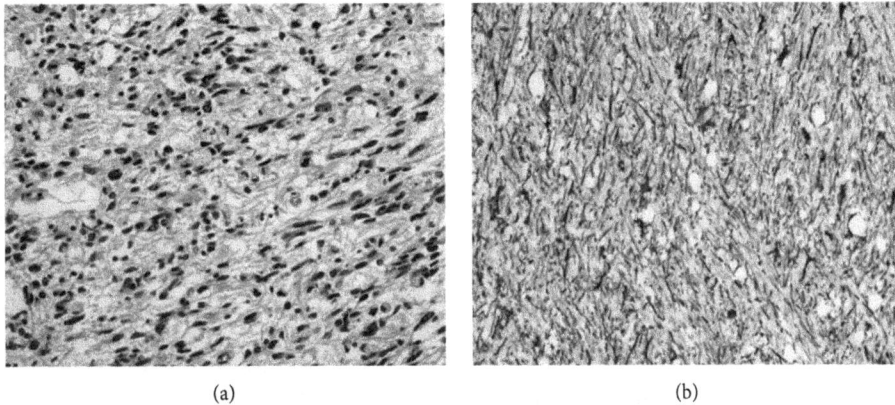

FIGURE 4: (a) Brain tissue. Diffuse infiltration of the white matter by neoplastic cells having elongate nuclei and fibrillary cytoplasm. The neuropile shows a finely fibrillary pattern (H&E, ×20). (b) Brain tissue. The neoplastic cells show a diffuse marked immunoreaction for glial fibrillary acidic protein. They are characterized by long branched cytoplasmic processes (antiglial fibrillary acidic protein-immunolabeling, ×10).

mononuclear pleocytosis is generally found at cerebrospinal fluid analysis [13, 29]. In our case mild mononuclear pleocytosis detected at CSF analysis was consistent with previous cases of GC in dogs in which normal or mild increased CSF cell count has been found [7, 12, 22]. Canine distemper meningoencephalitis has been reported in an adult dog showing diffuse bilaterally and symmetric T2 hyperintensity of the subcortical parietal and frontal white matter [30]. In that case the predominately white matter distribution of signal intensity changes was consistent with the extensive white matter involvement occurring in the chronic forms [30]. As in this previous report, in our case the negativity of the PCR analyses made chronic distemper encephalitis less likely; any way it did not allow us to rule out distemper definitely. Cerebral edema is generally T1-hypointense, T2-hyperintense and it does not enhance after contrast medium administration [28]. Moreover, edema tends to diffuse along white matter and may outline the corona radiata providing a typical spiked pattern and uniform signal changes [28]. However, extensive cerebral edema is generally associated with a primary brain lesion either vascular, inflammatory, or neoplastic [28]. None of these lesions were evident in our case. To the authors' knowledge none of the toxic-metabolic and degenerative diseases described in dogs show an imaging pattern of diffuse bilateral and symmetric T2 and FLAIR hyperintensities in the white matter. On the contrary, bilateral but selective focal involvement of different brain areas has been observed in thiamine deficiency [31, 32], hepatic encephalopathy [28, 33], osmotic myelinolysis [28], and L2-hydroxyglutaric aciduria (L2-HGA) [34]. A degenerative disease showing MRI patter comparable to that observed in this case is the adult cheetah leukoencephalopathy [35]. This is a diffuse and bilateral white matter disease of unknown etiology described in 1999 in a group of cheetahs, characterized by axonal and myelin degeneration and reactive astrocytosis [35]. However, there are no reports on a similar disease in dogs.

In this study the areas affected by neoplastic infiltration did not express contrast enhancement suggesting blood-brain integrity [36] as described for low-grade gliomas [26–28] and GC in humans [16, 37] as in dogs [9, 11, 22, 24].

In conclusion we describe a distinct MRI pattern of GC in a dog in which bilateral and symmetric T2 and FLAIR white matter hyperintensities were found in the parieto-occipital lobes and corpus callosum. The lesions were isointense on T1W images without contrast enhancement and mass effect. Our imaging findings, unusual for brain tumor, were confirmed as repeatable imaging pattern in canine GC. The most likely differential diagnoses based on MRI signal changes and anatomical preservation seem to be chronic canine distemper meningoencephalitis and NLE. To the authors' opinion GC should be considered in the list of differential diagnosis in a dog having a so peculiar MRI pattern.

## Abbreviations

GC:     Gliomatosis cerebri
MRI:    Magnetic resonance imaging
FLAIR:  Fluid attenuated inversion recovery
CSF:    Cerebrospinal fluid
PCR:    Polymerase chain reaction
GFAP:   Glial fibrillary acidic protein
CNS:    Central nervous system
NLE:    Necrotizing leukoencephalitis.

## Conflict of Interests

The authors declare that there is no conflict of interests regarding the publication of this paper.

## References

[1] P. L. Lantos and J. M. Bruner, "Gliomatosis cerebri in tumors of the nervous system," in *World Health Organization Classification of Tumours: Pathology and Genetics of Tumours of the Nervous System*, P. Kleihues and W. K. Cavenee, Eds., pp. 92–93, IARC Press, Lyon, France, 2000.

[2] G. N. Fuller and J. M. Kros, "Gliomatosis cerebri," in *WHO Classification of Tumours of the Central Nervous System*, D. N. Louis, H. Ohgaki, O. D. Wiestler, and W. K. Cavenee, Eds., pp. 50–52, IARC Press, Lyon, France, 4th edition, 2007.

[3] S. Nevin, "Gliomatosis cerebri," *Brain*, vol. 61, no. 2, pp. 170–191, 1938.

[4] S. Taillibert, C. Chodkiewicz, F. Laigle-Donadey, M. Napolitano, S. Cartalat-Carel, and M. Sanson, "Gliomatosis cerebri: a review of 296 cases from the ANOCEF database and the literature," *Journal of Neuro-Oncology*, vol. 76, no. 2, pp. 201–205, 2006.

[5] T. Inoue, T. Kumabe, M. Kanamori, Y. Sonoda, M. Watanabe, and T. Tominaga, "Prognostic factors for patients with gliomatosis cerebri: retrospective analysis of 17 consecutive cases," *Neurosurgical Review*, vol. 34, no. 2, pp. 197–208, 2011.

[6] G. E. Vates, S. Chang, K. R. Lamborn et al., "Gliomatosis cerebri: a review of 22 cases," *Neurosurgery*, vol. 53, no. 2, pp. 261–271, 2003.

[7] B. Porter, A. De Lahunta, and B. Summers, "Gliomatosis cerebri in six dogs," *Veterinary Pathology*, vol. 40, no. 1, pp. 97–102, 2003.

[8] F. J. F. de Sant'Ana and C. S. L. Barros, "Gliomatosis cerebri in a dog," *Brazilian Journal of Veterinary Pathology*, vol. 4, no. 1, pp. 58–61, 2011.

[9] A. Gruber, M. Leschnik, S. Kneissl, and P. Schmidt, "Gliomatosis cerebri in a dog," *Journal of Veterinary Medicine Series A: Physiology Pathology Clinical Medicine*, vol. 53, no. 8, pp. 435–438, 2006.

[10] T. Ide, K. Uchida, F. Kikuta, K. Suzuki, and H. Nakayama, "Immunohistochemical characterization of canine neuroepithelial tumors," *Veterinary Pathology*, vol. 47, no. 4, pp. 741–750, 2010.

[11] S. Ródenas, M. Pumarola, L. Gaitero, À. Zamora, and S. Añor, "Magnetic resonance imaging findings in 40 dogs with histologically confirmed intracranial tumours," *Veterinary Journal*, vol. 187, no. 1, pp. 85–91, 2011.

[12] A. Galán, S. Guil-Luna, Y. Millán, E. M. Martín-Suárez, M. Pumarola, and J. M. de las Mulas, "Oligodendroglial gliomatosis cerebri in a Poodle," *Veterinary and Comparative Oncology*, vol. 8, no. 4, pp. 254–262, 2010.

[13] A. de Lahunta and E. Glass, *Veterinary Neuroanatomy and Clinical Neurology*, Elsevier, St. Louis, Miss, USA, 3rd edition, 2009.

[14] B. Stierstorfer, B. Janowetz, and W. Schmahl, "Gliomatosis cerebri in a cat. A case report," *Tierarztl Prax Ausg K Kleintiere Heimtiere*, vol. 30, pp. 282–285, 2002.

[15] U. Braun, M. Hilbe, and F. Ehrensperger, "Clinical and pathological findings in a goat with cerebral gliomatosis," *The Veterinary Journal*, vol. 170, no. 3, pp. 381–383, 2005.

[16] M. Yip, C. Fisch, and J. B. Lamarche, "Gliomatosis cerebri affecting the entire neuraxis," *Radiographics*, vol. 23, no. 1, pp. 247–253, 2003.

[17] P. Peretti-Viton, H. Brunel, O. Chinot et al., "Histological and MR correlations in Gliomatosis cerebri," *Journal of Neuro-Oncology*, vol. 59, no. 3, pp. 249–259, 2002.

[18] M. E. Novillo López, A. Gómez-Ibáñez, M. Rosenfeld, and J. Dalmau, "Gliomatosis cerebri: review of 22 patients," *Neurologia*, vol. 25, no. 3, pp. 168–173, 2010.

[19] J. Schoenen, L. De Leval, and M. Reznik, "Gliomatosis cerebri: clinical, radiological and pathological report of a case with a stroke-like onset," *Acta Neurologica Belgica*, vol. 96, no. 4, pp. 294–300, 1996.

[20] G. J. Felsberg, S. A. Silver, M. T. Brown, and R. D. Tien, "Radiologic-pathologic correlation: gliomatosis cerebri," *The American Journal of Neuroradiology*, vol. 15, no. 9, pp. 1745–1753, 1994.

[21] J. G. Chi, "Gliomatosis cerebri: Comparison of MR and CT features," *The American Journal of Roentgenology*, vol. 161, no. 4, pp. 859–862, 1993.

[22] P. Martin-Vaquero, R. C. Da Costa, K. E. Wolk, C. Premanandan, and M. J. Oglesbee, "Mri features of gliomatosis cerebri in a dog," *Veterinary Radiology and Ultrasound*, vol. 53, no. 2, pp. 189–192, 2012.

[23] B. L. Plattner, M. Kent, B. Simon et al., "Gliomatosis cerebri in two dogs," *Journal of the American Animal Hospital Association*, vol. 48, no. 5, pp. 359–365, 2012.

[24] H. Fukuoka, J. Sasaki, H. Kamishina et al., "Gliomatosis cerebelli in a Saint Bernard dog," *The Journal of Comparative Pathology*, vol. 147, no. 1, pp. 37–41, 2012.

[25] J. Cambier, B. Lechevalier, F. Chapon, V. de La Sayette, F. Viader, and L. Devarrieux, "Diffuse cerebral gliomatosis: a clinico-pathological case," *Revue Neurologique*, vol. 148, no. 2, pp. 129–132, 1992.

[26] M. T. Mandara, C. Cantile, M. Baroni, and M. Bernardini, *Neuropatologia e Neuroimaging—Testo Atlante*, Poletto, Vermezzo, Italy, 2011.

[27] M. Vandevelde, R. J. Higgins, and A. Oevermann, *Veterinary Neuropathology—Essential of Theory and Practice*, Wiley-Blackwell, Oxford, UK, 2012.

[28] P. R. Gavin and R. S. Bagley, *Practical Small Animal MRI*, Wiley-Blackwell, Ames, Iowa, USA, 2009.

[29] M. J. Higginbotham, M. Kent, and E. N. Glass, "Noninfectious inflammatory central nervous system diseases in dogs," *Compendium: Continuing Education For Veterinarians*, vol. 29, no. 8, pp. 488–497, 2007.

[30] J. F. Griffin IV, B. D. Young, and J. M. Levine, "Imaging diagnosis—chronic canine distemper meningoencephalitis," *Veterinary Radiology and Ultrasound*, vol. 50, no. 2, pp. 182–184, 2009.

[31] L. S. Garosi, R. Dennis, S. R. Platt, F. Corletto, A. de Lahunta, and C. Jakobs, "Thiamine deficiency in a dog: clinical, clinicopathologic, and magnetic resonance imaging findings," *Journal of Veterinary Internal Medicine*, vol. 17, no. 5, pp. 719–723, 2003.

[32] M. Singh, M. Thompson, N. Sullivan, and G. Child, "Thiamine deficiency in dogs due to the feeding of sulphite preserved meat," *Australian Veterinary Journal*, vol. 83, no. 7, pp. 412–417, 2005.

[33] S.-J. Moon, J.-W. Kim, B.-T. Kang, C.-Y. Lim, and H.-M. Park, "Magnetic resonance imaging findings of hepatic encephalopathy in a dog with a portosystemic shunt," *Journal of Veterinary Medical Science*, vol. 74, no. 3, pp. 361–366, 2012.

[34] L. S. Garosi, J. Penderis, J. F. McConnell, and C. Jakobs, "L-2-hydroxyglutaric aciduria in a West Highland white terrier," *Veterinary Record*, vol. 156, no. 5, pp. 145–147, 2005.

[35] L. Munson, "Leukoencephalopathy in cheetahs (*Acinonyx jubatus*)," in *Report of Workshop on Ataxia in Cheetah Cubs*, J. J. Callanan, L. Munson, and N. Stronach, Eds., University College, Dublin, Ireland, 1999.

[36] M. Law, S. Yang, H. Wang et al., "Glioma grading: sensitivity, specificity, and predictive values of perfusion MR imaging and proton MR spectroscopic imaging compared with conventional MR imaging," *The American Journal of Neuroradiology*, vol. 24, no. 10, pp. 1989–1998, 2003.

[37] P. Ponce, M. V. Alvarez-Santullano, E. Otermin, M. A. Santana, and M. G. Ludeña, "Gliomatosis cerebri: findings with computed tomography and magnetic resonance imaging," *European Journal of Radiology*, vol. 28, no. 3, pp. 226–229, 1998.

# 24

# Development of Some Organs Derived from the Three Embryonic Germ Layer in a Degus Ectopic Pregnancy and Presence of a Cytotrophoblast That Mimics Human Chorionic Placenta

**C. Bosco, E. Díaz, J. González, and R. Gutierrez**

*Placenta and Fetal Development Laboratory, Anatomy and Developmental Biology Programme, Institute of Biomedical Sciences, Faculty of Medicine, University of Chile, Independencia 1027, Casilla Postal 70079, 8380453 Santiago, Chile*

Correspondence should be addressed to C. Bosco; cbosco@med.uchile.cl

Academic Editor: Isabel Pires

This report describes a case of abdominal pregnancy in an adult female degu from which we recovered two large tissular masses from the peritoneal cavity. The bigger one showed a number of thin vascular connections to the serosa layer of the small intestine. It was also directly connected to the smaller mass by a thin membranous process. The surface of the bigger mass facing the small intestine wall showed the presence of chorionic villous that resembled a villous human chorionic placenta, rather than the hemomonochorial labyrinthine placenta, characteristic of this species. This unusual finding leads us to postulate that in the degu's uterus the cytotrophoblast is exposed to a number of factors that will activate cascades of cellular and molecular events that ultimately will be signaling the cytotrophoblast to develop into a labyrinthine hemomonochorial placenta. In absence of the proper uterine environment, as is the case of the abdominal pregnancy in the peritoneal cavity reported here, the lack of signaling will lead the cytotrophoblast to develop into a villous chorionic placenta, similar to that observed in human.

## 1. Introduction

No uniform criterion for human or animal ectopic pregnancy classification exists. In order to facilitate a more didactic approach for the study of ectopic pregnancy, various criteria have been taken into consideration. Ectopic or extrauterine pregnancy denotes a pregnancy or an implantation event that occurs elsewhere rather than within the uterine cavity [1]. Although ectopic pregnancy has been reported in several species, its occurrence is considered a low incidence process [2].

Two main types of ectopic pregnancy have been described: (i) tubal and (ii) abdominal pregnancy [2, 3]. It is known that approximately 1.3% of the ectopic pregnancies are abdominal [4], and they occur through direct implantation into the peritoneal surface. This type of ectopic pregnancy is further divided into primary and secondary types. Primary abdominal pregnancy involves the extrusion of the ovum from the fimbriated end of the uterine tube into the peritoneal cavity, either after or possibly before fertilization [2], followed by its implantation and ulterior development within the abdominal cavity. The implantation has been described to occur in a variety of extrapelvic organs such as omentum, liver, spleen, and the walls of the small and large intestines [1, 5, 6]. Secondary abdominal pregnancy is usually a consequence of rupture of the uterus or oviducts and the release of the fertilized ovum or developing embryo into the abdominal cavity. In this case, the placentae and membranes may or may not be expelled from these organs [2].

## 2. Case Report

A four-year-old female *Octodon degus*, from the breeding colony maintained at the Anatomy and Developmental Biology Programme, Institute of Biomedical Sciences, Faculty of Medicine, University of Chile, was found dead overnight and was submitted to the diagnostic laboratory for necropsy. During the course of postmortem examination, two large tissue

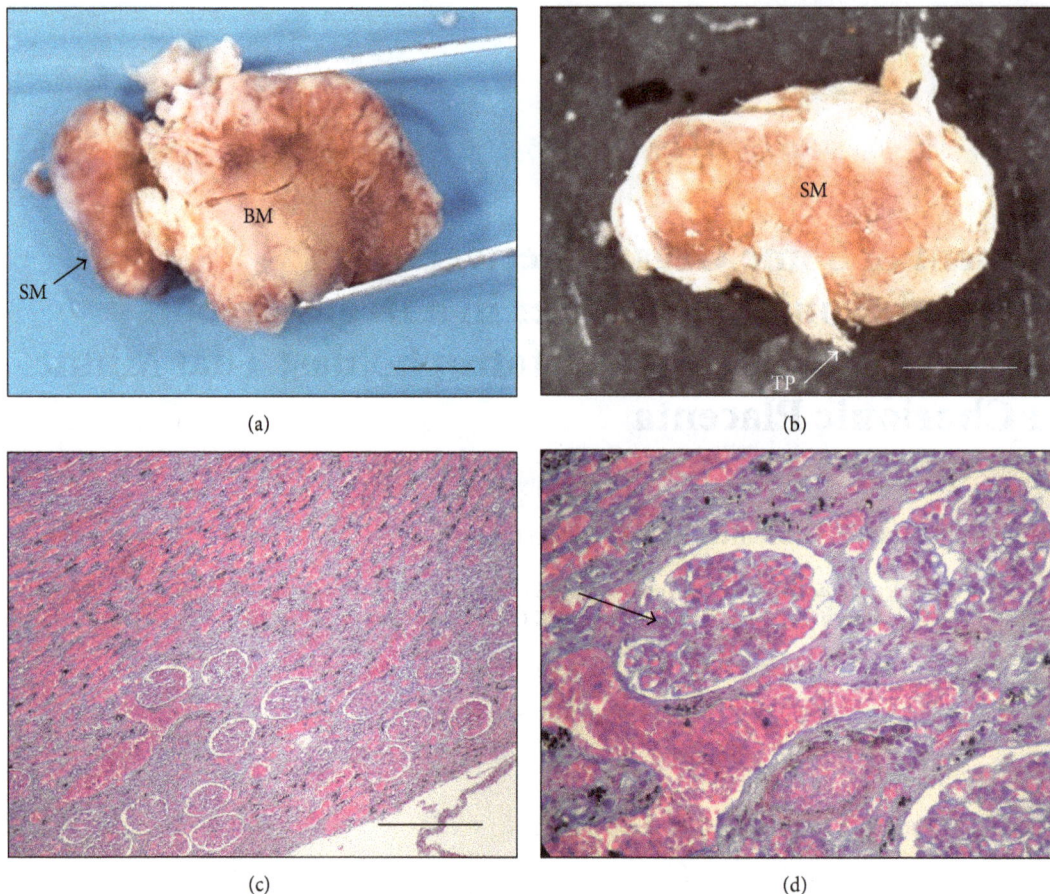

FIGURE 1: Macro- and microscopic views of the degu's intraperitoneal masses. (a) External aspect of the bigger (BM) and the smaller (SM) masses. They were enveloped by a thin translucent membrane and were profusely irrigated. The arrows depict the zone of the chorionic villus (CV) (see also Figure 5) and the zone of the apparent umbilical cord (UC) (see also Figure 3(d)). A remnant of the small intestine (SI) near the bigger mass is also observed. (b) Smaller mass showing the thin process (white arrow heads) that connects to the bigger mass. (c) Photomicrograph showing the kidney-like tissue formation towards the peripheral surface of the bigger mass. (d) Higher magnification of a selected region from (c) showing three glomerulus, one of them depicting a clear vascular pole (arrow). (c and d) Trichromic Masson staining. Calibration bars (a) = 1.5 cm; (b) = 3.2 cm; (c) = 198 $\mu$m; (d) = 52 $\mu$m.

masses were found and removed from the peritoneal cavity. There were no signs of hemorrhage, lesions, or anatomical abnormalities, and the remaining abdominal organs showed normal appearance. In this context, we postulated that these tissue masses could correspond to either a teratoma or an ectopic pregnancy and decided to perform further histological observations.

## 3. Material and Methods

The masses were carefully dissected, cut into 0,5 cm pieces, and immediately fixed by immersion into 10% buffered formalin solution for 24 hours. In order to assess the histological integrity of the tissues, other organs including heart, kidneys, brain, liver, spleen, oviducts, ovaries, and uterus were also dissected and fixed. All the samples were thoroughly dehydrated through graded alcohols before being embedded in paraffin wax.

Several sections 4 $\mu$m thick were obtained from each sample and mounted onto gelatinized slides. Due to the embryonic constitution of the tissue, some difficulties

aroused during the cutting process or the mounting of the sections.

Routine histological analysis was performed using hematoxylin-eosin (H/E), trichromic Masson-staining, and PAP techniques. All sections were observed and photographed under a Zeiss Axiolab light microscopy (Carl Zeiss, Germany).

## 4. Results

The two large tissular masses found in the degus peritoneal cavity are shown in Figures 1(a) and 1(b). They were round in shape, the bigger mass measuring $3 \times 3.5 \times 0.9$ cm and the smaller one $3 \times 1.9 \times 0.9$ cm. Both masses were enveloped by a thin translucent membrane and were profusely irrigated. Under microscopic observation, the others studied organs showed no signs of lesions or degenerative changes that are usually associated to the process of autolysis.

The two masses were united between them by a thin process (see Figure 1(b)) and the bigger one was connected

(a)

(b)

(c)

(d)

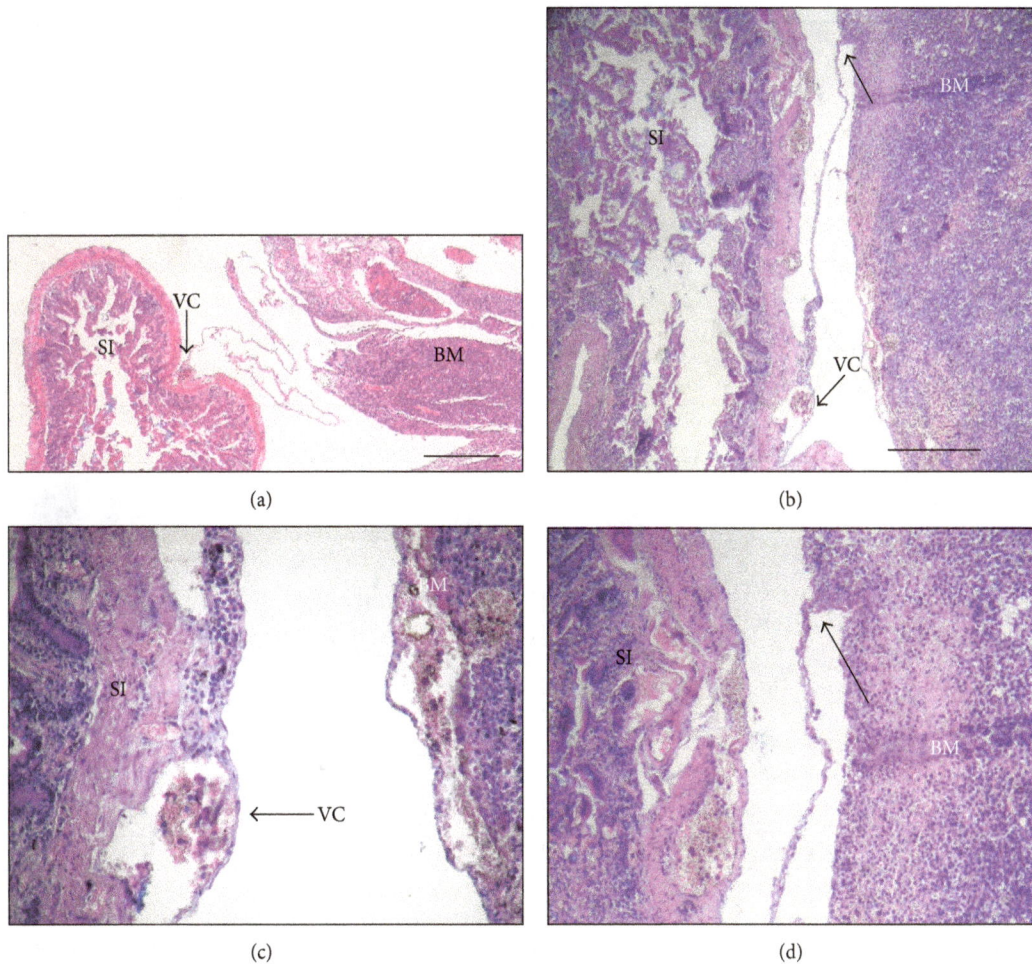

FIGURE 2: Vascular connections of the bigger mass to the small intestine. (a) Photomicrograph showing the vascular connection (VC, arrows) between the bigger mass (BM) and the serosa layer of the small intestine (SI). (b) Another vascular connection (arrows) between the same structures. H/E staining. Calibration bars: (a) = 223 μm; (b) = 223 μm.

to the serosa layer of the small intestine of the animal, as it was evidenced by microscopic observation (Figure 2).

Reproductive organs such as ovaries, oviducts, and both uterine horns displayed normal histological appearance (see Figures 3(a), 3(b), and 3(c)). In one of the ovaries, the presence of two functional corpora lutea was evident and they were surrounded by multiples degenerative corpora lutea (Figure 3(c)). The bicorneal uterus showed some traces of inflammatory secretion in the lumen (Figure 3(a)).

Inside both masses, areas of developing tissues were observed which showed characteristics of kidney (Figures 1(c) and 1(d)) and pancreas (Figure 4). Developing tissues showing characteristics of liver, striated muscle, bone, and suprarenal gland, as well as some fibrous tissue were also observed (not shown).

Histologically, the masses consisted of various tissues derived from all three embryonic germ layers, that is, ectoderm (nervous cells in the pancreas [7] and nerve fibers), mesoderm (kidney, striated muscle, and bone), and endoderm (glandular tissues such as liver and pancreas), but appendages of the skin were not found. Unexpectedly, we observed in the zone between the bigger mass and the small intestine the presence of some chorionic villus (Figure 5), whose aspect resembled that observed in the human placenta. Briefly, each villus consisted of a central core of loose connective tissue surrounded by a double layer of trophoblast, an outer syncytiotrophoblast and an inner cytotrophoblast. The core contained the fetal placental capillaries (Figures 5(b) and 5(d)) [8]. It must be emphasized that, in the degu's placental barrier, the fetal capillaries are separated from the maternal blood by a single layer of labyrinthine fine syncytium, derived from the cytotrophoblast of the subplacenta [9, 10]. In addition, a structure resembling an umbilical cord was observed inserted into the bigger mass (Figure 3(d)).

## 5. Discussion

This is the first time that the occurrence of an ectopic pregnancy in the degu is reported, although a direct placental attachment to the maternal viscera was not observed, probably due to scarse development of the subplacenta (cytotrophoblast) which disappear when it differentiates into

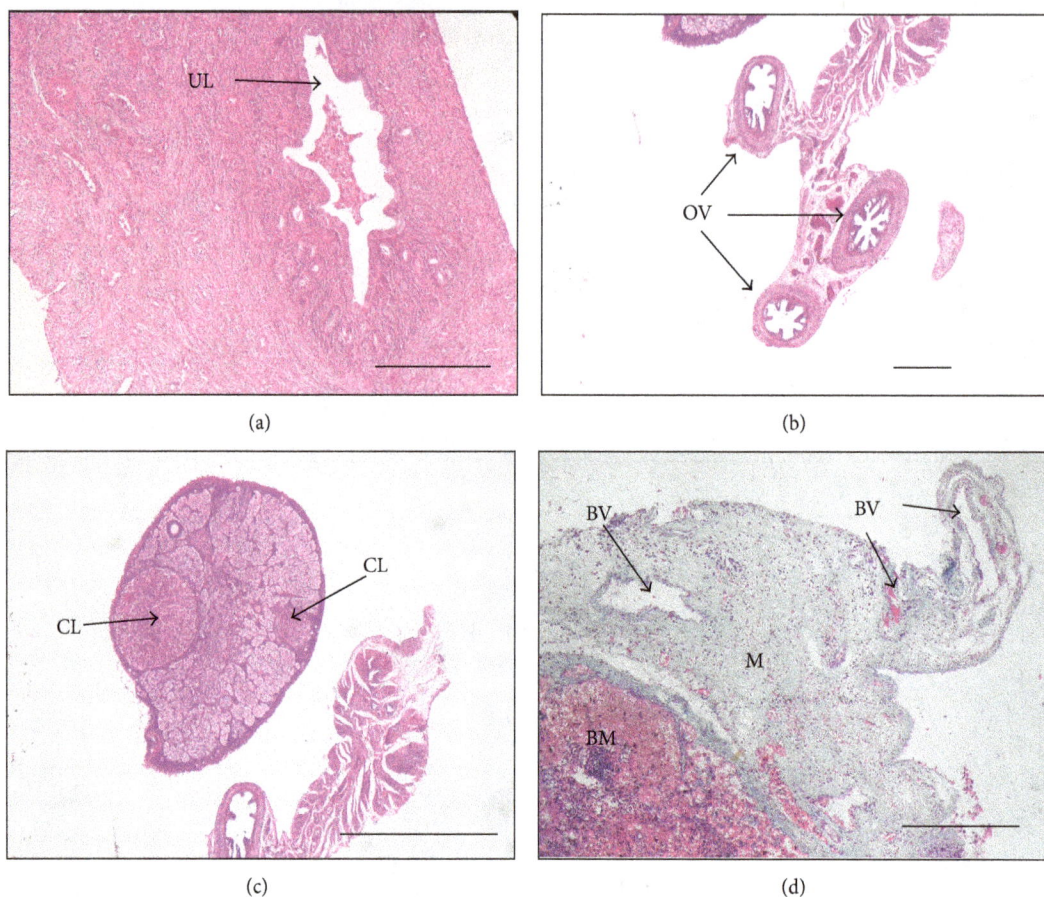

FIGURE 3: Normal aspect of the maternal reproductive organs. (a) The uterus evidences the endometrial, myometrial, and perimetrial layers. The lumen of the organ (UL) shows the presence of some type secretion. (b) Transversal sections of the oviduct (OV) displaying normal evaginations of the mucosa layer. (c) Transversal section of an ovary showing the presence of two functional corpora lutea (CL) surrounded by multiples degenerative corpora lutea. Figure 3(d) shows mesenchymal tissue (M) organized as a structure with large blood vessels (BV), with the appearance of an umbilical cord attached to the bigger mass (BM). (a, b, and c) H/E staining; (d) PAP staining; bars: (a) = 223 $\mu$m; (b) = 245 $\mu$m; (c) = 245 $\mu$m and (d) = 223 $\mu$m.

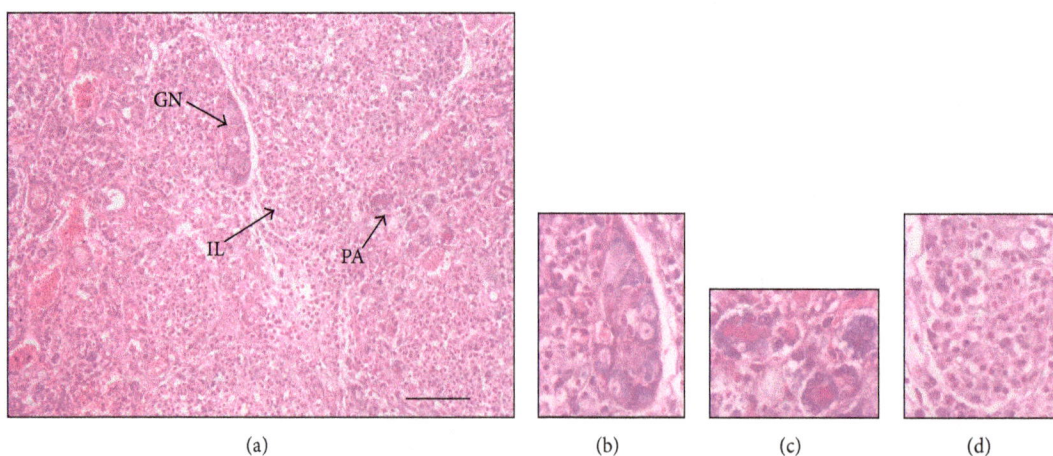

FIGURE 4: Developing pancreatic tissue in the bigger mass. (a) Low magnification microphotograph showing islets of Langerhans (IL) in the endocrine pancreatic tissue and pancreatic acini (PA) in the exocrine portion. A group of ganglionic neurons (GN) can also be observed. (b, c, and d) correspond to higher magnifications of the regions described in (a). H/E staining; bars (a) = 223 $\mu$m; (b) = 179 $\mu$m; (c) = 179 $\mu$m: (d) = 179 $\mu$m.

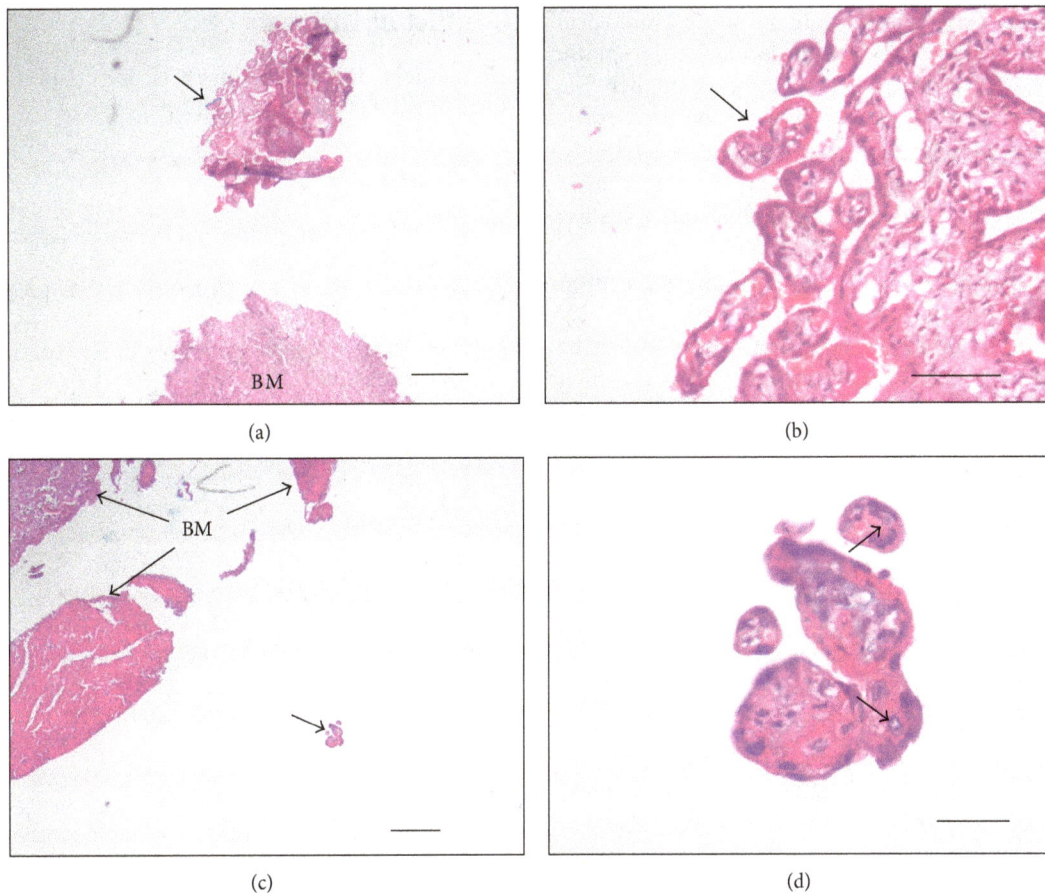

(a)    (b)    (c)    (d)

FIGURE 5: Chorionic villous-like structures observed in the vicinity of the bigger mass. (a) The bigger mass (BM) was found in relation to a number of chorionic villi (arrow) that at higher magnification resemble the human placenta. (b) High magnification of the chorionic villi showed in (a). These villi display a human placental appearance rather than degus. In fact, each villus has a central core of loose connective tissue surrounded by a double layer of trophoblast, an outer syncytiotrophoblast and an inner cytotrophoblast. Fetal placental capillaries in the central core are clearly observed. (c) Spatial relation of the bigger mass (BM) with another group of chorionic villi (CV) with the same human placental appearance as shown in (a and b). (d) Higher magnification of the chorionic villi (arrow) observed in (c) showing the presence of two inner cytotrophoblasts (arrows). H/E staining. Calibration bars: (a) = 245 $\mu$m; (b) = 1225 $\mu$m; (c) = 245 $\mu$m; (d) = 600 $\mu$m.

syncytiotrophoblast [10]. Clinically, there were no pathognomonic signs or symptoms of the presence of these masses in the peritoneal cavity and the animal death was probably the result of compression of surrounding structures such as heart and lungs. There was no apparent antemortem abdominal inflammation, neither fluid accumulation nor necrosis associated to the tissues.

Histologically, the masses consisted of tissues derived from all three embryonic germ layers, but appendages of the skin were not observed. It is well known that teratomas are tumors composed of tissues derived from the three germinal layers of the embryo, but in addition appendages of the skin such as hairs, sebaceous gland, and sweat glands, often associated with dermoid tissue, are frequently presented in teratomas. They may occur either as a cystic lesion, usually benign, or as a solid tumor, usually malignant [11]. Thus, the lack of appendages of the skin and the presence of some villous placental tissue in the findings reported here support the notion of a primary ectopic pregnancy in the degus.

In a guinea pig (other caviomorph rodents) study about ectopic pregnancy, placental attachment to the left peritoneal

wall was clearly identified, but unfortunately the authors failed to show or even describe a placental structure [12]. On the other hand, Buckley and Caine [13] showed in hamster that one out of four ectopic fetuses had a placenta attached to the abdominal surface of the diaphragm and that all the other three fetuses were lying free in the abdomen, with no associated placentae, as occurs in the smaller mass described in this study. The authors concluded that these cases of abdominal pregnancy were more likely to be of the secondary type, in which the placentae have been extruded from the uterus along with one fetus but not with the others. In the present study, we did not observe evidence of uterine rupture or remains of placental tissues in the uterine wall.

We showed that the bigger mass was attached to the serosa layer of the small intestine (Figures 4(a), 4(b), 4(c), and 4(d)) by a number of thin irrigated processes such as those observed by Norén and Lindblom [14] whom, in a human case of abdominal pregnancy, reported that only minimal vascular connection with the peritoneal surface was presented. These authors declared that this was the first report in the literature of an abdominal pregnancy without placental attachment to the maternal viscera. In our study, histological examination showed that there was no decidual-cell response of maternal stromal tissue in the small intestine and therefore the area of placental attachment could not be determined.

In the case reported here, only microscopic observations allowed us to demonstrate that between the bigger mass and the small intestine the degus' scarse chorionic villus has histological characteristics of human placenta.

It is important to note that the placenta of the degu is hemomonochorial and labyrinthine as in the guinea pig [9, 15] and that the degus cytotrophoblast develops from the subplacenta, from which the syncytial labyrinthine placental barrier is formed [10, 16]. On the other hand, Bland and Donovan [17] were able to induce abdominal implantation in guinea pig by introducing fertilized eggs into the peritoneal cavity. These authors found that trophoblast was produced in all cases, but the nontrophoblastic component of these implants was restricted to a mesenchyme-like tissue. They concluded that the higher rate of success (four out of seven animals) in induced abdominal implantation in guinea pigs may have been due to the greater ability of the guinea pig blastocyst to penetrate the peritoneum. In a histological micrograph, these authors showed a subplacenta and invasive trophoblast in the spleen but not the development of a real placental organ as we report in the present study. In addition, Bosco et al. [10, 16] demonstrated that in the degu the cytotrophoblast is found only in the subplacenta and not in the labyrinthine placental barrier as it is known to occur in the human villous placental barrier. In the human species, each villus consists of a central core of loose connective tissue surrounded by a double layer of trophoblast, an outer syncytiotrophoblast and an inner cytotrophoblast that differentiate to syncytiotrophoblast [8], as is the case in this report (see Figures 5(a), 5(b), 5(c), and 5(d)).

The evidence showed here strongly suggests that in the degu the uterine environment provides the cytotrophoblast with exposure to a number of factors that will activate signaling cascades that play a role in determining the developing of the cytotrophoblast into a labyrinthine hemomonochorial placenta. In the absence of uterine environment, as in the case of the peritoneal cavity, the lack of signaling will lead to the development of a villous chorionic placenta with human appearance.

Based on these results, we consider that our case report may motivate molecular biologists to determine the DNA base sequence of human cytotrophoblast in order to compare it with that from the degu subplacenta and thereby ascertain if they may share a common sequence. This would give a stronger support to our proposal of the degu as an experimental animal model for the study of preeclampsia in the early stages of placentation [10, 16].

Finally, we want to emphasize that the discovery of an ectopic pregnancy in a species other than human is often an incidental finding, as animals may show or not clinical signs of fever, lethargy, or anorexia. We want to note that our unexpected discovery corresponds to a serendipity case that allows our minds to observe, act, and propose ideas.

## Conflict of Interests

The authors declare that there is not conflict of interests regarding the publication of this paper.

## References

[1] R. Varma, L. Mascarenhas, and D. James, "Successful outcome of advanced abdominal pregnancy with exclusive omental insertion," *Ultrasound in Obstetrics and Gynecology*, vol. 21, no. 2, pp. 192–194, 2003.

[2] J. M. Corpa, "Ectopic pregnancy in animals and humans," *Reproduction*, vol. 131, no. 4, pp. 631–640, 2006.

[3] C. D. Buergelt and K. Russell, "Ectopic pregnancy in a dog," *Veterinary Medicine*, vol. 99, no. 3, pp. 225–226, 2004.

[4] J. Bouyer, J. Coste, H. Fernandez, J. L. Pouly, and N. Job-Spira, "Sites of ectopic pregnancy: a 10 year population-based study of 1800 cases," *Human Reproduction*, vol. 17, no. 12, pp. 3224–3230, 2002.

[5] A. N. Kalof, B. Fuller, and M. Harmon, "Splenic pregnancy: a case report and review of the literature," *Archives of Pathology & Laboratory Medicine*, vol. 128, no. 11, pp. e146–e148, 2004.

[6] M. A. Onan, A. B. Turp, A. Saltik, N. Akyurek, C. Taskiran, and O. Himmetoglu, "Primary omental pregnancy: case report," *Human Reproduction*, vol. 20, no. 3, pp. 807–809, 2005.

[7] C. Bosco, E. Díaz, R. Gutiérrez, J. González, and J. Pérez, "Ganglionar nervous cells and telocytes in the pancreas of *Octodon degus*: extra and intrapancreatic ganglionar cells and telocytes in the degus," *Autonomic Neuroscience: Basic and Clinical*, vol. 177, no. 2, pp. 224–230, 2013.

[8] C. Bosco, "Morphology of the capillaries in the alpha and beta zone of human term placenta: the relationship between capillary morphology and the trophoblastic layer," *Medical Science Research*, vol. 22, no. 2, pp. 115–117, 1994.

[9] C. Bosco, "Ultrastructure of the degu term placental barrier (*Octodon degus*): a labyrinthine hemomonochorial placental model," *Medical Science Research*, vol. 23, no. 1, pp. 15–18, 1997.

[10] C. Bosco, C. Buffet, M. A. Bello, R. Rodrigo, M. Gutierrez, and G. García, "Placentation in the degu (*Octodon degus*): analogies with extrasubplacental trophoblast and human extravillous trophoblast," *Comparative Biochemistry and Physiology A: Molecular and Integrative Physiology*, vol. 146, no. 4, pp. 475–485, 2007.

[11] A. Marcolongo, G. Divirgilio, G. Bettili et al., "Immature mesenteric teratoma in a male newborn infant: prenatal ultrasonographic diagnosis and surgical treatment," *Prenatal Diagnosis*, vol. 17, no. 7, pp. 686–688, 1997.

[12] C. C. Hong and M. L. Armstrong, "Ectopic pregnancy in 2 guinea-pigs," *Laboratory Animals*, vol. 12, no. 4, pp. 243–244, 1978.

[13] P. Buckley and A. Caine, "A high incidence of abdominal pregnancy in the Djungarian hamster (*Phodopus sungorus*)," *Journal of Reproduction and Fertility*, vol. 56, no. 2, pp. 679–682, 1979.

[14] H. Norén and B. Lindblom, "A unique case of abdominal pregnancy: what are the minimal requirements for placental contact with the maternal vascular bed?" *American Journal of Obstetrics and Gynecology*, vol. 155, no. 2, pp. 394–396, 1986.

[15] B. F. King and A. C. Enders, "The fine structure of the guinea pig visceral yolk sac placenta," *American Journal of Anatomy*, vol. 127, no. 4, pp. 394–414, 1970.

[16] C. Bosco and C. Buffet, "Immunohistochemical identification of the extravillous trophoblast during the placentation of the degu (*Octodon degus*)," *Journal of Experimental Zoology B*, vol. 310, no. 6, pp. 534–539, 2008.

[17] K. P. Bland and B. T. Donovan, "Experimental ectopic implantation of eggs and early embryos in guinea-pigs," *Journal of Reproduction and Fertility*, vol. 10, no. 2, pp. 189–196, 1965.

# 25

# Incidental Intracranial Aneurysm in a Dog Detected by 16-Multidetector Row Computed Tomography Angiography

## Giovanna Bertolini

*San Marco Veterinary Clinic, Diagnostic Imaging Division, Via Sorio 114/c, 35141 Padova, Italy*

Correspondence should be addressed to Giovanna Bertolini; bertolini@sanmarcovet.it

Academic Editors: C. Gutierrez, S. C. Rahal, and S. Stuen

This paper describes a small intracranial aneurysm incidentally found in a 24-month-old Nova Scotia Duck Tolling Retriever evaluated for a recent history of lethargy, fever, and cervical pain. The clinicopathological analysis revealed leukocytosis, and increased haptoglobin and C-reactive protein consistent with severe flogistic process. Nonenhanced computed tomography of the brain and cervical spine showed a diffuse encephalopathy and moderate cervical syringohydromyelia. Computed tomography angiography series of the brain showed a small saccular dilation at the joining point of the two rostral cerebral arteries consistent with a small aneurysm. Cerebrospinal fluid examination led to the final diagnosis of aseptic meningitis. The dog was discharge with a long-term corticosteroid therapy for the meningitis. At two-month follow-up evaluation, the cerebrospinal fluid examination was normal and the computed tomography of the brain showed no abnormalities except for the stable aneurysm. To our knowledge, this is the first description of a spontaneous cerebral aneurysm in dogs and serves to broaden the spectrum of cerebrovascular diseases in this species.

## 1. Introduction

A brain aneurysm is an abnormal, outward pouching of the artery wall caused by a weakness in the wall of an artery that supplies the brain. In humans, the prevalence of this condition is about 5%. Approximately, 85% of aneurysms develop in the anterior portion of the circulation of the brain and are asymptomatic until they rupture [1–3]. Cerebral aneurysms are classified based on a number of features including etiology, size, shape, the association with the specific intracranial branch, or according to their angioarchitecture features [2, 4–6].

To date, very little is known concerning the type and incidence of variants and anomalies of the cerebrovascular system in dogs and cats [7–9]. Historically, few cases of cerebral hemorrhage in dogs were thought to be correlated to aneurysm, but their existence could not be proved [10]. To the authors knowledge, this is the first description of a spontaneous cerebral aneurysm in dogs.

## 2. Case Presentation

A 24-month-old 22 kg intact male Nova Scotia Duck Tolling Retriever was evaluated for a recent history of lethargy, fever, and cervical pain. Medical history included another episode of cervical pain that has occurred one year before and rapidly improved with corticosteroid therapy for few days. At the time of presentation, the dog was receiving amoxicillin/clavulanic acid for 2 days (10 mg/kg PO q12).

At physical examination, the dog showed ventroflexion of the neck and was tachypneic (80 breath/min), with 39.3°C rectal temperature and normal heart rate (96 beats/min), increased blood pressure (120–180 mmHg, mean 145 mmHg), and normal mucous membrane appearance and capillary refill time (approximately 1 sec). Heart and thoracic auscultation were normal. Abdominal palpation revealed splenomegaly.

At neurological examination, the dog had cervical rigidity and cervical pain. Cranial nerve function, postural reaction testing, and segmental spinal reflexes were normal. The CBC showed leukocytosis accompanied by a "left shift" in the ratio of immature to mature neutrophils. Serum biochemistry profile showed increased haptoglobin and C-reactive protein. These clinicopathological results indicated a severe flogistic process.

Thoracic and cervical radiographs were normal. Abdominal ultrasound confirmed a diffuse subjective enlargement

(a)

(b)

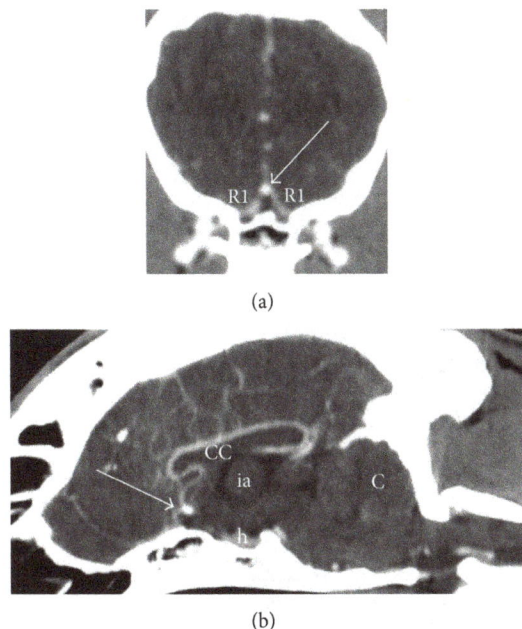

FIGURE 1: Multiplanar reformatted images (MPRs) of the neurocranium. (a) Transverse (slight oblique) view showing the small aneurysm (arrow) at the joining point of the two R1 segments of the left and right rostral cerebral arteries. (b) Mid-sagittal view of the same dog. The arrow indicates the aneurysm. CC: corpus callosum; ia: interthalamic adhesion; C: cerebellum; h: hypophysis.

FIGURE 2: Volume rendering (VR) of the skull, dorsal view. The vault of the skull has been removed to visualize the circulus arteriosus cerebralis (Circle of Willis). RCA: rostral cererbal artery; MCA: middle cerebral artery; ICA: internal carotid artery; CCA: caudal cerebral artery; CCoA: caudal communicating artery; BA: basilar artery; h: hypophysis. The arrow indicates the small aneurysm at the joining point of the two rostral cerebral arteries (RCAs).

of the spleen, but no other anomalies were noted. The dog was then placed under general anesthesia and underwent 16-multidetector-CT (GE Lightspeed 16, GE Medical Systems, Milwaukee, WI) examination of the neurocranium, cervical spine, and abdomen. For the neurocranium, unenhanced scans were obtained followed by an angiographic series. The acquisition, dose, and reconstruction parameters were axial modality, 2 s/rotation, caudal-to-rostral direction, 16 × 0.625 mm detector configuration, 120 kVp, 210 mAs, standard algorithm. For brain CTA, 640 mg I/kg of iodixanol (Visipaque320, Amersham Health, Princeton, HJ) was injected at 37°C at a rate of 4 mL/s using a power injector system, (Stellant, Medrad, Indianola, IA) through a 20 gauge catheter placed in the left cephalic vein. An injection-to-scan delay of 10 sec. was used. Original data sets of $512^2$ matrix size were transferred to a freestanding workstation (Advantage Workstation 4.1, GE Medical Systems, Milwaukee, WI) and postprocessed using multiplanar reformation (MPR), maximum intensity projection (MIP), and volume rendering (VR) techniques. Unenhanced CT of the neurocranium revealed a moderate diffuse hypoattenuation of the white matter. In the cervical spine, a slight dilation of the central canal was noted. These CT features were consistent with a diffuse encephalopathy and moderate cervical syringohydromyelia. The CTA series of the brain showed the two rostral cerebral arteries anastomosed with each other rostro-dorsally to the optic chiasm forming a single median artery. At the joining point there was a small saccular dilation, enhancing at the same degree of the arteries, consistent with a small aneurysm (Figures 1, 2, and 3). Measurements of the aneurysm were

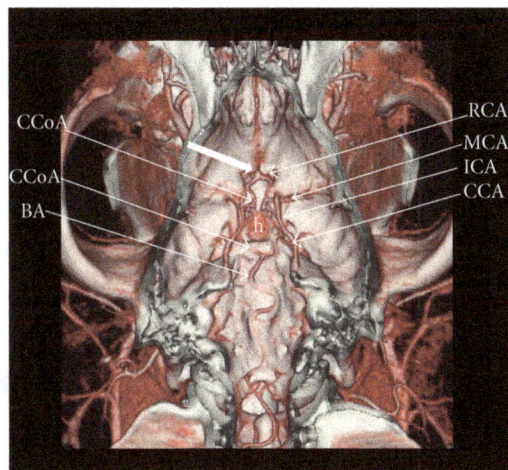

performed from magnified MPR images with an electronic caliper at the workstation. The aneurysm was 1.3 mm at the neck point, 2.0 mm in width, and 1.8 mm in height (Figure 4).

Contrast-enhanced abdominal CT revealed a saccular dilation of the prehepatic segment of the portal vein and a small dilation of the umbilical part of the left portal branch within the liver. These features were consistent with extrahepatic and intrahepatic portal vein aneurysms.

Cisternal cerebrospinal fluid (CSF) was collected at the end of the CT scans. CSF had 324 white blood cells/$\mu$L (reference range, ≤5 cells/$\mu$L), 142 red blood cells/$\mu$L, and 21 mg/dL protein (reference range, ≤25). Glucose concentration was 76 mg/dL (reference range, 53–104 mg/dL). The differential cell count indicated a neutrophilic and macrophagic pleocytosis (80% neutrophils and 20% macrophages).

Based on these findings, the final diagnosis was of aseptic meningitis. The dog was discharged with a long-term corticosteroid therapy. The owner reported that the dog had a rapid improvement, and at two-month follow-up evaluation, the cerebrospinal fluid examination was normal. CT of the neurocranium showed the rostral cerebral small aneurysm stable. The enhanced abdominal scan showed a large filling defect in the aneurysmal portal vein, consistent with thrombosed portal vein aneurysm. The small intrahepatic aneurysm was stable. Followup by CT scan and/or US of the abdomen was suggested.

## 3. Discussion

The overall schema of the blood supply to the cranial region and the brain, the histological structure of the walls of the arteries, and the basic pattern of the embryological development are essentially the same in dog as they are in man (Figure 5) [7, 11]. Many variations of the Circle of Willis have

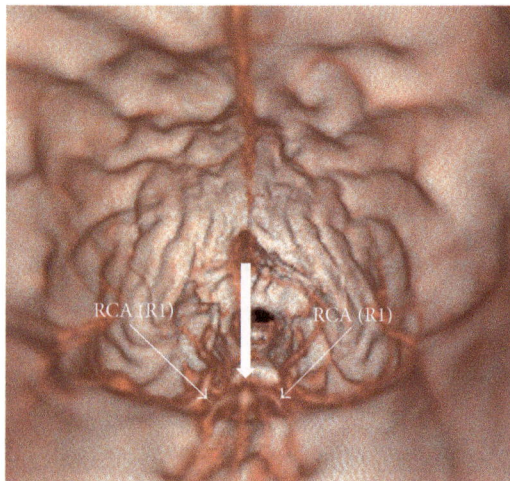

(a)

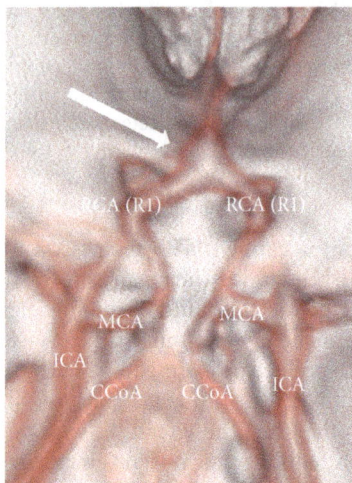

(b)

FIGURE 3: Virtual navigation through the cranial cavity. (a) Forward view, showing the small saccular aneurysm at the joining point of the two pre-joining segments (R1) of the left and right rostral cerebral arteries. (b) Dorsal backward view of the Circle of Willis showing the small aneurysm (arrow). RCA: rostral cerebral artery; R1: pre-joining segment; MCA: middle cerebral artery; ICA: internal carotid artery; CCoA: caudal communicating artery.

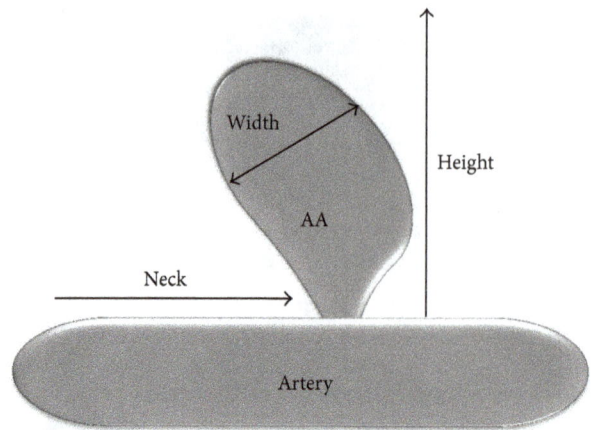

FIGURE 4: Drawing showing the measurement technique of the saccular aneurysm (AA).

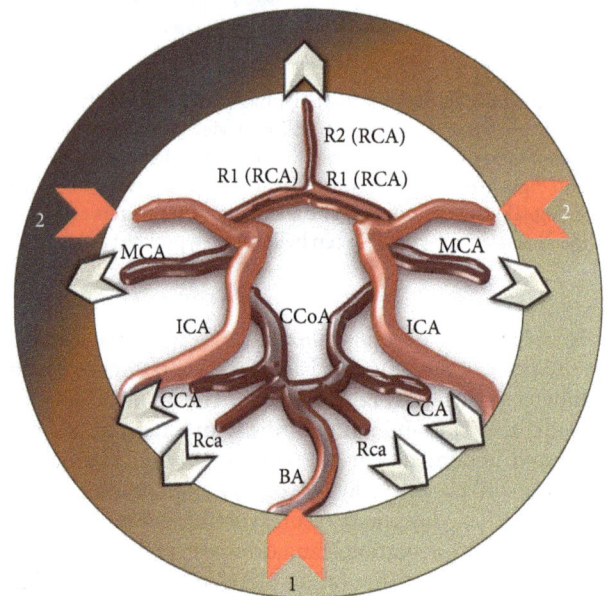

FIGURE 5: The drawing shows the blood flow to the Circle of Willis from the three vessels: 1, basilar artery (BA), and 2, internal carotid arteries (ICAs). From internal carotid arteries, blood flows from circle of Willis to the brain through the rostral cerebral arteries (RCA). The anterior communicating artery that connects the two anterior cerebral arteries in humans is rarely described in dogs. However, either the canine rostral cerebral artery can be subdivided into a pre-joining point (R1) and, generally, in a single median R2 segment (post-joining). Internal carotid artery gives off the median cerebral arteries (MCAs) and the caudal communicating arteries (CCoAs), that connect the circle with the basilar artery. In most dogs, the caudal cerebral artery (CCA) and the rostral cerebellar artery (RcAs) are from the caudal communicating artery.

been described in humans, and they play a significant role in the cerebral aneurysms formation, in terms of hemodynamic stress caused by variations [12, 13]. In contrast, variants of the Circle of Willis have been rarely described in dog so far [7, 14, 15]. In most dogs, the two rostral arteries form a common median trunk, as described in the present case.

In humans, various shear stresses (flow, turbulences, jet effects, and others) are known to produce aneurysms. These represent "luminal" aneurysmal vasculopathies in which it is postulated that these stresses induce pathogenetic changes in normal vessel walls. In contrast, structural vessel-wall diseases (inflammatory, infectious, collagen diseases, and others) are "abluminal" aneurysmal vasculopathies. In these, there is a primary abnormality of the vessel wall which is potentially aggravated by shear stresses [1, 3–6].

From the clinical point of view, most human patients have no symptoms or complaints until the aneurysm ruptures. Neurological signs in our patient were attributed to the meningitis. The meningitis of our Nova Scotia Duck

Tolling Retriever was diagnosed as aseptic meningitis, a noninfectious inflammatory disorder frequently diagnosed in this breed of dog [16]. Aetiological hypotheses of the cerebral aneurysm in our dog include congenital weakness or degenerative changes in vessel walls due to a connective tissue disorder or a local inflammatory process. This dog had simultaneous extrahepatic and intrahepatic portal vein aneurysms. Portal vein aneurysm is a rare condition we recently described in a series of dogs including the dog of this paper [17]. Aneurysm of the portal vein can be either congenital or acquired and thrombosis of the aneurysmal portal vein with its consequences is a possible complication. The development of more than one aneurysm at different site is an uncommon event in human patients [18, 19] and it has been reported once in a dog [20].

This incidentally discovered cerebral aneurysm broads the spectrum of cerebrovascular diseases in dogs. Intracranial vessels can now be routinely assessed in living animals using CT and magnetic resonance (MR) imaging [21–24]. With the widespread use of these advanced imaging technologies, the potential to identify variants of the Circle of Willis or anomalies of the cerebrovascular system in dogs can substantially increase. Moreover, the non- or minimally invasive nature of these techniques, combined with the ability to obtain information about the brain parenchyma within the same examination, represents a clear advantage of CT-angiography (CTA) and MR angiography (MRA) over all other imaging techniques [21–23].

# References

[1] T. Krings, D. M. Mandell, T. R. Kiehl et al., "Intracranial aneurysms: from vessel wall pathology to therapeutic approach," Nature Reviews Neurology, vol. 7, no. 10, pp. 547–559, 2011.

[2] M. B. Pritz, "Cerebral aneurysm classification based on angioarchitecture," Journal of Stroke and Cerebrovascular Diseases, vol. 20, no. 2, pp. 162–167, 2011.

[3] I. Loumiotis, A. Wagenbach, R. D. Brown Jr., and G. Lanzino, "Small (< 10-mm) incidentally found intracranial aneurysms, part 1: reasons for detection, demographics, location, and risk factors in 212 consecutive patients," Neurosurg Focus, vol. 31, no. 6, p. E3, 2011.

[4] F. Bonneville, N. Sourour, and A. Biondi, "Intracranial aneurysms: an overview," Neuroimaging Clinics of North America, vol. 16, no. 3, pp. 371–382, 2006.

[5] M. A. Castro, C. M. Putman, M. J. Sheridan, and J. R. Cebral, "Hemodynamic patterns of anterior communicating artery aneurysms: a possible association with rupture," American Journal of Neuroradiology, vol. 30, no. 2, pp. 297–302, 2009.

[6] T. J. Grobelny, "Brain aneurysms: epidemiology, treatment options, and milestones of endovascular treatment evolution," Disease-a-Month, vol. 57, no. 10, pp. 647–655, 2011.

[7] K. Kapoor, V. K. Kak, and B. Singh, "Morphology and comparative anatomy of circulus arteriosus cerebri in mammals." Anatomia, Histologia, Embryologia, vol. 32, no. 6, pp. 347–355, 2003.

[8] W. R. Hause, M. L. Helphrey, R. W. Green, and P. C. Stromberg, "Cerebral arteriovenous malformation in a dog," Journal of the American Animal Hospital Association, vol. 18, pp. 601–607, 1982.

[9] W. B. Thomas, R. O. Scheuler, and J. N. Kornegay, "Surgical excision of a cerebral arteriovenous malformation in a dog," Progress in Veterinary Neurology, vol. 6, pp. 20–23, 1995.

[10] J. T. McGrath, Neurologic Examination of the Dog with Clinico-Pathologic Observations, Lea & Febiger, Philadelphia, Pa, USA, 2nd edition, 1960.

[11] O. Shaller, Illustrated Veterinary Anatomic Nomenclature, Georg Thieme, 2nd edition, 2007.

[12] A. F. van Raamt, W. P. Mali, P. J. van Laar, and Y. van der Graaf, "The fetal variant of the circle of Willis and its influence on the cerebral collateral circulation.," Cerebrovascular Diseases, vol. 22, no. 4, pp. 217–224, 2006.

[13] K. Kapoor, B. Singh, and L. I. J. Dewan, "Variations in the configuration of the circle of Willis," Anatomical Science International, vol. 83, no. 2, pp. 96–106, 2008.

[14] W. E. Stehbens, "Cerebral aneurysms of animals other than man," The Journal of Pathology and Bacteriology, vol. 86, pp. 160–168, 1963.

[15] R. Frankhauser, H. Luginbuhl, and J. T. McGrath, "Cerebrovascular disease in various animal species," Annals of the New York Academy of Sciences, vol. 127, no. 1, pp. 817–860, 1965.

[16] K. P. Anfinsen, M. Berendt, F. J. H. Liste et al., "A retrospective epidemiological study of clinical signs and familial predisposition associated with aseptic meningitis in the Norwegian population of Nova Scotia duck tolling retrievers born 1994–2003," Canadian Journal of Veterinary Research, vol. 72, no. 4, pp. 350–355, 2008.

[17] G. Bertolini and M. Caldin, "Computed tomography findings in portal vein aneurysm of dogs," The Veterinary Journal, vol. 193, no. 2, pp. 475–480, 2012.

[18] W. J. Henry, "Multiple aneurysm formation in a young man: a case report," Annals of surgery, vol. 158, pp. 1043–1046, 1963.

[19] Y. Ito, K. Tarao, S. Tamai et al., "Portal vein aneurysm in the liver associated with multiple vascular malformations," Journal of Gastroenterology, vol. 29, no. 6, pp. 776–781, 1994.

[20] K. R. Salmeri, J. R. Bellah, N. Ackerman, and B. Homer, "Unilateral congenital aneurysm of the jugular, linguofacial, and maxillary veins in a dog," Journal of the American Veterinary Medical Association, vol. 198, no. 4, pp. 651–654, 1991.

[21] M. Sager, J. Assheuer, H. Trümmler, and K. Moormann, "Contrast-enhanced magnetic resonance angiography (CE-MRA) of intra- and extra-cranial vessels in dogs," Veterinary Journal, vol. 179, no. 1, pp. 92–100, 2009.

[22] P. Martin-Vaquero, R. C. da Costa, R. L. Echandi, C. L. Tosti, M. V. Knopp, and S. Sammet, "Time-of-flight magnetic resonance angiography of the canine brain at 3.0 Tesla and 7.0 Tesla," American Journal of Veterinary Research, vol. 72, no. 3, pp. 350–356, 2011.

[23] A. S. Tidwell and I. D. Robertson, "Magnetic resonance imaging of normal and abnormal brain perfusion," Veterinary Radiology and Ultrasound, vol. 52, no. 1, supplement 1, pp. S62–S71, 2011.

[24] O. D. Jacqmot, F. R. Snaps, N. M. Maquet, M. P. Heinen, and A. E. Gabriel, "Arterial head vascularization cartographies of normal metencephalic dogs using magnetic resonance angiography," The Anatomical Record, vol. 294, no. 11, pp. 1834–1841, 2011.

# 26

# Unicameral Bone Cyst in the Proximal Humerus with Secondary Infection in an 18-Month-Old Foal

**Maria C. Fugazzola, Christoph Klaus, and Christoph Lischer**

*The Department of Veterinary Clinical Sciences, Unit of Equine Medicine and Surgery, University of Teramo (Fugazzola); V.le Crispi-Loc. Cartecchio, 64100 Teramo and Klinik für Pferde, Free University of Berlin (Klaus and Lischer) Oertzenweg 19b, 14163 Berlin, Germany*

Correspondence should be addressed to Maria C. Fugazzola; maria.fugazzola@gmail.com

Academic Editor: Jeffrey Lakritz

An 18-month-old warmblood filly was 4/5 lame on the front right limb at referral and showed severe swelling of the right shoulder region and pain during manipulation of the shoulder region. Radiography revealed a roundish 5 × 7 cm radiolucent area with defined borders within the greater tubercle and the presence of a fracture of the lateral tubercle associated with the cyst. Cellular blood count was 27,500 WBC/μL and serum biochemical analyses revealed fibrinogen of 855 mg/dL. The fractured bone was removed surgically; the cyst debrided and filled with autologous cancellous bone graft. Three and five weeks after surgery the filly was reoperated on because of an osseous sequestrum and a periostal defect on the distal dorsolateral aspect of the pastern of the right hind limb and a septic synovitis of the DFTS of the left hind limb. Fifteen month after surgery the filly was not lame and was introduced to training. Unicameral bone cysts (UBC) are well described lesions, often associated to pathologic fracture in the proximal humerus of children but, until present, no scientific report exists of UBC in the foal. The prompt surgical management had a favorable outcome.

## 1. Case Details

An 18-month-old warmblood filly which was kept on pasture with other foals was referred to the clinic for horses of the Free University of Berlin because of sudden onset of severe lameness of the right front limb and a swelling in the shoulder region.

At presentation the horse was 4/5 lame (AAEP scale) on the front right limb showing a severe firm swelling of the shoulder region. Palpation revealed an increased skin temperature and elicited a painful response. All vital parameters were within normal range.

## 2. Diagnostic Imaging

A lateromedial and a cranio 45° medial-caudolateral oblique view of the scapulohumeral joint and a cranioproximal-craniodistal oblique view of the humeral tubercles revealed a roundish 5 × 7 cm radiolucent area with defined, unreactive borders within the greater tubercle; the lesion was visible in all three projections. A 4 cm long partly detached bony fragment lateral to the radiolucent area could be detected in the cranioproximal-craniodistal oblique projection (Figure 1).

The epiphyseal growth plate of the proximal humerus was visible distal to the greater tubercle in the lateromedial projection at the level of the radiolucent area (Figure 2).

The ultrasonographic examination confirmed effusion of the bicipital bursa with no evidence of pathological changes of the bicipital tendon. Furthermore, a fracture associated with the insertion of the infraspinatus tendon was diagnosed in the dorsolateral aspect of the proximal humerus (Figure 3).

Fluid retrieved from the bicipital bursa had a brown discolored appearance and contained 9600 nucleated cells/μL and 5 gr/dL proteins (reference values: <1000 cells/μL and 0,5–1 g/dL total protein). Cellular blood count was 27,500 WBC/μL and serum biochemical analyses

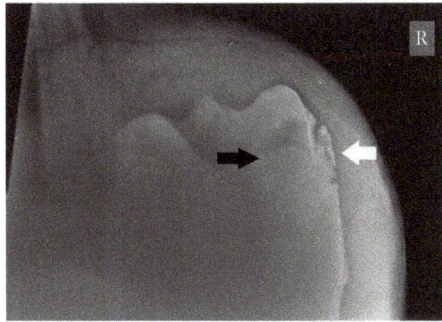

FIGURE 1: Cranioproximal-craniodistal oblique projection on the humeral tubercles: a 4 cm long partly detached bony fragment (white arrow) lateral to the radiolucent area (black arrow) is visible.

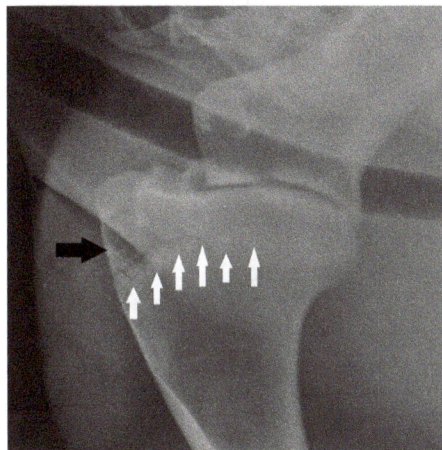

FIGURE 2: Lateromedial projection of the humerus: the epiphyseal growth plate of the proximal humerus (white arrows) is visible distal to the greater tubercle at the level of the radiolucent area (black arrow).

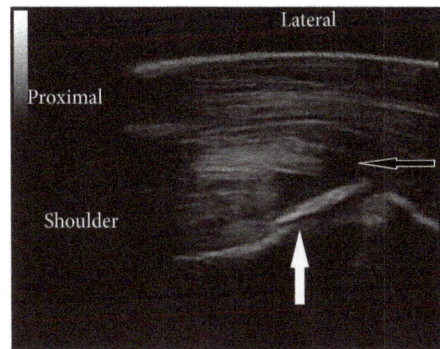

FIGURE 3: Ultrasound image of the lateral aspect of the greater tubercle of the humerus: a bony fragment (white arrow) associated with the insertion of the infraspinatus tendon (white empty arrow) on the distal aspect of the greater tubercle is visible.

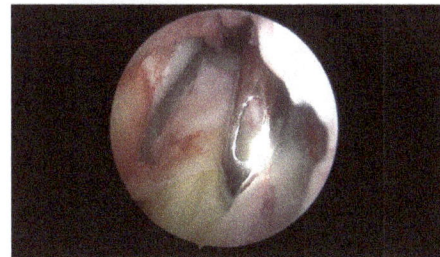

FIGURE 4: Bursoscopic image of the bicipital bursa: small amounts of fibrin pannus were found adherent to the bursal wall.

revealed 855 mg/dL of fibrinogen (reference values: 4,000–12,000 WBC/$\mu$L and <300 mg/dL fibrinogen). All other CBC and biochemical parameters were within reference range.

The severe lameness, the probably septic bursitis of the intertubercular bursa, and the presence of the fracture close to the bone cyst determined the decision to treat the case surgically.

Under general anesthesia the filly was placed in lateral recumbency with the affected limb uppermost. The bicipital bursa was flushed during bursoscopy and small amounts of fibrin pannus were found adherent to the bursal wall, which was partially torn on its lateral aspect (Figure 4). No cartilaginous lesions could be detected in the intertubercular grooves.

A 15 cm long incision was performed in a proximodistal direction over the caudal eminence of the lateral tubercle, slightly distal to the infraspinatus tendon insertion. Dissection was performed bluntly until bone was exposed. The fractured bone was found in close proximity to the infraspinatus tendons attachment to the lateral tubercle and was removed. A cystic lesion of the tubercle became visible underlying the fragment, containing yellowish discolored fluid and fibrous

material that was evacuated and sent for histopathologic and microbiologic examination. After thorough debridement (Figure 5) and flushing with a disinfectant the bony defect was packed with autologous cancellous bone graft previously harvested from the ipsilateral tuber coxae.

Surgical closure was performed in 3 layers and the site was protected with a stent bandage until the day after surgery. Recovery from anesthesia was uneventful and an antibiotic therapy with ceftiofur sodium at 2,2 mg/kg (IM, q24h) was administered for 5 days postoperatively and then shifted to sulfonamide 25 mg/kg and trimethoprim 5 mg/kg (PO q12h) for 5 additional days. Anti-inflammatory medication consisted of phenylbutazone 2,2 mg/kg (PO q12h) that was discontinued when clinical symptoms had ceased.

CBC and plasma fibrinogen values were monitored every second day until discharge and showed a steady decrease with return to reference range by day 12 after surgery.

Histopathology of the cystic content revealed purulent-necrotic trabecular bone with fibrotic lining. Microbial culture revealed a severe gram positive *Staphylococcus (Sp. S. aureus)* infection with sensitivity among others to trimethoprim sulfonamide and ceftiofur.

Within two weeks the swelling of the shoulder had almost resolved completely and the filly was not lame at walk in the right front but showed a mild lameness on the hind right limb. Radiographically the cyst of the humerus showed a sclerotic rim (Figure 6). The hind right pastern region showed a warm,

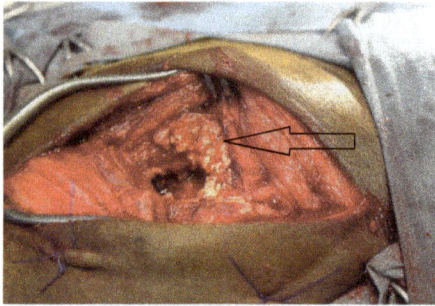

FIGURE 5: View of the bone cyst opening after debridement: proximal to the right and distal to the left. The debrided infraspinatus fibres (black arrow) are visible dorsal to the cyst opening.

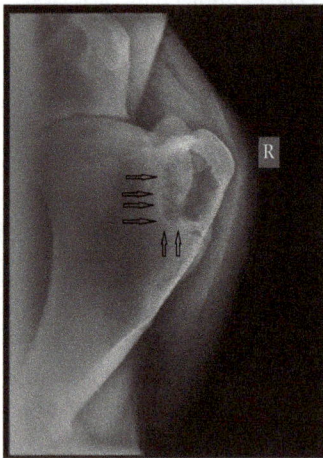

FIGURE 6: Cranial 45° medial-caudolateral view of the humerus two weeks after surgery: the radiolucent area shows a sclerotic rim (black arrows).

painful swelling and the hind left digital flexor tendon sheath was mildly distended.

The dorsomedial-plantarolateral radiographic view of the right hind pastern showed osseous modelling of the periosteal surface of the distal dorsolateral aspect of the proximal phalanx, which could be confirmed by ultrasound. The proximal interphalangeal joint was not distended and synovial fluid could not be retrieved. Due to the strong suspect of a septic process spreading to the pastern, regional limb perfusion with 2 gr of amikacin was performed twice in the following 4 days. Oral antibiotic administration of sulfonamide 25 mg/kg and trimethoprim 5 mg/kg, q12h was resumed.

As after two weeks of antibiotic therapy no clinical improvement of the condition could be observed, diagnostic imaging of the right hind pastern was repeated showing progression of the periosteal reaction, in addition to the presence of a sequestrum and an osteolytic defect on the distal dorsolateral aspect of the proximal phalanx. Based on the assumption of an osteomyelitic process, the decision was made to remove the sequestrum and debride the site under general anesthesia. Due to the close proximity to the proximal interphalangeal joint a CT scan of the region was performed

preceding the surgery (Figures 7(a) and 7(b)), in order to allow a precise localization and surgical approach. Before the skin incision was performed, the synovial fluid from the still notably distended hind left DFTS was analyzed. Values at this point were within reference ranges (cell number: 700 cells/$\mu$L, protein: 0,8 gr/dL). A skin incision was made at the area of the sequestrum, which could be located and removed. An irregular osseous defect 1 cm long was debrided and flushed thoroughly. The proximal interphalangeal joint was opened during the procedure, since the joint capsule had its proximal attachment to the proximal phalanx in correspondence of the osteolytic site. Regional limb perfusion with 2 gr of amikacin was repeated during surgery and two days after surgery.

Histopathologic examination of parts of proximal interphalangeal joint capsule of the hind right showed a subacute capsulitis and synovitis with predominant lymphocytic and less neutrophilic infiltration; the cancellous bone that was removed through debridement of the osteomyelitic site on the distal aspect of the proximal phalanx showed only minimal lymphocytic infarction. Culture revealed colonies of *Staphylococcus aureus* two days later.

To identify a potential primary source of infection, ultrasonography of the heart, the lung, and the abdomen was performed with no relevant findings.

Six weeks after admission, the filly became lame on the left hind limb (grade 2/5); the distention of the DFTS in this limb had not regressed. Radiographic views of the left hind pastern showed no detectable abnormalities and synoviocentesis revealed a septic synovitis (protein 3 g/dL, 17400 cells/$\mu$L with 92% of neutrophils). Flushing of the tendon sheath was performed under general anesthesia. Oral administration of sulfonamide 25 mg/kg and trimethoprim 5 mg/kg, q12h was continued until 5 days after the tenovaginoscopy. Ten days after flushing the tendon sheath the lameness of the hind left had resolved.

Two months after admission to the clinic, the filly was discharged with grade 1/5 lameness on the right hind limb.

A clinical and radiographic follow-up examination was performed 6 and 15 months after admission to the clinic. The mare was not lame at trot. Radiographically the bone defect of the greater tubercle of the humerus showed radiopaque content within a sclerotic rim (Figure 8). The periostal defect of the hind right pastern showed an irregular dorsolateral osseous profile but no radiolucencies were visible any more. The mare started training successfully two months later.

## 3. Discussion

In pediatric medicine UBC is a single-chambered lesion that occurs mostly in the proximal humerus of skeletally immature individuals [1]. When such cysts are immediately adjacent to a growth plate, they are referred to as active cysts, whilst when they are distant from the growth plate they are considered to be latent cysts [1]. It is estimated that approximately 75% of children with unicameral bone cysts present pathological fractures involving the cyst location due to weakening of the bone [2]. In our case location of the cyst within the proximal aspect of the humerus, skeletal immaturity, and fracture involving the cyst match presentation

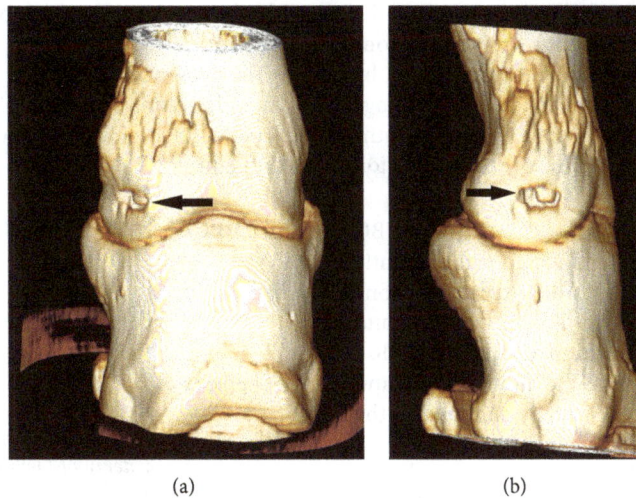

(a)                                                 (b)

FIGURE 7: (a) and (b) 3D reconstruction of a CT scan of the hind right proximal interphalangeal joint area from a dorsal and lateral view. The osteolytic defect and the sequestrum (arrow) on the distal dorsolateral aspect of the proximal phalanx are visible.

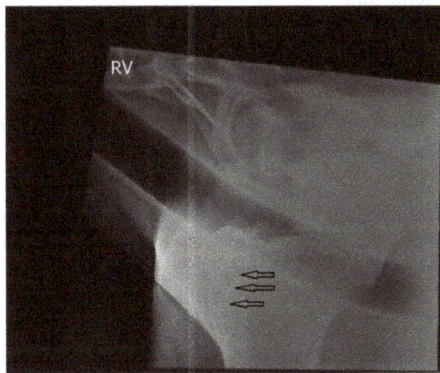

FIGURE 8: Lateromedial projection of the humerus 15 months after surgery: the bone defect of the humeral greater tubercle shows radiopaque content within a sclerotic rim.

criteria of a UBC. The characteristic radiographic appearance with absence of sclerotic rim and the involvement of the proximal growth-plate of the humerus represent a further typical feature which was evident also in the filly. Most cysts in pediatric medicine are an incidental finding when radiographs are taken for other reasons, proving that unless fractured they may be asymptomatic [1, 3]. The symptoms of UBC are most often brought on by trauma [2]. In the present case the filly was kept with other yearling on pasture and was referred to be moderately lame from one day to the other. The most probably explanation for this would be a traumatic event that caused the humeral tubercle to fracture in the weakened location. During this trauma an undetected penetrating wound could then explain the infection with *Staphylococcus aureus* and explain the rapid worsening of the clinical symptoms, including swelling of the bicipital bursa in the following days preceding referral. The secondary spreading from the cyst to two distant sites would consequently be hematogenous. Alternatively the presence of septicemia, previously to the trauma, could have caused an infection of

the cyst and a consequent hematogenous spreading to the hind right pastern and the hind left DFTS. UBC are fluid filled chambers with a fibrous membrane [2]. The infective process of the cyst explains the more extensive quantity of fibrous and purulent material found additionally to the fluid content in our case. *Staphylococcus aureus* represents a major cutaneous saprophyte in the horse enforcing the hypothesis of the infection of the preexisting bone cyst coming through undetected cutaneous trauma. The anatomic proximity to the epiphyseal growth plate of the humerus and of the greater tubercle which ossify after 24 months of age [4] could explain also the subsequent outbreak involving the right hind pastern bone and the DFTS of the hind left through a haematogenous pathway.

The humeral tubercles are an uncommon localization for osseous cyst-like lesions and only two case reports [5, 6] and one 5-case-series [7] have been reported in equine medicine. In one case the lesion was localized within the lateral tubercle of the humerus whilst in the others it was in the intermediate tubercle. The bicipital bursa was involved in 5 cases and in none of the cases a fracture of the tubercles could be detected. Follow-up was available in seven cases, of which one was submitted to euthanasia due to poor outcome [6] whilst all the horses of the 5-case-series underwent successful conservative therapy [7]; the last case was treated with surgical debridement of the cyst [5].

Unlike the present report, in the aforementioned cases no further complications arose, with resolution of the primary lesion after conservative (5 cases) or surgical (1 case) management. The infection of the cyst in our case most likely was the cause for the subsequent hematogenous spreading to the pastern bone and DFTS. The presented case also differs regarding the age of the horses. In the reported cases horses were of mean age of 10 (SD ± 4) years whilst our filly was 18 months old. In the 5-case series, altered biomechanics of the shoulder, as a result of trauma, lameness in other sites of the limb, or bicipital bursitis was suggested to be responsible for abnormal fibrocartilage wear patterns [7].

---

The pathogenesis was suggested to be microtrauma of the osteochondral surface leading to osseous cyst-like lesions through breakthrough of synovial fluid into the defect by hydraulic action [8, 9]. The horses involved had a mean age of 10 years and were active in training; our filly was 18 months old and not broken. It is therefore unlikely that the lesion resulted from altered biomechanics.

Another possible differential diagnosis besides a UBC could be a primary bone infection, which subsequently caused the cyst to develop. Such lesions include a bone abscess, known as Brodie's Abscess in human literature and described in the equine proximal third metatarsal bone [10], first phalanx [11], lateral epicondyle of the humerus [12], and proximal tibia [13]. These lesions are usually confined to the diaphysis or metaphysis of long bones and are characterized by presence of a sclerotic rim [14]. Location of our lesion and absence of bone reaction of the cysts borders make this pathogenesis remote.

A primary osteomyelitis due to septicemia could have also been the cause of cyst development, although it is unlikely that such process would cause lameness in such an acute manner as in our case. In order for the infectious process to reach such extension within the bone a longer time span would have been necessary. Furthermore *Staphylococcus aureus* is a commonly isolated bacterium in human pediatric and adult horses' osteomyelitis [15, 16], but it is rare in foals [17]. The spreading of a primary bone infection to distant sites in young horses has been described. In a report of multiple bone infection in foals, Bennett et al. [18] retrieved *Staphylococcus aureus* always in proximity to physeal growth plates. As in our case, the multiple bone infection was assumed to spread by hematogenous pathway, either through septicaemia or by dissemination of infected emboli (septic emboli). There was involvement of other sites which were not suspected on initial clinical examination similar to our case. Although ossification of the physeal growth plate in the distal pastern bone occurs within the first month of life, the lesion in our case was in exact correspondence of where it once had been, whilst the proximal humeral growth plate was still open and was therefore probably the primary portal of the infection to the bloodstream.

A further pathogenesis could have been an overwhelming septicemia that seeded to the shoulder, the proximal phalanx of the right hind limb, and the DFTS of the left hind limb. In this case the infection of the cyst after the trauma would have been hematogenous.

The surgical removal of the fractured bone and the transosseous evacuation of the cystic content resolved the humeral lesion by decreasing intraosseous pressure, removing the cystic lining, and reducing inflammatory mediator release into the bursa as described by von Rechenberg et al. [19]. Similar procedure is nowadays the treatment of choice for unicameral bone cysts [20].

Plasma fibrinogen concentration has been recently shown to be a useful indicator of physeal or epiphyseal osteomyelitis in foals [21]. Our outcome is in line with these results and constant measurement of plasma fibrinogen throughout the hospitalization reflected the constant decrease along

with clinical improvement of the condition after surgical treatment.

The present case reports for the first time the presence of a unicameral bone cyst in an 18-month-old foal. The favorable outcome was similar to that described in pediatric orthopedics [20].

## Conflict of Interests

The authors declare that there is no conflict of interests regarding the publication of this paper.

## References

[1] R. M. Wilkins, "Unicameral bone cysts," *The Journal of the American Academy of Orthopaedic Surgeons*, vol. 8, no. 4, pp. 217–224, 2000.

[2] J. H. Beaty and J. R. Kasser, "Pathologic fractures associated with tumors and unique conditions of the musculoskeletal system," in *Rockwood & Wilkins' Fractures in Children*, J. P. Dormans and J. M. Flynn, Eds., pp. 136–137, Lippincott Williams & Wilkins, 6th edition, 2006.

[3] J. Cohen, "Etiology of simple bone cyst," *Journal of Bone and Joint Surgery. American Volume*, vol. 52, no. 7, pp. 1493–1497, 1970.

[4] S. J. Dyson, "The elbow, brachium and shoulder," in *Diagnosis and Management of the Lameness in the Horse*, M. W. Ross and S. J. Dyson, Eds., p. 456, Elsevier, 2nd edition, 2011.

[5] C. E. Arnold, M. K. Chaffin, C. M. Honnas, M. A. Walker, and W. K. Heite, "Diagnosis and surgical management of a subchondral bone cyst within the intermediate tubercle of the humerus in a horse," *Equine Veterinary Education*, vol. 20, no. 6, pp. 310–315, 2008.

[6] P. H. L. Ramzan, "Osseous cyst-like lesion of the intermediate humeral tubercle of a horse," *The Veterinary Record*, vol. 154, no. 17, pp. 534–536, 2004.

[7] D. Little, W. R. Redding, and M. P. Gerard, "Osseous cyst-like lesions of the lateral intertubercular groove of the proximal humerus: a report of 5 cases," *Equine Veterinary Education*, vol. 21, no. 2, pp. 60–66, 2009.

[8] L. B. Jeffcott, S. E. Kold, and F. Melsen, "Aspects of the pathology of stifle bone cysts in the horse," *Equine veterinary Journal*, vol. 15, no. 4, pp. 304–311, 1983.

[9] F. Verschooten and A. de Moor, "Subchondral cystic and related lesions affecting the equine pedal bone and stifle," *Equine Veterinary Journal*, vol. 14, no. 1, pp. 47–54, 1982.

[10] J. M. White, K. J. Hughes, C. Scruton, J. Morris, A. W. Philbey, and C. J. Lischer, "Intramedullary abscess of the proximal third metatarsal bone in a 4-year-old Thoroughbred horse," *Equine Veterinary Education*, vol. 19, no. 6, pp. 291–296, 2007.

[11] J. A. Hanson, H. J. Seeherman, C. A. Kirker-Head, and M. W. O'Callaghan, "The role of computed tomography in evaluation of subchondral osseous lesions in seven horses with chronic synovitis," *Equine Veterinary Journal*, vol. 28, no. 6, pp. 480–488, 1996.

[12] M. J. Huber and G. R. Grisel, "Abscess on the lateral epicondyle of the humerus as a cause of lameness in a horse," *Journal of the American Veterinary Medical Association*, vol. 211, no. 12, pp. 1558–1561, 1997.

[13] B. D. Young, D. A. Hendrickson, and R. D. Park, "What is your diagnosis? Mixed lytic-proliferative lesion in the left tibia,"

*Journal of the American Veterinary Medical Association*, vol. 221, no. 9, pp. 1251–1252, 2002.

[14] T. D. Lopes, W. R. Reinus, and A. J. Wilson, "Quantitative analysis of the plain radiographic appearance of Brodie's abscess," *Investigative Radiology*, vol. 32, no. 1, pp. 51–58, 1997.

[15] J. Dartnell, M. Ramachandran, and M. Katchburian, "Haematogenous acute and subacute paediatric osteomyelitis," *Journal of Bone and Joint Surgery B*, vol. 94, no. 5, pp. 584–595, 2012.

[16] G. W. Trotter, "Osteomyelitis," in *Equine Fracture Repair*, A. J. Nixon, Ed., p. 359, Saunders, Philadelphia, Pa, USA, 1st edition, 1996.

[17] R. M. Moore, R. K. Schneider, J. Kowalski, L. R. Bramlage, L. M. Mecklenburg, and C. W. Kohn, "Antimicrobial susceptibility of bacterial isolates from 233 horses with musculoskeletal infection during 1979–1989," *Equine Veterinary Journal*, vol. 24, no. 6, pp. 450–456, 1992.

[18] D. Bennett, "Pathological features of multiple bone infection in the foal." *Veterinary Record*, vol. 103, no. 22, pp. 482–485, 1978.

[19] B. von Rechenberg, H. Guenther, C. W. McIlwraith et al., "Fibrous tissue of subchondral cystic lesions in horses produce local mediators and neutral metalloproteinases and cause bone resorption in vitro," *Veterinary Surgery*, vol. 29, no. 5, pp. 420–429, 2000.

[20] F. Canavese, J. G. Wright, W. G. Cole, and S. Hopyan, "Unicameral Bone Cysts: comparison of percutaneous curettage, steroid, and autologous bone marrow injections," *Journal of Pediatric Orthopaedics*, vol. 31, no. 1, pp. 50–55, 2011.

[21] J. M. Newquist, G. M. Baxter, R. Sangeeta, and F. Olea-Popelka, "Evaluation of plasma fibrinogen concentration as an indicator of physeal or epiphyseal osteomyelitis in foals: 17 cases (2002–2007)," *Journal of the American Veterinary Medical Association*, vol. 235, no. 4, pp. 415–419, 2009.

# 27

# Canine Oral Eosinophilic Granuloma Treated with Electrochemotherapy

**Matías Nicolás Tellado,**[1] **Sebastián Diego Michinski,**[2,3] **Nahuel Olaiz,**[3] **Felipe Maglietti,**[3] **and Guillermo Marshall**[3]

[1] *Facultad de Ciencias Veterinarias, Universidad de Buenos Aires, Avenida Chorroarín 280, C1427CWO Ciudad de Buenos Aires, Argentina*
[2] *Instituto Tecnológico de Buenos Aires, Avenida Eduardo Madero 399, C1106ACD Ciudad de Buenos Aires, Argentina*
[3] *Laboratorio de Sistemas Complejos, Facultad de Ciencias Exactas y Naturales, Universidad de Buenos Aires, Intendente Guiraldes 2160, Pabellon I, C1428EGA Ciudad de Buenos Aires, Argentina*

Correspondence should be addressed to Guillermo Marshall; marshallg@arnet.com.ar

Academic Editor: Isabel Pires

A case of a canine oral eosinophilic granuloma in a 14-year-old female crossbred is described. The dog was presented with a history of ptyalism, halitosis, local pain, decreased appetite, and blood staining noted on food and water bowls. Clinical, hematologic, and biochemical examinations, abdominal ultrasonography, and 3-view chest radiographs were performed, and no metastases were found. Histopathologic examination of two 6 mm punch biopsies from the oral lesion revealed the presence of eosinophilic granulomatous lesions in the submucosa. After treatment with corticosteroids and wide spectrum antibiotics no significant changes in clinical signs and lesion size were observed. Electrochemotherapy (ECT), a novel tumor treatment routinely used for cutaneous and subcutaneous tumors in human patients in the European Union since 2006, was used to treat the eosinophilic granuloma. The procedure was performed under general anesthesia, followed by intravenous administration of bleomycin. Six weeks after treatment a complete response with disappearance of the mass and improvement of clinical signs were observed.

## 1. Introduction

Canine eosinophilic granuloma is an eosinophilic disease reported as a rare lesion characterized by nodules and plaques in the mouth, tonsils, or skin. The exact cause is unknown, but infectious agents as bacteria, parasites, or fungal organisms have been implicated in the pathogenesis. Siberian Huskies and Cavalier King Charles Spaniels are most commonly affected [1, 2]. Few studies have documented the disease in older crossbred dogs. Oral lesions are characterized by plaques or proliferative masses. These are most commonly found on the palate and the lateral or ventral side of the tongue. Oral lesions may be painful and halitosis is usually the presenting complaint.

The etiology of these lesions remains unknown, although an underlying allergic condition is likely. This disease occurs in dogs as a collagen tissue degeneration [1, 3–5]. In humans, some reports have proposed several mechanisms of pathogenesis as vasculitis, microangiopathies, fibromatosis, phagocytic dysfunction, and cell mediated immune-response dysfunction [6].

Standard treatments are made with the aim of reducing the size of the granuloma and to improve the general condition of the patient. A treatment with antibiotic and corticosteroid therapy has been reported with a partial response and occurrence of side effects such as gastritis, enteritis, and chronic renal failure due to prolonged use of high doses of corticosteroids in older patients [3]. The surgical excision followed by immunosuppressive therapy with corticosteroids or azathioprine might achieve best local results, but in patients with large masses aggressive procedure is necessary. Also, a high rate of recurrence was observed after a short treatment period [2, 3, 7].

ECT is a novel treatment modality consisting in the use of an electric field to increase tissue permeability to certain drugs [8, 9]. Bleomycin is usually the drug of choice, which works as an endonuclease, cutting the DNA strands and thus interfering with cell division. This provides a sort of selectivity towards dividing cells, sparing the quiescent ones and thus allowing the tissue to heal with minimum scaring. It has been used in the European Union since 2006, for the treatment of cutaneous and subcutaneous tumors [10, 11], particularly for the treatment of melanoma nodules. Cemazar et al. reviewed the use of electrochemotherapy for treating tumors in veterinary oncology [12].

In this case report we show for the first time the use of electrochemotherapy for the treatment of a canine eosinophilic granuloma, a nononcological disease.

## 2. Case Presentation

A case of a 14-year-old canine female crossbred is described. The dog was presented with a history of ptyalism, halitosis, mild weight loss, local pain, decreased appetite, and blood staining noted on food and water bowls.

*2.1. Clinical Examination.* The patient's general condition was good on the physical exam; hypersalivation, halitosis, and uncomfortable chewing were the main clinical signs. A $3.8 \times 2.2 \times 1.2$ cm bloody mass was found on the lower right side of the mouth (Figure 1). We also detected a right submandibular lymph node enlargement; thus a fine needle aspiration was performed. Complete laboratory analysis, abdominal ultrasound, and 3-view thoracic radiographs were performed as a first clinical staging. The blood count revealed mild anemia (29% hematocrit, reference range 35–55%), mild leukocytosis ($36 \times 10^3$ leukocytes/$\mu$L, reference range $6.0$–$12.0 \times 10^3$ leukocytes/$\mu$L), an increased percentage of segmented neutrophilic granulocytes (83%, reference range 60–75%), 13% lymphocytes (reference range 15–30%), 4% eosinophils (reference range 0–6%), and slight thrombocytopenia ($250 \times 10^3$ platelets/$\mu$L, reference range $300$–$500 \times 10^3$ platelets/$\mu$L). The routine biochemical parameters were within the normal range. The cytology from the fine needle aspiration showed a reactive lymph node, likely due to the oral inflammation and infection. No metastatic signs were observed on the imaging studies; therefore two samples of 6 mm punch biopsy were taken from the mass to be referred to the pathologist.

Two formalin fixed samples were embedded in paraffin wax and then stained with hematoxylin and eosin (HE). The histopathology samples revealed a chronic eosinophilic granuloma consisting of densely eosinophilic material representing remnants of fragmented collagen bundles and degenerate eosinophils which have released their granules to the interstitium. At the periphery of the granuloma, mainly differentiated fibrovascular tissue can be seen with some eosinophilic granulocytes intermingled with small numbers

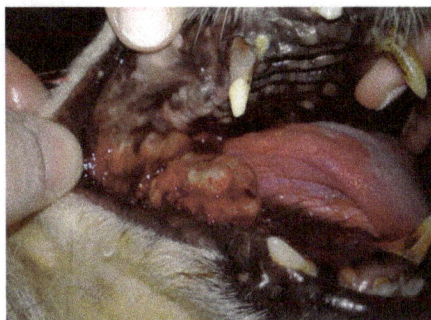

FIGURE 1: Picture taken on day 1, before the ECT treatment. On the right side of the mouth a $3.8 \times 2.2 \times 1.2$ cm bloody mass can be seen corresponding to an eosinophilic granuloma.

of lymphocytes, macrophages, plasma cells, and neutrophils (Figure 2).

*2.2. Treatment.* After a treatment with prednisolone 2 mg/kg/sid and amoxicillin/clavulanic acid 62.5 mg/kg/bid, no significant changes in clinical signs and lesion size were observed.

A wide-margin surgical excision was indicated to ensure that all eosinophilic granuloma is removed, but this indication was not accepted by pet owners. For this reason, ECT was the therapeutic modality chosen and an informed consent was signed. Local regulations were followed (Argentina, law N° 14,072) [13].

The treatment was performed under general anesthesia. The patient was induced with intravenous bolus of propofol (3 mg/kg) and diazepam (0.5 mg/kg) and maintained after tracheal intubation with isoflurane and intravenous fentanyl (2 $\mu$g/kg). This scheme of anesthesia guarantees an adequate comfort of the patient during the treatment. Prophylactic antibiotics were administered.

A single dose of bleomycin (15,000 IU/m²) was administered in bolus, and the electric pulses were delivered 8 minutes later, applying 8 pulses of 800 V/cm and 100 $\mu$sec long at a repetition frequency of 10 Hz, covering the whole lesion surface, using a pulse generator BTX ECM 830, Harvard Apparatus, Boston, USA. We used a 6-needle electrode (Figure 3), as the area covered with the electrode is $0.8 \times 0.8$ cm; 15 applications were needed to cover the lesion and superposition was avoided. After the procedure, oral meloxicam (0.1 mg/kg/sid) was administered for pain and local swelling control.

To determine the dose of bleomycin the body surface of the dog was estimated using the following formula [14]:

$$\text{body surface in m}^2 = \frac{10.1 \times (\text{weight in grams})^{2/3}}{10\,000}. \quad (1)$$

The weight was 8.9 kg; thus the calculated body surface was $0.434 \text{ m}^2$.

*2.3. Followup.* Four days after ECT, the patient showed mild inflammation of the gingiva, but no significant changes in food and water intake were observed by the pet owner.

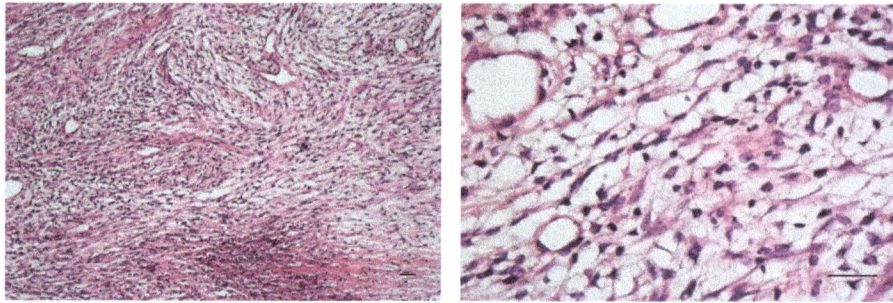

FIGURE 2: Histopathology samples stained with hematoxylin and eosin revealed a chronic eosinophilic granuloma consisting of densely eosinophilic material representing remnants of fragmented collagen bundles and degenerate eosinophils which have released their granules to the interstitium. At the periphery of the granuloma, mainly differentiated fibrovascular tissue can be seen with some eosinophilic granulocytes intermingled with small numbers of lymphocytes, macrophages, plasma cells, and neutrophils (scale bars = 100 $\mu$m).

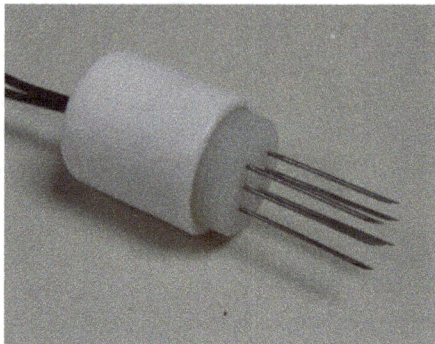

FIGURE 3: Six-needle electrode used to treat the patient. It consists of two rows of 3 needles. The separation of the rows is 0.8 cm; the separation between the needles in the same row is 0.4 cm. Each needle is 2 cm long and 1.2 mm in diameter.

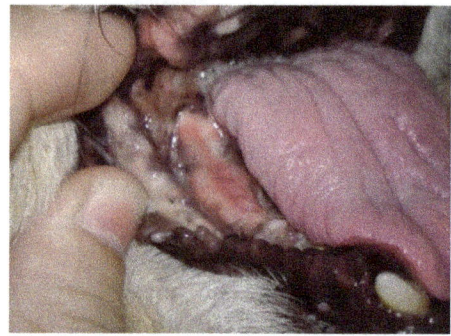

FIGURE 4: Picture taken 45 days after the ECT treatment. A complete response was achieved.

14 days after ECT, no signs of inflammation or a clear improvement in general condition due to the partial reduction of the mass were observed. Meloxicam was discontinued due to lack of inflammation.

45 days after treatment (Figure 4) improvement of life quality was observed to be likely related to absence of pain; also decreased sialorrhea and halitosis were obvious. In accordance with the World Health Organization response criteria [15], a complete remission with a 100% reduction of the lesion size was observed.

After day 45, one month of corticosteroid therapy with prednisolone 1.5 mg/kg/sid and omeprazole 1 mg/kg/sid was indicated to prevent local recurrence.

## 3. Conclusions and Discussion

The standard treatment for the eosinophilic granuloma has a very low efficacy and most of its side effects may seriously affect the quality of life of the patient. We conclude that, in this case of canine oral eosinophilic granuloma, ECT was a very good treatment option with excellent results. This result confirms that one of the most remarkable aspects of ECT is its effectiveness against any histological type of tumor [12, 16, 17]. As ECT kills proliferating cells mainly by apoptosis, quiescent cells are preserved. In this case, ECT was a logical treatment option since it will affect the replicating cells in the lesion without affecting the others, even though they were not oncological cells.

Although intratumoral administration of bleomycin is usually recommended in human treatments [17], we decided to use a systemic administration whereas this disease consists of an heterogeneous tissue; thus, the local injection of bleomycin would probably not provide a uniform distribution inside the granuloma in our case.

Our data also confirm that ECT is very useful when the patient's clinical condition impedes a more aggressive treatment. ECT is a cancer treatment modality that has not been used routinely in nononcological diseases [18]. In this case, this modality of treatment achieved excellent results treating eosinophilic granuloma. The patient regained its general condition after a few days, with a rapid overall improvement. The low doses of bleomycin (11 to 30 times lower dose than the one reported as toxic [19]) had no undesired effects. However, the treatment provoked a mild swelling of the gingiva and oral discomfort after the ECT. The situation ceased in less than seven days, controlled with nonsteroidal anti-inflammatory drugs (NSAIDs). It must be noticed that, prior to the ECT treatment, the lesion itself made the food and water intake very difficult. Thus, this side effect was quite limited in time and it was actually compensated by the efficacy of the ECT.

The ECT proves to be very useful in cases of a large size granuloma that cannot be reduced considerably by standard treatments based on immunosuppression. The major advantage of ECT could be for treating cases where the owner rejects the radical surgical excision or in those cases where high dose corticosteroids therapy is not a viable option.

## Conflict of Interests

The authors declare that there is no conflict of interests regarding the publication of this paper.

## Acknowledgments

The authors are grateful to Dr. Minatel for the histopathologic processing samples. F. Maglietti and N. Olaiz have fellowships from Consejo Nacional de Investigaciones Cientificas y Tecnicas (CONICET), S. Michinski has a fellowship from Instituto Tecnológico de Buenos Aires (ITBA), and G. Marshall is Member of CONICET. This work is supported by grants from CONICET (PIP 1087/05) and Universidad de Buenos Aires (UBACyT X132/08) and CONICET STAN 599/11.

## References

[1] W. P. Bredal, G. Gunnes, I. Vollset, and T. L. Ulstein, "Oral eosinophilic granuloma in three Cavalier King Charles spaniels," *Journal of Small Animal Practice*, vol. 37, no. 10, pp. 499–504, 1996.

[2] B. R. Madewell, A. A. Stannard, L. T. Pulley, and V. G. Nelson, "Oral eosinophilic granuloma in Siberian Husky dogs," *Journal of the American Veterinary Medical Association*, vol. 177, no. 8, pp. 701–703, 1980.

[3] J. M. Sykes IV, M. M. Garner, L. L. Greer et al., "Oral eosinophilic granulomas in tigers (Panthera tigris)-a collection of 16 cases," *Journal of Zoo and Wildlife Medicine*, vol. 38, no. 2, pp. 300–308, 2007.

[4] M. J. Lommer, "Oral inflammation in small animals," *Veterinary Clinics of North America: Small Animal Practice*, vol. 43, no. 3, pp. 555–571, 2013.

[5] V. A. Fadok, "Granulomatosis dermatitis in dogs and cats," *Seminars in Veterinary Medicine & Surgery*, vol. 2, no. 3, pp. 186–194, 1987.

[6] S. J. Key, C. J. O'Brien, K. C. Silvester, and S.-J. Crean, "Eosinophilic granuloma: Resolution of maxillofacial bony lesions following minimal intervention. Report of three cases and a review of the literature," *Journal of Cranio-Maxillofacial Surgery*, vol. 32, no. 3, pp. 170–175, 2004.

[7] K. A. Potter, R. D. Tucker, and J. L. Carpenter, "Oral eosinophilic granuloma in Siberian huskies," *Journal of the American Animal Hospital Association*, vol. 16, no. 4, pp. 595–600, 1980.

[8] L. M. Mir, "Bases and rationale of the electrochemotherapy," *European Journal of Cancer, Supplement*, vol. 4, no. 11, pp. 38–44, 2006.

[9] T. Kotnik, P. Kramar, G. Pucihar, D. Miklavčič, and M. Tarek, "Cell membrane electroporation—part 1: the phenomenon," *IEEE Electrical Insulation Magazine*, vol. 28, no. 5, pp. 14–23, 2012.

[10] M. L. Yarmush, A. Golberg, G. Serša, T. Kotnik, and D. Miklavčič, "Electroporation-based technologies for medicine: principles, applications, and challenges," *Annual Review of Biomedical Engineering*, vol. 16, pp. 295–320, 2014.

[11] M. Marty, G. Sersa, J. Garbay et al., "Electrochemotherapy—an easy, highly effective and safe treatment of cutaneous and subcutaneous metastases: results of ESOPE (European Standard Operating Procedures of Electrochemotherapy) study," *European Journal of Cancer Supplements*, vol. 4, pp. 3–13, 2006.

[12] M. Cemazar, Y. Tamzali, G. Sersa et al., "Electrochemotherapy in veterinary oncology," *Journal of Veterinary Internal Medicine*, vol. 22, no. 4, pp. 826–831, 2008.

[13] Local normative law in Argentina, (Law no. 14,072), http://www.infoleg.gob.ar/infolegInternet/anexos/55000-59999/56727/norma.htm.

[14] Weight to body surface area conversion, http://www.merckvetmanual.com/mvm/htm/bc/tref9.htm.

[15] *WHO Handbook for Reporting Results of Cancer Treatment*, WHO Offset Publications no. 48, World Health Organization, Geneva, Switzerland, 1979.

[16] L. G. Campana, S. Mocellin, M. Basso et al., "Bleomycin-based electrochemotherapy: clinical outcome from a single institution's experience with 52 patients," *Annals of Surgical Oncology*, vol. 16, no. 1, pp. 191–199, 2009.

[17] B. Mali, T. Jarm, M. Snoj, G. Sersa, and D. Miklavcic, "Antitumor effectiveness of electrochemotherapy: a systematic review and meta-analysis," *European Journal of Surgical Oncology*, vol. 39, no. 1, pp. 4–16, 2013.

[18] Y. Tamzali, J. Teissie, and M. P. Rols, "Cutaneous tumor treatment by electrochemotherapy: preliminary clinical results in horse sarcoids," *Revue de Medecine Veterinaire*, vol. 152, no. 8-9, pp. 605–609, 2001.

[19] R. W. Fleischman, J. R. Baker, G. R. Thompson et al., "Bleomycin-induced interstitial pneumonia in dogs," *Thorax*, vol. 26, no. 6, pp. 675–682, 1971.

# 28

# Surgical Treatment of a Chronically Recurring Case of Cervical Mucocele in a German Shepherd Dog

**Davoud Kazemi,[1] Yousef Doustar,[2] and Gholamreza Assadnassab[1]**

[1] *Department of Veterinary Clinical Sciences, Faculty of Veterinary Medicine, Tabriz Branch, Islamic Azad University, Tabriz, Iran*
[2] *Department of Veterinary Pathobiology, Faculty of Veterinary Medicine, Tabriz Branch, Islamic Azad University, Tabriz, Iran*

Correspondence should be addressed to Davoud Kazemi, dkazemi@iaut.ac.ir

Academic Editors: R. M. Jerram and G. Stoica

A-six-year old male German shepherd dog with swelling and enlargement of the intermandibular and cervical region with a duration of nearly one year was referred to the small animal veterinary hospital, Islamic Azad University of Tabriz. Based on the history, clinical findings, and laboratory investigations, the animal was diagnosed as having cervical mucocele with the involvement of the left sublingual and mandibular salivary glands. Surgical treatment consisting of the excision of the involved gland/duct complex was immediately undertaken with definitive results. Clinical and histopathologic features of this chronic case of canine salivary mucocele are presented in this paper.

## 1. Introduction

A salivary mucocele or sialocele is an abnormal accumulation of saliva in the subcutaneous tissue adjacent to a damaged salivary gland or duct and is surrounded by granulation tissue. The saliva originates from a ruptured salivary gland or duct. The sublingual and mandibular salivary glands are most commonly affected [1–4]. In the present paper, an unusually large and chronic case of cervical mucocele is described in a German shepherd dog.

## 2. Case Presentation

A six-year-old male German shepherd dog was referred to the small animal veterinary hospital, Islamic Azad University of Tabriz with obvious swelling and enlargement of the cervical and intermandibular region. According to the dog's owner, the swelling had first appeared almost a year ago, and during this period the dog had no other abnormalities. The gradually enlarging swelling had been drained on several occasions by a private sector veterinarian during this time, and dilute povidone iodine solution had been injected into the swelling without clinical success.

On clinical examination, a very large fluctuant, non-painful fluid filled mass was evident in the cervical and inter-mandibular region. Palpation of the mass caused drooling of saliva from the mouth. Body temperature, pulse, and respiration were within normal range and slight anemia, and increased neutrophil and band cells were detected on a complete blood count (CBC). Ultrasonographic evaluation revealed a hypoechoic region with a more echogenic border indicating a fluid filled cavity surrounded by a well-defined thick border. Based on the history and clinical findings, cervical mucocele was suspected. Aspiration of the mass under aseptic conditions was performed (Figure 1), and a thick mucoid, yellow blood tinged fluid which reacted positively with periodic acid schiff (PAS) stain (Figure 2) confirmed the presence of saliva and a diagnosis of mucocele. Because of the chronic nature of the disease, surgery was immediately undertaken to excise the involved gland and mass.

After premedication with acepromazine (Alfasan, Woerden, Holland), 0.05 mg/kg and atropine (Iran Pharmaceutical Development and Investment Co., Tehran, Iran), 0.02 mg/kg, anesthesia was induced with 2.5% solution of thiopental (Sandoz GmbH, kundl, Austria) and maintained

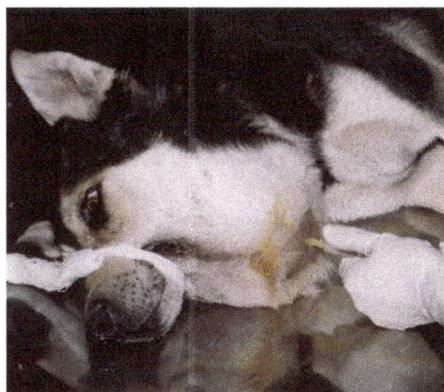

FIGURE 1: Aspiration of the cervical swelling under aseptic conditions. Note the extent and size of the swelling in the cervical and intermandibular region.

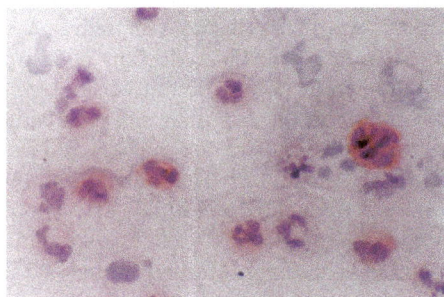

FIGURE 2: Periodic acid Schiff (PAS) staining of the aspirated fluid. The blue staining indicates that the fluid is saliva and confirms the diagnosis of mucocele. Note the presence of the inflammatory cells (×400).

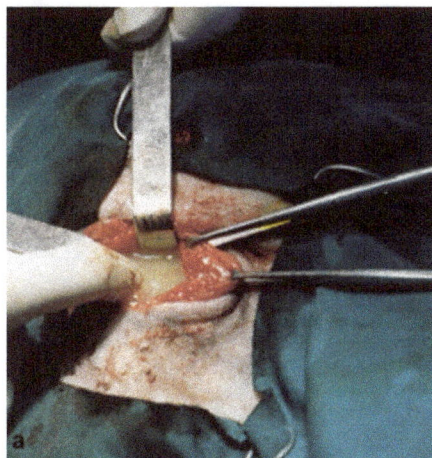

(a)

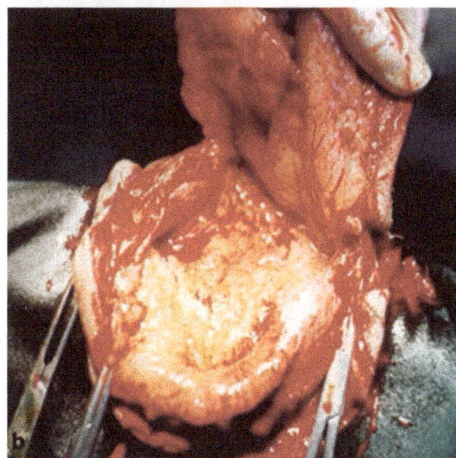

(b)

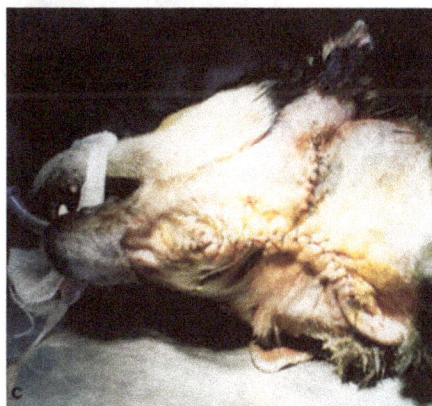

(c)

FIGURE 3: Intraoperative and postoperative views of the surgical procedure. Saliva was encountered at the incision site (a) and the surrounding reactive connective tissue is being excised (b). The cervical region resumes normality following the surgery (c).

with halothane. The affected side was determined to be the left side by placing the animal in dorsal recumbency. The left mandibular and sublingual salivary glands were excised by making an incision over the mandibular gland region just caudal to the ramus of the mandible with the animal in right lateral recumbency (Figure 3(a)). After incising skin, subcutaneous tissues, and the platysma muscle, the capsule of the mandibular salivary gland was identified and incised to expose the gland. Dissection was continued rostrally to include the mandibular duct and closely associated sublingual gland. After complete removal, the incised muscular and subcutaneous tissues were sutured with absorbable sutures and the skin was routinely closed with nonabsorbable sutures. The mucocele was drained through a stab incision in the most ventrally dependant area, and approximately 1 litre of fluid was withdrawn. Due to cosmetic reasons, the large pendulous mass was also removed surgically (Figures 3(b) and 3(c)). The animal recovered uneventfully and skin sutures were removed after 10 days.

On histopathologic examination, mild atrophy of the excised glands was observed (Figures 4(a) and 4(b)). The mucocele wall consisted of an outer highly vascularised layer of immature connective tissue and an inner zone of loosely arranged fibroblasts. A pleocellular inflammatory reaction was evident in the central area, which also contained much amorphous acidophilic or amphophilic debris. The inflammatory cells were mainly mononuclear and plasma cells (Figures 4(c) and 4(d)).

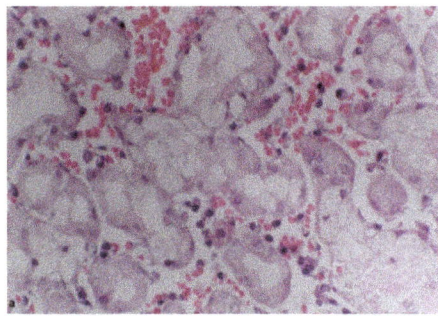

(a)

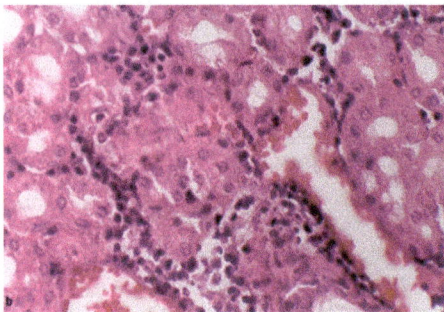

(b)

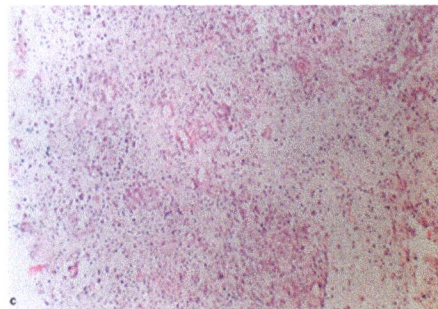

(c)

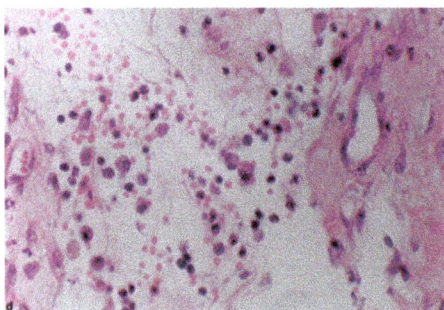

(d)

FIGURE 4: Histopathologic sections of the excised sublingual (a) and mandibular (b) salivary glands indicating mild atrophy and hemorrhage (Hematoxylin and Eosin, ×100). The mucocele wall consisting of connective tissue lining and inflammatory cells is clearly evident (c) (Hematoxylin and Eosin, ×40) alongside the presence of red blood cells and blood vessels (d) (Hematoxylin and Eosin, ×100).

The case was closely followed for a period of six months after the surgery, and there was no recurrence of the condition.

## 3. Discussion

Although diseases of the salivary glands are rare in small animals, mucocele is the most common clinically recognized disease of these structures in the dog, and the incidence of occurrence has been reported as fewer than 20 in 4000 dogs [5]. In most cases, the inciting cause of a salivary mucocele is usually unknown although blunt trauma, salivary gland or duct foreign bodies, sialoliths, and dirofilariasis have been suggested [1, 2, 5–7]. Clinically, a salivary mucocele is observed as an abnormal swelling containing saliva. The swelling is commonly observed in the cranial cervical or intermandibular, sublingual, or pharyngeal tissues hence cervical, sublingual, or pharyngeal mucoceles are used to describe these abnormal collections of saliva. A very rare form of this condition is the collection of saliva ventral to the globe known as zygomatic mucocele [1–6, 8]. Dogs are more commonly affected than cats and although all breeds are susceptible, there are reports indicating that poodles, German shepherds, dachshunds, and Australian silky terriers are frequently affected [1–3]. The diagnosis of salivary mucocele is based on the history, clinical signs and histopathologic findings. Affected animals are presented with soft and fluctuant swellings which are painless except in the acute phase of the inflammatory response. Definitive treatment of this condition requires resection of the affected gland/duct complex. Repeated drainage or injection of cauterizing or anti-inflammatory agents will not only fail to eliminate the mucocele but will complicate the surgical procedure because of subsequent abscessation or fibrosis [1–3, 8].

In the case described in this report, blunt trauma in the form of choke chain was the most probable inciting cause in this dog. The continuous pressure exerted by a very tight choke chain around the neck appeared to have damaged the sublingual and mandibular salivary gland/duct complex leading to gradually increasing accumulation of saliva manifested as cervical mucocele.

It has been observed that cervical mucocele is the most common form of this condition [9]. Previous studies have also pointed out that resection of the mandibular and sublingual salivary glands alongside drainage and excision of the redundant tissues is the most definitive treatment of this condition [9, 10] although in a high percentage of cases (42%) drainage alone was employed for treatment of the affected animals which resulted in the recurrence of the condition within the next 48 hours [9]. This scenario was also observed in the present case, and, as stated by the dog's owner, the only form of treatment the animal had received before surgery consisted of drainage and injection of povidone iodine solution as a cauterizing agent which had merely complicated the situation. The basis for nonsurgical treatment of mucocele lies in the belief that mucocele is a true cyst with secretory lining but the fact that it is not a cyst but a reactive encapsulating structure has prompted the surgical removal of the affected salivary gland/duct complex with definitive results [5].

Sialography has been described as a method for the diagnosis of sialoceles [1–5], but it is technically difficult and in most cases like the present one it is unnecessary and, therefore, not often performed because the diagnosis can generally be accurately made by careful observation and palpation.

Salivary mucoceles are not cysts because they lack luminal epithelium and contain granulation tissue lining which originates from inflammatory reaction to free saliva [7, 11–13]. It has been stated that the histopathologic appearance of salivary mucoceles varies according to their stage of development. In long standing cases, saliva is surrounded by mature dense connective tissue with abundant vessels, and the lumen of the sialocele contains eosinophilic amorphous material and desquamated cells indicating that the process of saliva secretion and mucocele formation is still continuous [7, 11]. These features were also observed in the present case indicating the long standing and chronic nature of the condition in this particular animal.

# References

[1] C. S. Hedlund and T. W. Fossum, "Surgery of the oral cavity and oropharynx," in *Small Animal Surgery*, T. W. Fossum, Ed., pp. 339–372, Mosby, St. Louis, Mo, USA, 3rd edition, 2007.

[2] D. Dunning, "Oral cavity," in *Textbook of Small Animal Surgery*, D. Slatter, Ed., pp. 553–572, Saunders, Philadelphia, Pa, USA, 3rd edition, 2003.

[3] C. D. Knecht, "Salivary glands," in *Current Techniques in Small Animal Surgery*, M. J. Bojrab, Ed., pp. 183–186, Williams & Wilkins, Baltimore, Md, USA, 4th edition, 1998.

[4] K. M. Tobias, *Manual of Small Animal Soft Tissue Surgery*, Wiley-Blackwell, Ames, Iowa, USA, 2010.

[5] M. M. Smith, "Oral and salivary gland disorders," in *Textbook of Veterinary Internal Medicine*, S. J. Ettinger and E. C. Feldman, Eds., pp. 1290–1297, Elsevier, 6th edition, 2005.

[6] C. P. Sturgess, "Diseases of the alimentary tract," in *Textbook of Small Animal Medicine*, J. K. Dunn, Ed., pp. 371–447, W. B. Saunders, 2000.

[7] C. C. Brown, D. C. Baker, and I. K. Barker, "Alimentary system," in *Jubb, Kennedy, and Palmer's Pathology of Domestic Animals*, M. Grant Maxie, Ed., vol. 2, pp. 1–237, Elsevier, 2007.

[8] S. Manfra Marretta, "Dentistry and diseases of the oropharynx," in *Saunders manual of Small Animal Practice*, pp. 609–635, Saunders, St. Louis, Mo, USA, 3rd edition, 2006.

[9] C. R. Bellenger and D. J. Simpson, "Canine sialocoeles-60 clinical cases," *Journal of Small Animal Practice*, vol. 33, no. 8, pp. 376–380, 1992.

[10] W. J. Weber, H. P. Hobson, and S. R. Wilson, "Pharyngeal mucoceles in dogs," *Veterinary Surgery*, vol. 15, no. 1, pp. 5–8, 1986.

[11] H. Yasonu, H. Nagai, Y. Ishimura et al., "salivary mucocele in a laboratory beagle," *Journal of Toxicologic Pathology*, vol. 24, pp. 131–135, 2011.

[12] H. J. van Kruiningen, "Gastrointestinal system," in *Thomson's Special Veterinary Pathology*, W. W. Carlton and M. D. McGavin, Eds., pp. 1–80, Mosby, St. Louis, Mo, USA, 2nd edition, 1995.

[13] H. B. Gelberg, "Alimentary system," in *Pathologic Basis of Veterinary Disease*, M. D. McGavin and J. F. Zachary, Eds., pp. 301–391, Mosby, 4th edition, 2007.

# 29

# Dermatitis due to Mixed *Demodex* and *Sarcoptes* Mites in Dogs

**B. Sudhakara Reddy,**[1] **K. Nalini Kumari,**[2] **S. Sivajothi,**[3] **and R. Venkatasivakumar**[4]

[1] Teaching Veterinary Clinical Complex (Veterinary Medicine), College of Veterinary Science, Sri Venkateswara Veterinary University, Proddatur, Andhra Pradesh 516360, India
[2] Department of Veterinary Medicine, College of Veterinary Science, Sri Venkateswara Veterinary University, Tirupati, Andhra Pradesh 517502, India
[3] Department of Veterinary Parasitology, College of Veterinary Science, Sri Venkateswara Veterinary University, Proddatur, Andhra Pradesh 516360, India
[4] Department of Veterinary Medicine, College of Veterinary Science, Sri Venkateswara Veterinary University, Proddatur, Andhra Pradesh 516360, India

Correspondence should be addressed to B. Sudhakara Reddy; bhavanamvet@gmail.com

Academic Editor: Franco Mutinelli

In dogs, dermatitis due to mixed mite infestation is rare. During the five-year period of study, two dogs were identified suffering from dermatitis due to mixed *Demodex* and *Sarcoptes* mites. Upon clinical examination dogs had primary and secondary skin lesions on face, around the ears, chin, neck, fore limbs and lateral abdomen. Microscopic examination of skin scrapings revealed *Demodex* and *Sarcoptes* mites. Both dogs were treated with daily oral ivermectin at 100 to 400 $\mu$g/kg body weight as incremental doses, external application of amitraz and supportive treatments with topical antimicrobial shampoo. After completion of forty-two days of therapy, dogs were recovered from the dermatitis.

## 1. Introduction

Canine demodicosis is a dermatologic disease that occurs when mites colonize the hair follicles and sebaceous glands [1]. *Demodex canis* was the main causative agent of canine demodicosis and it is characterized by the presence of large numbers of *Demodex* mites. The three recognized canine *Demodex* mites are *Demodex canis*, *Demodex injai*, and *Demodex cornei* [2–4]. Scabies is a transmissible and zoonotic ectoparasitic skin infection caused by tiny mites of the species *Sarcoptes scabiei*. It is transmitted readily among the animals, often even throughout an entire household, by skin to skin contact. The parasite commonly affects young dogs and dogs with poor nutrition but can affect healthy dogs that are exposed to the mites [5]. Literatures related to the individual types of mange mites in different animals were available from the last decade. There are no reports about the mixed infection of *Demodex* and *Sarcoptes* in dogs. This paper reports the rare occurrence of mixed demodectic and sarcoptic mange in dogs and their therapy.

## 2. Materials and Methods

Present case reports were recorded at College Hospital of College of Veterinary Science, Tirupati and Teaching Veterinary Clinical Complex, Proddatur during the five-years period from January 2009 to January 2014 of clinical study on dermatological cases. Dogs with dermatological problems were regularly screened for the ectoparasites and underlying factors for development of dermatological illness at major Veterinary Hospitals in four different districts of Andhra Pradesh. Superficial and deep skin scrapings, tape impression smears and hair plucks were collected from the affected dogs for laboratory examination. Scrapings were collected with scalpel blade dipped in liquid paraffin and collection of scrapings was continued until there was slight ooze of blood from dermal capillaries. Material was suspended in a few drops of liquid paraffin on a microscopic slide, a coverslip was applied and the preparation was examined under low and high magnifications (10X, 40X) of microscope. The acetate tape impression smears were used to investigate

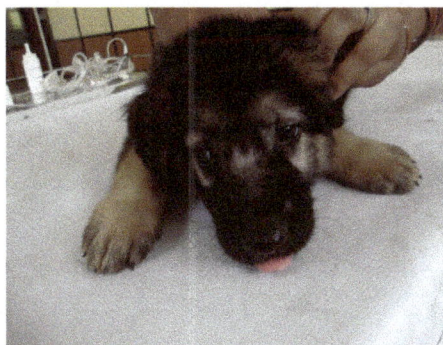

FIGURE 1: Dog with lesions at face and neck regions (Case 1).

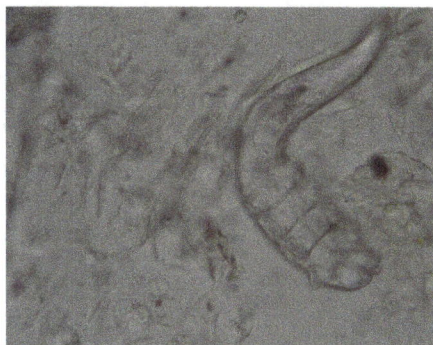

FIGURE 2: Dog with chronic generalized dermatitis (Case 2).

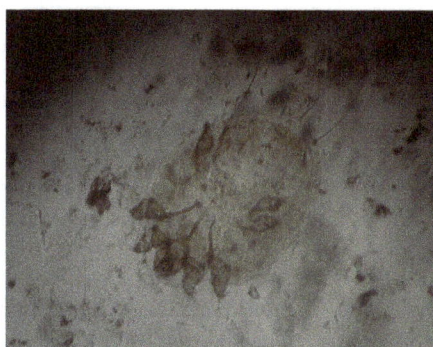

FIGURE 3: Scraping containing *Demodex* mites (40X).

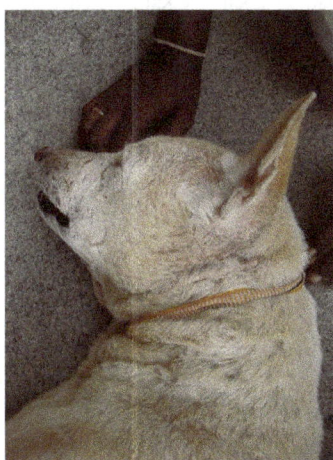

FIGURE 4: Scraping containing sarcoptic mites (40X).

superficial mites [6]. Out of 1200 dogs examined with dermatological problems during the study two dogs were found to be affected with mixed demodectic and sarcoptic mange mites. From the two dogs blood was collected in 10% EDTA coated vials. Blood was processed for packed cell volume (PCV), haemoglobin (Hb), total leucocyte count (TLC), total erythrocyte count (TEC) and stained peripheral blood smears were for differential count (DLC) to know about the haematological abnormalities and to screen for any other infections.

*Case 1.* A three-month-old German Shepherd dog was presented with a history of skin lesions associated with pruritus from one month. Upon clinical examination, dog exhibited papules, pustules, erythema, alopecia, erosions on the face, around the eyes, ears, chin and neck regions (Figure 1).

*Case 2.* A three-year-old mongrel (local breed) dog was brought with a history of skin lesions associated with pruritus from one week onwards. Dog was recently kept at dog care center for about two weeks. Mild lesions were detected on the ears, face, nasolabial area, chin, neck, flank, abdominal skin, elbow and legs. Upon clinical examination, dog exhibited papules, pustules, erythema, alopecia, hyperpigmentation, erosions, lichenification and cellulitis. Distribution of lesions was observed on face, around the ears and overall the body (Figure 2).

## 3. Results and Discussion

Skin scrapings collected from the two dogs revealed different stages of *Demodex* mites along with *Sarcoptes* mites (Figures 3 and 4). Hair pluck examination revealed 3 to 6 number of *Demodex* mites around the hair follicle. Based on the history, lesions and laboratory findings, the present condition was diagnosed as generalized dermatitis due to two different types of mites. Both the dogs were treated with oral ivermectin at 100 to 400 $\mu$g/kg body weight as incremental doses and they were kept on observation for any adverse symptoms [7]. Treatment was continued till two consequent negative skin scrapings were obtained at an interval of two weeks. External application was advised with amitraz (2 mL in 1 liter of water) twice a week as topical application followed by bath with benzyl peroxide shampoo up to the recovery period.

Both the dogs were subjected to scoring for relevant clinical signs of demodectic and sarcoptic mange (papules, pustules, erythema, pruritus, alopecia, hyperpigmentation and crusting). Clinical dermatological assessments (severity of the lesions and recovery degree) were made on days 0, 7, 14, 21, 28, 42, and 56 after therapy. Parasitological examination was conducted to test the response to the therapy. The data were recorded on the presence or absence of live mites. Efficacy of therapy was assessed based on the reversal of symptoms and parasitological examination. Response to therapy was graded as excellent, good, fair, and poor by assessing the clinical symptoms and lesions [8].

TABLE 1: Therapeutic response to ivermectin in both the dogs.

| Posttreatment evaluation days | Case 1 | | | | | Case 2 | | | | |
|---|---|---|---|---|---|---|---|---|---|---|
| | Demodex | | Sarcoptes | | Clinical response | Demodex | | Sarcoptes | | Clinical response |
| | Live | Dead | Live | Dead | | Live | Dead | Live | Dead | |
| 0th day | +++ | Nil | +++ | Nil | ⋯ | ++++ | Nil | ++ | Nil | ⋯ |
| 7th day | ++ | + | + | ++ | F | ++ | + | + | ++ | F |
| 14th day | + | ++ | Nil | + | F | ++ | ++ | + | +++ | F |
| 21st day | + | +++ | Nil | Nil | G | + | ++ | Nil | Nil | F |
| 28th day | Nil | + | Nil | Nil | E | Nil | + | Nil | Nil | G |
| 42nd day | Nil | Nil | Nil | Nil | E | Nil | Nil | Nil | Nil | E |

Clinical response:
E: excellent, complete remission of clinical signs of dermatitis and point of recovery,
G: good, most primary lesions have resolved but mild secondary lesions such as erythema, crusts, and scales are still evident,
F: fair, some response to treatment but primary and secondary lesions are still evident.

Complete clinical response was recorded in Table 1. One week after therapy, scales had disappeared and dogs had mild pruritus. Two weeks after treatment, the number of mites gradually decreased and the dogs were free from pruritus, erythema, erosions, and ulcers. One month after treatment, the general skin condition was improved; absence of pruritus was noticed and number of mites was also decreased. Complete disappearance of mites and regrowth of hair were noticed after forty two days of therapy. Haematological abnormalities included reduced total erythrocyte count ($6.2 \pm 0.10 \times 10^6$/cumm), haemoglobin concentration ($11.2\pm0.27\%$), leukocytosis ($1220\pm850$/cumm), neutrophilia ($9420 \pm 1221$/cumm), and eosinophilia ($1200 \pm 782$/cumm). Haematological abnormalities recorded in this study were in agreement with the previous studies on dogs with different types of mange [9, 10]. The anaemia due to loss of skin proteins and leukocytosis might be due to allergic reaction caused by mites or their products of inflammatory reactions [11].

In previous studies sarcoptic mange, mange due to two types of demodicosis, was reported in individual dogs [5, 12, 13]. Different types of mange mites were treated with oral ivermectin at different dose rates in dogs and cats [7, 11]. According to the authors' knowledge this is the first attempt to report and treat the mixed infection in dogs. Life cycle of Sarcoptes scabiei presumes that development from egg to adult may require 9–13 days and maturation of the egg takes 3-4 days, following which the larva hatches from the egg [14]. It is also known that survival on the host is up to 10 days or lesser. Avermectin compounds have no ovicidal activity on the eggs of mites and repetition of the treatment was advised to dogs with sarcoptic mange to prevent recurrence of this condition [15]. Therapy continued till two consequent negative skin scrapings and showed the ability to kill adult mites, besides killing any larvae hatching from eggs, as well as to prevent reinfection of mites of the host. To control recurrence of infection, once a week house premises were also sprayed with amitraz (4 mL in 1 liter of water).

## Conflict of Interests

The authors declare that there is no conflict of interests regarding the publication of this paper.

## References

[1] D. W. Scott, W. M. Miller, and C. E. Griffin, "Chapter 6. Parasitic skin disease," in Muller and Kirk's Small Animal Dermatology, C. di Berardino, Ed., pp. 423–516, W.B. Saunders Company, Philadelphia, Pa, USA, 6th edition, 2001.

[2] C. E. Desch and A. Hillier, "Demodex injai: a new species of hair follicle mite (Acari: Demodecidae) from the domestic dog (Canidae)," Journal of Medical Entomology, vol. 40, no. 2, pp. 146–149, 2003.

[3] B. S. Reddy, K. N. Kumari, V. C. Rayulu, and S. Sivajothi, "Demodex cornei causing demodicosis in dogs," Indian Journal of Veterinary Medicine, vol. 31, no. 2, pp. 100–102, 2011.

[4] S. Sivajothi, B. S. Reddy, K. N. Kumari, and V. C. Rayulu, "Morphometry of demodex canis and demodex cornei in dogs with demodicosis in India," International Journal of Veterinary Health Science & Research, vol. 1, article 301, 2013.

[5] B. S. Reddy and K. N. Kumari, "Canine scabies—its therapeutic management and zoonotic importance," Intas Polivet, vol. 14, no. 2, pp. 292–294, 2013.

[6] W. Rosenkrantz, "Cutaneous cytology—A quick review of an indispensable test," Veterinary Medicine Supplement, pp. 20–21, 2008.

[7] B. S. Reddy and K. N. Kumari, "Demodicosis and its successful management in dogs," Indian Journal of Field Veterinarians, vol. 6, no. 2, pp. 48–50, 2010.

[8] B. S. Reddy, K. N. Kumari, V. V. Rao, and V. C. Rayulu, "Efficacy of cefpodoxime with clavulanic acid in the treatment of recurrent pyoderma in dogs," ISRN Veterinary Science, vol. 2014, Article ID 467010, 5 pages, 2014.

[9] B. S. Reddy, K. N. Kumari, and S. Sivajothi, "Haemato-biochemical findings and thyroxin levels in canine demodicosis," Comparative Clinical Pathology, 2014.

[10] B. S. Reddy, K. N. Kumari, and S. Sivajothi, "Thyroxin levels and haematological changes in dogs with sarcoptic mange," *Journal of Advances in Parasitology*, vol. 1, no. 2, pp. 27–29, 2014.

[11] B. S. Reddy and S. Sivajothi, "*Notoedric* mange associated with *Malassezia* in Cats," *International Journal of Veterinary Health Science & Research*, vol. 2, p. 101, 2014.

[12] S. Sivajothi, B. S. Reddy, and V. C. Rayulu, "Management of *Sarcoptic mange* in rabbits," *International Research Journal of Life Sciences*, vol. 1, no. 1, pp. 21–25, 2013.

[13] S. Sivajothi, B. S. Reddy, and V. C. Rayulu, "Demodicosis caused by *Demodex canis* and *Demodex cornei* in dogs," *Journal of Parasitic Diseases*, 2013.

[14] R. Wall and D. Shearer, *Veterinary Ectoparasites: Biology, Pathology and Control*, Blackwells Science, Oxford, UK, 2nd edition, 2001.

[15] B. Pan, M. Wang, F. Xu, Y. Wang, Y. Dong, and Z. Pan, "Efficacy of an injectable formulation of eprinomectin against *Psoroptes cuniculi*, the ear mange mite in rabbits," *Veterinary Parasitology*, vol. 137, no. 3-4, pp. 386–390, 2006.

# 30

# Primary Corneal Squamous Cell Carcinoma in a Dog: Clinical and Histopathological Evaluation

**Giovanni Barsotti,[1] Lorenzo Ressel,[2] Riccardo Finotello,[3] Veronica Marchetti,[1] and Francesca Millanta[2]**

[1] Department of Veterinary Clinics, Faculty of Veterinary Medicine, University of Pisa, Via Livornese Lato Monte, San Piero a Grado, 56122 Pisa, Italy
[2] Department of Animal Pathology, Faculty of Veterinary Medicine, University of Pisa, Delle Piagge 2 Avenue, 56100 Pisa, Italy
[3] Small Animal Teaching Hospital, University of Liverpool, Leahurst, Liverpool, Leahurst Campus Chester High Road, Neston, Wirral CH64 7TE, UK

Correspondence should be addressed to Giovanni Barsotti, gbarsott@vet.unipi.it

Academic Editor: M. Bugno-Poniewierska

An 8-year-old male pug with a 12-month history of a progressive nonpainful mass on the left cornea was evaluated. Ocular examination showed a severe bilateral keratoconjunctivitis sicca, pigmentary keratitis, and an exophytic irregular pink mass occupying approximately 75% of the total corneal surface of the left eye. A squamous cell carcinoma (SCC) was suspected on cytology, and clinical investigations showed no evidence of metastases. A transpalpebral enucleation was therefore performed, and the diagnosis of SCC was confirmed on histopathology. Immunohistochemical investigations showed that the neoplastic cells were pan-cytokeratin positive and vimentin negative. Additionally, nuclei immunoreactive to Ki-67 antigen were detected. Tumor cells were also negative to p53. Immunoreactivity to COX-2 was found in less than 10% of the neoplastic cells. No adjuvant therapies were instituted, and no evidence of local recurrence or distance metastasis was identified during the 24-month follow-up period.

## 1. Introduction

Neoplasms of the cornea occur uncommonly in dogs although various primary and secondary tumors have been described in veterinary literature [1, 2]. Corneal squamous cell carcinoma (SCC) is considered rare in the dog and often represents a secondary extension of a primary limbal or conjunctival neoplasia [1, 3, 4]. A number of cases of canine primary SCC of the cornea have been described especially in recent years [5–10], and some authors report an increased occurrence of the tumor in this period [11]. Only three canine SCCs have been characterized by the use of immunohistochemistry, and p53 protein was generally investigated with varying results [7, 9]. Cyclooxygenase (COX) overexpression has been identified in various neoplastic tissues in humans [12–18] and domestic animals [19–26]. COX-2 has been found to be strongly expressed in all the cases of canine SCC of the cutis [27].

Since the etiopathogenesis of ocular SCC is still unclear, some authors have evaluated the expression of COX, especially COX-2, in corneal neoplastic tissues of horses and have suggested a possible role of the enzyme in oncogenesis and/or progression of this type of corneal tumor [23, 24].

The aim of the present study was to describe the clinical and histopathological appearance of a primary corneal SCC in an 8 year-old male pug dog, to report its histopathological findings, and to characterise the tumour using antivimentin and antipan cytokeratin antibodies and evaluate the expression of cyclooxygenase-2, p53 protein, and Ki-67 antigen in the neoplastic cornea by the use of immunohistochemical (IHC) techniques.

## 2. Case Presentation

An 8 year-old, 8 kg, intact male Pug was examined for 12-month history of a progressive nonpainful lesion of the

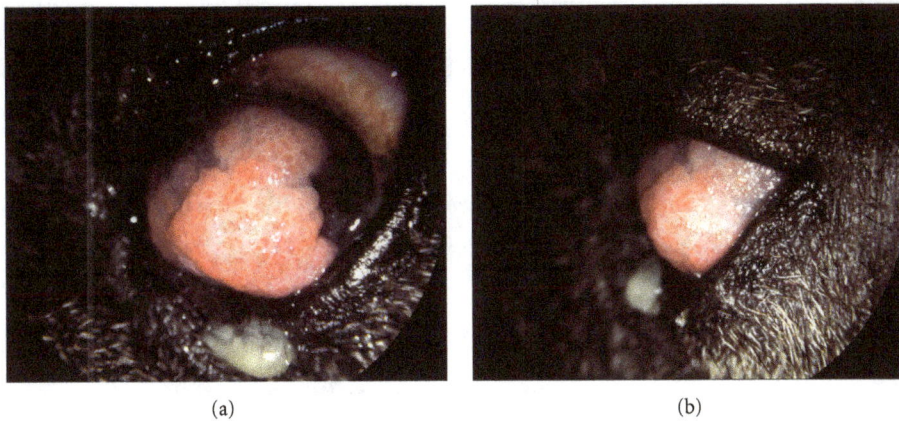

(a)                                                                          (b)

FIGURE 1: (a) Photograph of the left eye of an 8-year-old male Pug demonstrating an exophytic, irregular reddish-pink mass occupying approximately 75% of the total corneal surface. The cornea surrounding the mass is pigmented and vascularized. (b) Lateral view of the eye. Note the highly deformed profile of the cornea.

left cornea. The past medical record of the dog excluded any major illnesses, vaccinations were routinely performed, and the dog was on heartworm prophylaxis. Serology for *Leishmania infantum* was performed every year with negative results. Physical examination revealed no other abnormal findings.

Gross ocular examination showed a bilateral nasal fold trichiasis, a bilateral ocular discharge, an exophytic reddish-pink mass arising from the cornea of the left eye, and a complete corneal, pigmentation of the right eye. Schirmer I tear test readings obtained using commercially available test strips (Dina strip Schirmer-Plus; GECIS sarl, France) were 3 and 4 mm/min OS and OD, respectively. Palpebral, corneal and dazzle reflexes were present in both eyes (OU), whereas menace response was negative in both eyes. Because of the complete opacity of the cornea of both eyes, it was no possible to evaluate direct and indirect pupillary light reflexes. The intraocular pressure was assessed by means of applanation tonometry (Tonopen-XL; Mentor, MA, USA) following a topical administration of 0.4% oxybuprocaine chlorhydrate (Benoxinato chlorhydrate Intes; Alfa Intes Industria Terapeutica Splendore S.r.l., Italy) and was found to be 18 mmHg in the right eye. The highly deformed profile of the left cornea did not allow us to obtain reliable intraocular pressure values from the left eye. Slit-lamp biomicroscopy (Kowa SL-14, Kowa company, Japan) showed conjunctival hyperemia and mild chemosis OU, a complete pigmentation of the right cornea with neovascularization and an exophytic, irregular reddish-pink mass occupying approximately 75% of the total corneal surface of the left eye (Figure 1). The growth was also firm, moderately friable, and bled easily on manipulation. The peripheral cornea, not involved by the lesion, was pigmented and vascularized, and the limbus and sclera were unaffected. The anterior chamber, the iris, the vitreous, and the fundus were not examined OU because of the complete opacity of both corneas.

An initial diagnosis of a suspected corneal tumor of the left eye, bilateral keratoconjunctivitis sicca, and pigmentary keratitis was formulated.

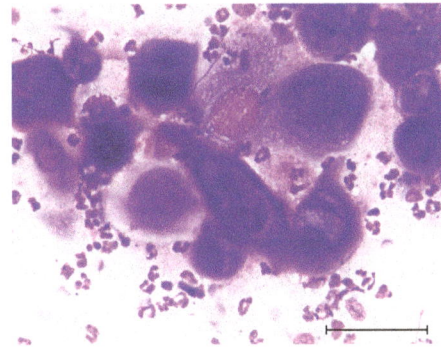

FIGURE 2: Cytological features. Pleomorphic squamous epithelium with marked anisokaryosis, hyperbasophilic cytoplasm, and perinuclear vacuolation associated with neutrophilic inflammation (magnification bar = 50 microns, May-Grunwald Giemsa stain).

Differential diagnosis of the mass included primary corneal tumor and nonneoplastic corneal lesions such as granulation tissue and chronic proliferative keratitis.

The diagnostic workup included CBC, blood smear evaluation, serum biochemical profile, coagulation profile, urinalysis, and fine needle aspiration biopsy (FNAB) of the mass. CBC, serum biochemical profile, coagulation profile, and urinalysis results were unremarkable.

Cytologic specimens were stained with May-Grunwald Giemsa and showed a moderate blood contamination and rounded, spindled, and angulated cells. Cells with hyperbasophilic keratinized cytoplasm displayed anisokaryosis and perinuclear vacuolization. Nondegenerate neutrophils were also present (Figure 2). The cytological pattern was compatible with an epithelial tumour and strongly suspicious of a squamous cell carcinoma.

The dog was then staged to evaluate the presence of distance metastases. An ocular ultrasound of the left eye, performed to rule out any orbital and intraocular involvement, was negative. Chest X-ray in three standard projections and abdominal ultrasonography were performed, revealing no evidence of disease.

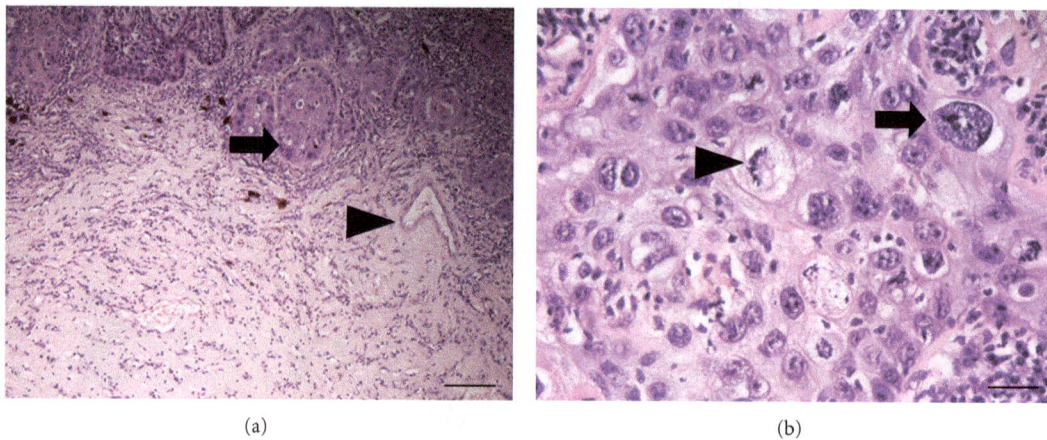

(a)                                                      (b)

FIGURE 3: Histopathological features. (a) Proliferation and invasion of the stroma by epithelial neoplastic cells (arrow). A blood vessel is present in the stroma (arrowhead) (magnification bar = 100 microns, haematoxylin and eosin stain). (b) Neoplastic epithelial cells are characterized by atypical anisokaryotic nuclei (arrow) and frequent mitotic figures (arrowhead) (magnification bar = 25 microns, haematoxylin and eosin stain).

Considering the clinical aspect of the lesion, the results of the FNAB and the concurrent severe keratoconjunctivitis sicca, a transpalpebral enucleation of the left eye was performed. After surgery, the dog recovered well from anaesthesia, and no adjuvant therapies were instituted. Followup every six months did not reveal any sign of orbital recurrence or metastatic disease. The dog appeared to be sound at the last clinical staging performed 24 months after surgery.

The enucleated eye was fixed in a 10% formalin solution before being routinely processed and paraffin-wax embedded. Sections were stained with haematoxylin and eosin (HE). Microscopically, the corneal epithelium was focally affected by an unencapsulated proliferation of squamous epithelial corneal cells infiltrating the underlying connective tissue (Figure 3(a)). Neoplastic cells were arranged in nests (Figure 3(a), arrow) and in multifocally formed foci of intraepithelial keratinisation. Neoplastic cells were round to polygonal, pleomorphic with abundant cytoplasm, with irregularly shaped immature nuclei characterized by a high grade of anisokaryosis and multiple nucleoli (Figure 3(b), arrow). Mitotic figures were frequent (45 per 10 HPFs), and often bizarre (Figure 3(b), arrowhead). The neoplasia showed an inflammatory cell infiltrate composed of lymphocytes and neutrophils, and the infiltrated stroma was characterized by the presence of newly formed blood vessels (Figure 3(a), arrowhead).

To perform IHC analysis, the sections were deparaffinized in Bio-Clear (Bio-Optica, Milan, Italy) and hydrated with grade ethanol concentration until distilled water. Antigen retrieval was performed by calibrated water bath capable of maintaining the epitope retrieval solution in a 10 mM sodium citrate buffer (pH 6.0) at 97°C for 30 min. The sections were allowed to cool down at room temperature (RT) for 20 min. To block endogenous peroxidase activity, the slides were treated with 3.0% hydrogen peroxide in distilled water for 10 min and washed with phosphate-buffered saline (PBS; Dako, Denmark) two or three times.

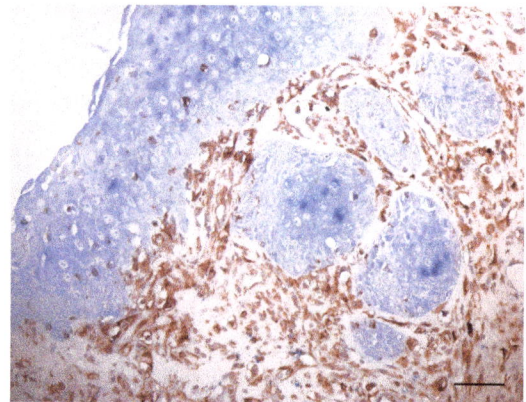

FIGURE 4: Immunohistochemical staining. Neoplastic epithelial cells express Pan-Cytokeratin (blue stain) and invade the stroma (brown stain) (magnification bar = 25 microns, double immunohistochemistry).

After blocking nonspecific antigen with normal horse serum (UltraVision; LabVision, CA, USA), the following was used as primary commercial antibodies: anti-COX-2 (goat polyclonal; Santacruz biotech, CA, USA) at 1 : 100 dilution, anti-Ki-67 (clone MIB-1; Neomarkers, CA, USA) at 1 : 100 dilution, anti-Pan-Cytokeratin (rabbit polyclonal; CKp Novocastra Laboratories, Newcastle upon Tyne, UK), antivimentin (clone V9; Dako, Denmark) at 1 : 100 dilution, and anti-p53 (mouse monoclonal clone DO7; Dako, Denmark) at dilution 1 : 25. The incubation of the primary antibodies was performed at room temperature for 60 minutes. The IHC analyses were performed using the streptavidin-biotin alkaline phosphatase complex (UltraVision; LabVision, CA, USA), and the peroxidase reaction was developed for 10 min with 3,3′-diaminobenzidine (DAB; Vector Laboratories Inc., CA, USA) and stopped with deionised water. The sections were counterstained with Mayer's hematoxylin. Negative controls were performed by substituting the primary antibody with a nonimmune serum at the same concentration.

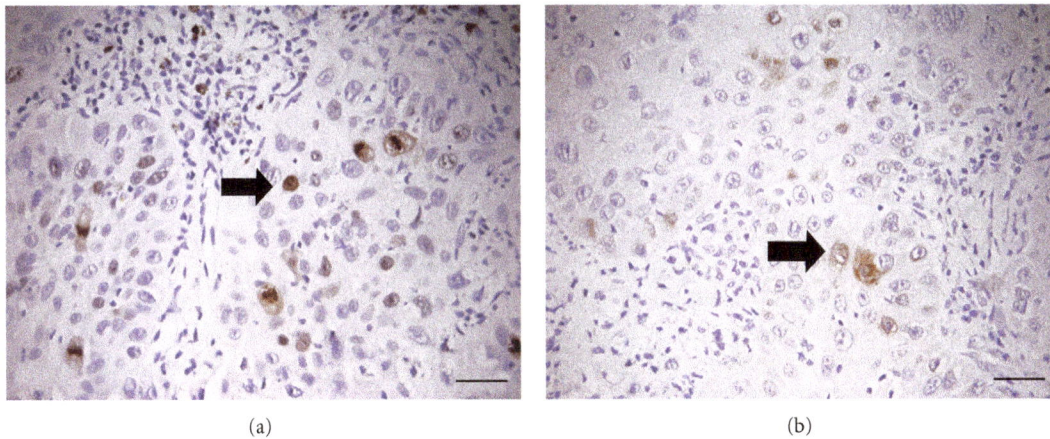

(a)

(b)

FIGURE 5: Immunohistochemical staining. (a) Ki67-positive cells (arrow) in the context of epithelial neoplastic cells (magnification bar = 25 microns, immunohistochemistry). (b) A small percentage of neoplastic cells express COX-2 (arrow) (magnification bar = 25 microns, immunohistochemistry).

COX-2 immunoexpression was quantified according to previously established guidelines [22]. The labeling index of Ki-67 was quantified as previously described [28]. Double immunohistochemistry was performed to investigate pan-cytokeratin and vimentin simultaneous expression using Multivision system (Thermo Scientific, MA, USA), following manufacturer's instructions.

Double immunostaining for pan-cytokeratin and vimentin showed a pan-cytokeratin positive/Vimentin negative pattern of tumor cells (Figure 4) and allowed their differentiation from stromal cells that expressed Vimentin alone. Cell proliferation, assessed by Ki-67 labelling index, was 8 positive nuclei/1000 cells at 400x (Figure 5(a)). Less than 10% of neoplastic cells were positive for COX-2 immunostaining (Figure 5(b)), and thus the tumor was considered as non-COX-2 overexpressing. No immunoreactivity to p53 was observed.

## 3. Discussion

Primary corneal squamous cell carcinoma (SCC) is considered rare in dogs [1, 2], indeed, until 2008, only four cases of this type of tumor had been described [5, 6]. Nevertheless, in the last two years, some case reports ($n = 6$) [7–10] and a case series ($n = 26$) [11] of canine primary corneal SCC have been published, and occurrence of this type of tumor seems to be increasing [11]. Most of the dogs presenting with corneal SCC had had a history of chronic keratitis [11], such as keratoconjunctivitis sicca [6], pigmentary keratitis [6, 9] or keratitis secondary to eyelid abnormalities [7], or trauma [5]. Only a few dogs did not show any concurrent ocular surface disease at the time of the diagnosis [8, 11]. Considering the clinical evidence of chronic keratitis in most cases, a continuous ocular surface inflammation seems to play a crucial role in the development of primary corneal SCC in dogs. Likewise, the object of this study presented a severe bilateral keratoconjunctivitis sicca and pigmentary keratitis with a 2-year history of mucous ocular discharge and corneal opacity with no record of topical treatment.

With respect to breed predisposition, brachycephalic dogs, especially pugs, with a history of chronic keratitis seem to be predisposed to developing this type of tumor. Out of 36 dogs presenting a primary corneal SCC described in veterinary literature [5–11], 13 were pugs, as is the dog of the present case report. Pugs exhibit a certain degree of exophthalmos, macroblepharon, and lagophthalmos, and this combination of anatomic features causes inadequate blinking and leads to exposure keratopathy syndrome. In addition, many pugs show a nasal fold trichiasis and a mild medial entropion of the lower eyelid. The severe corneal irritation secondary to its exposure, to eyelid defects, and to the presence of facial folds might explain the high prevalence of primary SCC cases in this breed.

Some authors have reported a possible relationship between the occurrence of corneal SCC and the use of topical immunosuppressants [11], but it is important to note that all the dogs who received this type of drug also showed a chronic keratitis. Thus, it is difficult to establish which is the most likely predisposing factor (chronic corneal inflammation versus immunosuppressant drugs) in the development of neoplastic disease.

Primary corneal SCC might be a related consequence of ultraviolet radiation exposure as reported by Montiani-Ferreira et al. [7]. In fact the IHC results of their study detected a strong p53 expression that is considered suggestive of p53 gene mutation which is likely to be a consequence of ultraviolet radiation exposure [29]. P53 is a nuclear phosphoprotein that is normally present in various tissues. The wild type of this protein is characterized by a short half-life (20–30 min) [30] and is usually undetectable with IHC [31]. If a somatic mutation occurs, the p53 half-life increases (2 hours) and the protein becomes detectable with IHC methods [30]. P53 mutation is a common feature of many neoplasms in both human and veterinary medicine, and p53 changes have also been observed in ocular SCC of domestic animals [32–35], and human beings [36].

Our results showed the absence of p53 immunoreactivity, in accordance with Takiyama et al. [9] who described two cases of canine primary corneal SCC in which nuclear p53 immunoreactivity was not detected. The adopted antibody, the same as used by Takiyama et al., was the monoclonal (MAb) mouse antihuman p53 protein clone DO-7. Instead, Montiani-Ferreira et al. [7] observed a strong p53 expression in the neoplastic tissue using a rabbit polyclonal (PAb) antihuman p53 protein. Differences between the results of Montiani-Ferreira et al. [7], and Takiyama et al. [9] and ours could be related to the use of different antibodies and staining protocols. Another possible cause explaining the negativity for p53 staining is a deletion of the p53 gene resulting in the absence of p53 protein in neoplastic cells. On the other hand, the negativity for p53 could also be related to no mutation of this protein, and thus, in our case, p53 gene mutation due to UV overexposure may not be a predisposing factor in the occurrence of the primary corneal SCC. It is important to note that Italy has UV index ranges 1–3 in January and 7–9 in July, slightly higher than Japan's [9] but lower than Brazil's, where the monthly average UV index goes from 3.5 in February to 13.4 in July [7]. In Italy, as in Japan, there is a lower UV exposure risk and probably a lower UV influence in corneal SCC development. This latter hypothesis may also explain the low Ki-67 labelling index observed. The lack of p53 mutations may, in fact, not have altered the cell-cycle regulation. It is well known that Ki-67 is a nonhistone nuclear protein which is expressed in all the phases of the cell cycle except G0 and G1, and that it is, therefore, widely used to assess the cell proliferation [37].

COX-2 is the inducible form of COX and catalyzes the production of prostaglandins from arachidonic acid. Of these prostaglandins, $PGE_2$ is the one primarily responsible for several tumorigenic effects, such as the increase of cell proliferation, inhibition of apoptosis, and neoangiogenesis. Our case showed a weak and focal immunoreactivity to COX-2 in less than 10% of neoplastic cells and was considered as a non-COX-2-overexpressing tumor [22, 38–40]. Previous studies have described COX-2 expression in SCC of the cornea in horses [23, 24]. Since the methodologies, as well as the scoring methods, adopted are different, it is still unclear whether COX-2 plays a role in the development and progression of this type of corneal tumor. A recent study performed by Smith et al. [25] has shown that COX-2 was expressed in a low percentage of tumor cells and at low intensity in equine ocular SCC.

Our results do not lend themselves as a rationale to consider COX-2 pharmacological inhibition as an adjuvant tool in the treatment of corneal SCC in dogs, as previously suggested by Smith et al. [25] in ocular SCC in horses.

In the case of dogs with normal function of the eye affected by corneal SCC, a superficial keratectomy alone [4, 6, 9] or associated with adjuvant therapies (cryosurgery [5] or topical mitomycin C [8]) has been described with good results.

In our dog we performed a transpalpebral enucleation without adjuvant therapies, and we did not consider any treatment to preserve the affected eye because of the wide extension of the neoplasia above the cornea, but especially because of the concurrent presence of a severe keratoconjunctivitis sicca, which could have delayed corneal healing with postoperative complications.

In conclusion, surgical treatment must be considered the best therapeutic approach for ocular SCC in dogs. Further studies would be useful to better understand the role of COX-2 expression and its therapeutic implication in corneal SCC of the dog, especially in dogs where the conservative surgical treatment, superficial keratectomy, is chosen.

# References

[1] C. A. Fischer, D. M. Lindley, W. C. Carlton, and H. van Hecke, "Tumors of the cornea and sclera," in *Ocular Tumors in Animals and Humans*, R. L. Peiffer Jr and K. B. Simons, Eds., pp. 149–202, Blackwell Publishing, Ames, Iowa, USA, 1st edition, 2002.

[2] B. C. Gilger, E. Bentley, and F. J. Ollivier, "Disease and surgery of the cornea and sclera," in *Veterinary Ophthalmology*, K. N. Gelatt, Ed., pp. 690–752, Blackwell Publishing, Ames, Iowa, USA, 4th edition, 2007.

[3] D. A. Ward, K. S. Latimer, and R. M. Askren, "Squamous cell carcinoma of the corneoscleral limbus in a dog," *Journal of the American Veterinary Medical Association*, vol. 200, no. 10, pp. 1503–1506, 1992.

[4] C. Busse, J. Sansom, R. R. Dubielzig, and A. Hayes, "Corneal squamous cell carcinoma in a Border Collie," *Veterinary Ophthalmology*, vol. 11, no. 1, pp. 55–58, 2008.

[5] K. S. Latimer, R. L. Kaswan, and J. P. Sundberg, "Corneal squamous cell carcinoma in a dog," *Journal of the American Veterinary Medical Association*, vol. 190, no. 11, pp. 1430–1432, 1987.

[6] M. E. Bernays, D. Flemming, and R. L. Peiffer, "Primary corneal papilloma and squamous cell carcinoma associated with pigmentary keratitis in four dogs," *Journal of the American Veterinary Medical Association*, vol. 214, no. 2, pp. 215–217, 1999.

[7] F. Montiani-Ferreira, M. Kiupel, P. Muzolon, and J. Truppel, "Corneal squamous cell carcinoma in a dog: a case report," *Veterinary Ophthalmology*, vol. 11, no. 4, pp. 269–272, 2008.

[8] K. Karasawa, H. Matsuda, and A. Tanaka, "Superficial keratectomy and topical mitomycin C as therapy for a corneal squamous cell carcinoma in a dog: case report," *Journal of Small Animal Practice*, vol. 49, no. 4, pp. 208–210, 2008.

[9] N. Takiyama, E. Terasaki, and M. Uechi, "Corneal squamous cell carcinoma in two dogs," *Veterinary Ophthalmology*, vol. 13, no. 4, pp. 266–269, 2010.

[10] F. S. Prando, F. G. Jannuzzi, M. Rosa, C. G. Lieberknecht, C. F. Lieberknecht, and J. S. Pereira, "Squamous cell carcinoma in the pug cornea-report of two cases (abstract)," *Veterinary Ophthalmology*, vol. 13, no. 5, p. 408, 2010.

[11] R. R. Dubielzig, C. S. Schobert, and J. Dreyfus, "Superficial corneal squamous cell carcinoma occurring in dogs with chronic keratitis," *Veterinary Ophthalmology*, vol. 14, no. 3, pp. 161–168, 2011.

[12] O. Gallo, E. Masini, B. Bianchi, L. Bruschini, M. Paglierani, and A. Franchi, "Prognostic significance of cyclooxygenase-2 pathway and angiogenesis in head and neck squamous cell carcinoma," *Human Pathology*, vol. 33, no. 7, pp. 708–714, 2002.

[13] B. Singh, J. A. Berry, A. Shoher, V. Ramakrishnan, and A. Lucci, "COX-2 overexpression increases motility and invasion of breast cancer cells," *International Journal of Oncology*, vol. 26, no. 5, pp. 1393–1399, 2005.

[14] T. C. Tang, R. T. Poon, C. P. Lau, D. Xie, and S. T. Fan, "Tumor cyclooxygenase-2 levels correlate with tumor invasiveness in

human hepatocellular carcinoma," *World Journal of Gastroenterology*, vol. 11, no. 13, pp. 1896–1902, 2005.

[15] R. Miao, N. Liu, Y. Wang et al., "Coexpression of cyclooxygenase-2 and vascular endothelial growth factor in gastrointestinal stromal tumor: possible relations to pathological parameters and clinical behavior," *Hepato-Gastroenterology*, vol. 55, no. 88, pp. 2012–2015, 2008.

[16] J. A. G. Filho, C. F. W. Nonaka, M. C. D. C. Miguel, R. D. A. Freitas, and H. C. Galvão, "Immunoexpression of cyclooxygenase-2 and p53 in oral squamous cell carcinoma," *American Journal of Otolaryngology*, vol. 30, no. 2, pp. 89–94, 2009.

[17] R. Kawata, S. Hyo, M. Araki, and H. Takenaka, "Expression of cyclooxygenase-2 and microsomal prostagalandin E synthase-1 in head and neck squamous cell carcinoma," *Auris Nasus Larynx*, vol. 37, no. 4, pp. 482–487, 2010.

[18] H. U. Kasper, E. Konze, H. P. Dienes, D. L. Stippel, P. Schirmacher, and M. Kern, "COX-2 expression and effects of COX-2 inhibition in colorectal carcinomas and their liver metastases," *Anticancer Research*, vol. 30, no. 6, pp. 2017–2023, 2010.

[19] K. N. M. Khan, D. W. Knapp, D. B. Denicola, and R. K. Harris, "Expression of cyclooxygenase-2 in transitional cell carcinoma of the urinary bladder in dogs," *American Journal of Veterinary Research*, vol. 61, no. 5, pp. 478–481, 2000.

[20] K. N. M. Khan, K. M. Stanfield, D. Trajkovic, and D. W. Knapp, "Expression of cyclooxygenase-2 in canine renal cell carcinoma," *Veterinary Pathology*, vol. 38, no. 1, pp. 116–119, 2001.

[21] M. Kleiter, D. E. Malarkey, D. E. Ruslander, and D. E. Thrall, "Expression of cyclooxygenase-2 in canine epithelial nasal tumors," *Veterinary Radiology and Ultrasound*, vol. 45, no. 3, pp. 255–260, 2004.

[22] F. Millanta, S. Citi, D. D. Santa, M. Porciani, and A. Poli, "COX-2 expression in canine and feline invasive mammary carcinomas: correlation with clinicopathological features and prognostic fmolecular markers," *Breast Cancer Research and Treatment*, vol. 98, no. 1, pp. 115–120, 2006.

[23] C. L. McInnis, E. A. Giuliano, P. J. Johnson, and J. R. Turk, "Immunohistochemical evaluation of cyclooxygenase expression in corneal squamous cell carcinoma in horses," *American Journal of Veterinary Research*, vol. 68, no. 2, pp. 165–170, 2007.

[24] K. M. Rassnick and B. L. Njaa, "Cyclooxygenase-2 immunoreactivity in equine ocular squamous-cell carcinoma," *Journal of Veterinary Diagnostic Investigation*, vol. 19, no. 4, pp. 436–439, 2007.

[25] K. M. Smith, T. J. Scase, J. L. Miller, D. Donaldson, and J. Sansom, "Expression of cyclooxygenase-2 by equine ocular and adnexal squamous cell carcinomas," *Veterinary Ophthalmology*, vol. 11, no. 1, pp. 8–14, 2008.

[26] F. L. Queiroga, I. Pires, L. Lobo, and C. S. Lopes, "The role of Cox-2 expression in the prognosis of dogs with malignant mammary tumours," *Research in Veterinary Science*, vol. 88, no. 3, pp. 441–445, 2010.

[27] E. M. P. de Almeida, C. Piché, J. Sirois, and M. Doré, "Expression of cyclo-oxygenase-2 in naturally occurring squamous cell carcinomas in dogs," *Journal of Histochemistry and Cytochemistry*, vol. 49, no. 7, pp. 867–875, 2001.

[28] F. Millanta, G. Lazzeri, M. Mazzei, I. Vannozzi, and A. Poli, "MIB-1 labeling index in feline dysplastic and neoplastic mammary lesions and its relationship with postsurgical prognosis," *Veterinary Pathology*, vol. 39, no. 1, pp. 120–126, 2002.

[29] V. O. Melnikova, A. Pacifico, S. Chimenti, K. Peris, and H. N. Ananthaswamy, "Fate of UVB-induced p53 mutations in SKH-hr1 mouse skin after discontinuation of irradiation: relationship to skin cancer development," *Oncogene*, vol. 24, no. 47, pp. 7055–7063, 2005.

[30] B. Vojtěšek, J. Bàrtek, C. A. Midgley, and D. P. Lane, "An immunochemical analysis of the human nuclear phosphoprotein p53. New monoclonal antibodies and epitope mapping using recombinant p53," *Journal of Immunological Methods*, vol. 151, no. 1-2, pp. 237–244, 1992.

[31] K. Cooper and Z. Haffajee, "bcl-2 and p53 protein expression in follicular lymphoma," *Journal of Pathology*, vol. 182, no. 3, pp. 307–310, 1997.

[32] S. J. Dugan, C. R. Curtis, S. M. Roberts, and G. A. Severin, "Epidemiologic study of ocular/adnexal squamous cell carcinoma in horses," *Journal of the American Veterinary Medical Association*, vol. 198, no. 2, pp. 251–256, 1991.

[33] S. J. Dugan, S. M. Roberts, C. R. Curtis, and G. A. Severin, "Prognostic factors and survival of horses with ocular/adnexal squamous cell carcinoma: 147 cases (1978–1988)," *Journal of the American Veterinary Medical Association*, vol. 198, no. 2, pp. 298–303, 1991.

[34] J. P. Teifke and C. V. Löhr, "Immunohistochemical detection of P53 overexpression in paraffin wax-embedded squamous cell carcinomas of cattle, horses, cats and dogs," *Journal of Comparative Pathology*, vol. 114, no. 2, pp. 205–210, 1996.

[35] G. Sironi, P. Riccaboni, L. Mertel, G. Cammarata, and D. E. Brooks, "p53 protein expression in conjunctival squamous cell carcinomas of domestic animals," *Veterinary Ophthalmology*, vol. 2, no. 4, pp. 227–231, 1999.

[36] J. Reszec, M. Sulkowska, M. Koda, L. Kanczuga-Koda, and S. Sulkowski, "Expression of cell proliferation and apoptosis markers in papillomas and cancers of conjunctiva and eyelid," *Annals of the New York Academy of Sciences*, vol. 1030, pp. 419–426, 2004.

[37] J. Gerdes, L. Li, C. Schlueter et al., "Immunobiochemical and molecular biologic characterization of the cell proliferation-associated nuclear antigen that is defined by monoclonal antibody Ki-67," *American Journal of Pathology*, vol. 138, no. 4, pp. 867–873, 1991.

[38] G. Singh-Ranger and K. Mokbel, "The role of cyclooxygenase-2 (COX-2) in breast cancer, and implications of COX-2 inhibition," *European Journal of Surgical Oncology*, vol. 28, no. 7, pp. 729–737, 2002.

[39] C. S. Williams, M. Mann, and R. N. DuBois, "The role of cyclooxygenases in inflammation, cancer, and development," *Oncogene*, vol. 18, no. 55, pp. 7908–7916, 1999.

[40] S. I. Mohammed, D. Dhawan, S. Abraham et al., "Cyclooxygenase inhibitors in urinary bladder cancer: in vitro and in vivo effects," *Molecular Cancer Therapeutics*, vol. 5, no. 2, pp. 329–336, 2006.

# 31

# Canine Bilateral Conjunctivo-Palpebral Dermoid: Description of Two Clinical Cases and Discussion of the Relevance of the Terminology

O. Balland,[1] I. Raymond,[2] I. Mathieson,[3] P. F. Isard,[4]
Emilie Vidémont-Drevon,[4] and T. Dulaurent[4]

[1]Centre Hospitalier Vétérinaire, 95 rue des Mazurots, 54710 Ludres, France
[2]Department of Clinical Sciences, National Veterinary School, 23 chemin des Capelles, BP 87614, 31076 Toulouse Cedex 3, France
[3]Eyevet Referrals, 41-43 Halton Station Road, Sutton Weaver, Cheshire WA7 3DN, UK
[4]Centre Hospitalier Vétérinaire, 275 route Impériale, 74370 Saint-Martin Bellevue, France

Correspondence should be addressed to O. Balland; balland@lorrainevet.fr

Academic Editor: Paola Roccabianca

Two young dogs were presented for the evaluation of an abnormally haired appearance of both eyes since adoption. In one dog, the lesions were symmetrical and appeared as disorganized skin tissue located on the cutaneous aspect of the lateral portion of both lower eyelids, and continuing to the palpebral and the bulbar conjunctiva, thus forming continuous lesions. In the other dog, a similar lesion was present in the right eye (OD), but the lesion of the left eye (OS) was of discontinuous, disorganized skin tissue located midway on the lower eyelid and on the lateral bulbar conjunctiva. The lesions were surgically removed and routinely processed for histopathological analysis. Definitive diagnosis was conjunctivo-palpebral dermoids for each dog. Dermoids are usually considered to be choristoma (normal tissue in an abnormal location) when they are located on the ocular surface (cornea and/or conjunctiva) and as hamartoma when located on the palpebral skin. The lesion presentation in these two dogs reveals that names of "choristoma" alone or "hamartoma" alone are not accurate to depict the continuous, composite, conjunctivo-palpebral dermoids. These cases suggest that choristoma and hamartoma might develop subsequently from the same abnormal event during the embryonic development, which means that the lesion location might be the only difference between the two terms.

## 1. Introduction

Dermoids result from the formation of histologically normal cutaneous tissue in an abnormal location during embryonic development [1–3]. These developmental anomalies are usually classified in the choristoma group [1]. The dermoid tissue has all of the characteristics of skin: an epidermis, dermis, fat tissue, sebaceous glands, hair follicles, and hairs [1]. Numerous types of ocular surface dermoid have been described in dogs [4–7], cats [8, 9], horses [10–12], and anecdotally in various other species [13–19]: corneal dermoid [4–7, 15, 19, 20], conjunctivo-corneal dermoid [9, 10, 16, 17], conjunctivo-palpebral dermoid [3, 20], and dermoid of the nictitating membrane [10]. Human ocular dermoids have also been described. They can be isolated lesions or a component of Goldenhar syndrome, which also affects other organs [21–24]. In dogs, the most frequent form is the conjunctivo-corneal dermoid [3]. However, the conjunctival-palpebral dermoid, for which a genetic predisposition has been identified, is a rare finding [3]. The predisposed breeds are German Shepherd, Dalmatian, and Saint-Bernard dogs [3]. In the latter breed, the presence of a dermoid is thought to be associated with other developmental anomalies such as eyelid coloboma [25]. The small number of cases described in the literature does not allow any particular sexual predisposition to be identified.

## 2. Clinical Cases

*2.1. Case 1.* A 4-month-old male German Shepherd dog presented with development of corneal pigmentation in both eyes (OU). The dog's owners reported an abnormal ocular appearance in OU, associated with a copious mucopurulent discharge, since the dog's adoption several weeks earlier. Medical treatment instituted by the referring veterinarian, of topical administration of fusidic acid ointment (Fucithalmic Vet, Léo) BID led to a temporary improvement in the dog's symptoms. The general physical examination was unremarkable. An abundant mucopurulent ocular discharge was present bilaterally (Figure 1). Vision testing gave unreliable results. The pupillary response to light was difficult to establish due to the poor visibility of intraocular structures. Adnexal examination revealed the presence of haired skin tissue in the lateral conjunctival fornix. These hairs were numerous, approximately 3 cm long, and straight and were matted together by the chronic ocular discharge and oriented towards the external canthus. The lesion was approximately 8 mm in length, and was slightly elevated and separated from the corneo-scleral limbus by a 2 mm wide strip of bulbar conjunctiva in the temporal canthal region. It continued to reach the cutaneous aspect of the lateral lower eyelid and resulted in the absence of the lid margin in this area. The identified lesions were bilateral and symmetrical (Figure 2). The palpebral length was measured with calipers (Castroviejo compass): the upper eyelid length was 29 mm and the lower eyelid was 28 mm (4 mm laterally and 24 mm medially from the skin tissue) in length. Corneal examination with a slit lamp (SL 15, Kowa, Düsseldorf, Germany) revealed diffuse pigmentation of low density in the temporal quadrant of OU. Schirmer's tear test (STT, MSD Santé Animal, Clermont-Ferrand, France) was within the normal range of OU. The rest of the ocular examination was unremarkable. The epidemiological data, combined with the characteristic clinical presentation, led us to the diagnosis of bilateral conjunctivo-palpebral dermoids. The corneal pigmentation, associated with signs of ocular discomfort and chronic ocular discharge, was considered a consequence of the irritation produced by the hairs growing from the dermoid.

*2.1.1. Surgical Procedure.* Surgical removal of the dermoid was undertaken. General anaesthesia was induced using intravenous administration of medetomidine (Domitor ND, Sogeval, Laval, 40 μg/kg), ketamine (Imalgene 1000 ND, Merial SAS, Villeurbanne, France, 5 mg/kg), and morphine hydrochloride (Morphine 10 mg, Lavoisier, Paris, France, 0.05 mg/kg). Anaesthesia was maintained using inhaled isoflurane (Isoflo ND, Axience, Pantin, France, 1.8%) and oxygen following endotracheal intubation. The eyelids were routinely prepared using a povidone-iodine solution (Vetedine ND, Vetoquinol SA, Lures, France, diluted to 2%) after the hair was carefully cut.

The conjunctival dermoid was incised around its periphery, at the limit of the lateral palpebral conjunctiva adjoining the external canthus and the bulbar conjunctiva close to the corneoscleral limbus. The excision was continued ventrally on the cutaneous aspect of the eyelid with a V-shape incision,

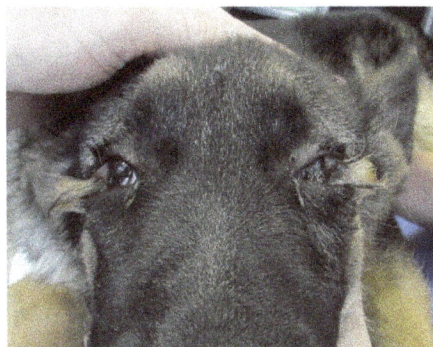

Figure 1: Case 1 appearance at initial presentation. Abnormal haired tissue and copious mucoid ocular discharge in OU.

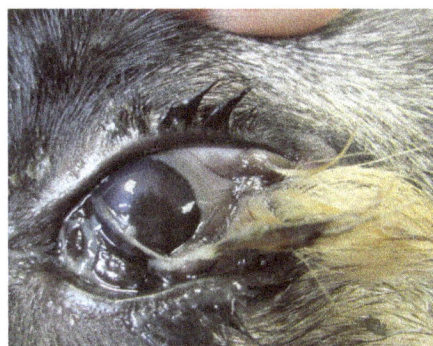

Figure 2: Case 1 appearance OS. Hair is present in the conjunctival fornix and extends beyond the lateral canthus. Ocular discharge and corneal pigmentation are also identified.

in order to achieve full excision of the dermoid and reconstruction of the lower palpebral margin. The resulting conjunctival defect was sutured in a simple continuous suture pattern using polyglactin 6-0 (Vicryl 6-0, Elanco, Neuilly-sur-Seine, France). A two-layered closure of the lower eyelid was performed. The palpebral conjunctiva was sutured using a simple continuous pattern of polyglactin 6-0 (Vicryl 6-0, Elanco, Neuilly-sur-Seine, France). The skin was then sutured with a simple interrupted pattern of nylon 5-0 (Prolene 5-0, Elanco, Neuilly-sur-Seine, France). The palpebral margin was restored by means of a "figure-of eight" suture, using the same suture material. The same procedure was followed on each side.

The postoperative medical treatment consisted of topical administration of chloramphenicol ointment (Ophtalon ND, TVM, Lempdes, France) TID OU for a period of 2 weeks. The wearing of an Elizabethan collar was prescribed for one week, together with strict precautions related to the animal's convalescence (short sanitary walks on a leash).

*2.2. Case 2.* A 1-year-old male French bulldog was referred with an abnormal ocular appearance in OU. The dog's owners reported chronic profuse bilateral ocular discharge, an abnormally haired eyelid appearance, and a whitish lesion of the left eye since his adoption. Topical chloramphenicol ointment (Ophtalon pommade, TVM, Lempdes, France) prescribed by the referring veterinarian for 2 weeks resulted in a slight reduction of the discharge.

The general physical examination was normal. Ophthalmic examination of the dog revealed slightly elevated haired tissue arising from the temporal palpebral conjunctival fornix OD, continuous with disorganised hair implantation on the adjacent skin. The palpebral margin was absent at the junction of the conjunctival and the cutaneous portion of the disorganised skin tissue. Pigmentary keratitis of the corneal region adjacent to the haired lesion was secondary to chronic irritation (Figure 3). A similar lesion was identified on the ventrolateral portion of the bulbar conjunctiva OS, with an area of disorganised skin tissue in the central portion of the lower eyelid, also involving the lid margin. The rest of the ocular examination revealed a corneal leukoma and anterior synechia OS, a consequence of a prior corneal perforation (Figure 4). Menace responses and dazzle reflexes were absent in OS and present in OD. The direct pupillary light reflex (PLR) was absent in OS and present in OD, and the indirect PLR was absent in OD and present in OS. The STT was within normal limits in OU. Intraocular pressure was 16 mm Hg OD and 15 mm Hg OS, as measured with a rebound tonometer (Tonovet, Icare, Helsinki, Finland). The clinical diagnosis was a conjunctival-palpebral dermoid affecting both eyes. The corneal scar OS was unrelated to these adnexal lesions.

*2.2.1. Surgical Procedure.* The anaesthesia and preparation of the patient were as described in Case 1. As the OD dermoid did not affect the bulbar conjunctiva, the surgery consisted of the removal of the temporal conjunctival fornix and the adjacent aberrant palpebral conjunctiva and skin. The reconstruction was carried out as described in Case 1. For the OS lesion, the disorganised skin tissue affecting the conjunctiva and the cutaneous palpebral aspect was not continuous and it required separated excisions. The abnormal tissue affecting the cutaneous aspect of the eyelid was resected with a simple V-shaped, full thickness incision to ensure removal of all hair follicles. The incision was closed in 2 layers with a continuous pattern (polyglactin 6-0 for the conjunctival repair and nylon 5-0 for the cutaneous repair). The palpebral margin was restored with a "figure-of-eight" suture using polyglactin 6-0. The isolated bulbar conjunctival lesion was removed by gentle dissection and then complete resection with straight Castroviejo scissors was carried. The bulbar conjunctiva was repaired using a continuous suture pattern of polyglactin 7-0. The excised tissues were routinely processed for histopathological analysis.

### 3. Histopathological Diagnosis (Figure 5)

The evaluated surgical excised samples consisted of fully differentiated skin tissue, regardless of their location (palpebral skin or conjunctiva) and were composed of multiple piloadnexal units, embedded in a fibrous connective tissue and deep adipose lobules. Overlying squamous stratified epithelium exhibited focal basal pigmentation, more pronounced in the conjunctival location, and variable amount of superficial

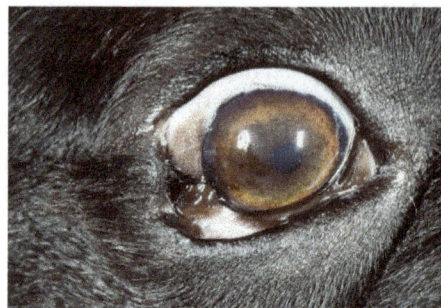

FIGURE 3: Case 2 appearance at initial presentation. Abnormal haired tissue is present in the lateral canthus OD and affects both the cutaneous and conjunctival aspects of the eyelid. Corneal pigmentation is also present.

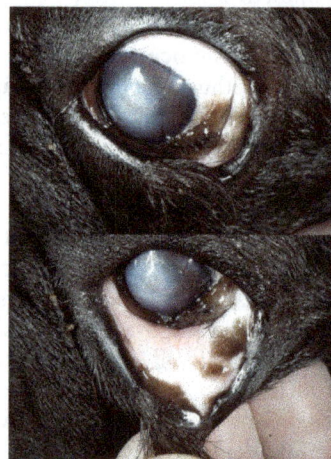

FIGURE 4: Case 2 appearance at initial presentation. Disorganized skin tissue is present on both the lower eyelid and the inferotemporal region of the bulbar conjunctiva. Gentle traction on the lower eyelid reveals that the lesions are distinct and that the conjunctival aspect of the eyelid is not affected.

keratinisation. These observations fully supported the microscopic diagnosis of conjunctivo-palpebral dermoid.

### 4. Follow-Up

Two weeks after surgery, the skin sutures were removed. A discreet cutaneous oedema limited to the lateral canthus was noticed on each side for both dogs. The palpebral margin of the lower eyelid was continuous. The owners noted that the dogs' behaviour had improved and their behaviour was more playful and less irritable. A steroidal anti-inflammatory ointment (Fradexam ointment, TVM, Lempdes, France) was prescribed BID OU for 2 weeks. Four weeks after surgery, the patients showed no signs of discomfort. The dogs' owners were satisfied with the cosmetic result (Figure 6) and the functional result, with complete resolution of any signs of ocular pain or irritation and a reduction in the degree of corneal pigmentation. There was no progression of the corneal leukoma OS of the second dog following surgery (Figure 7).

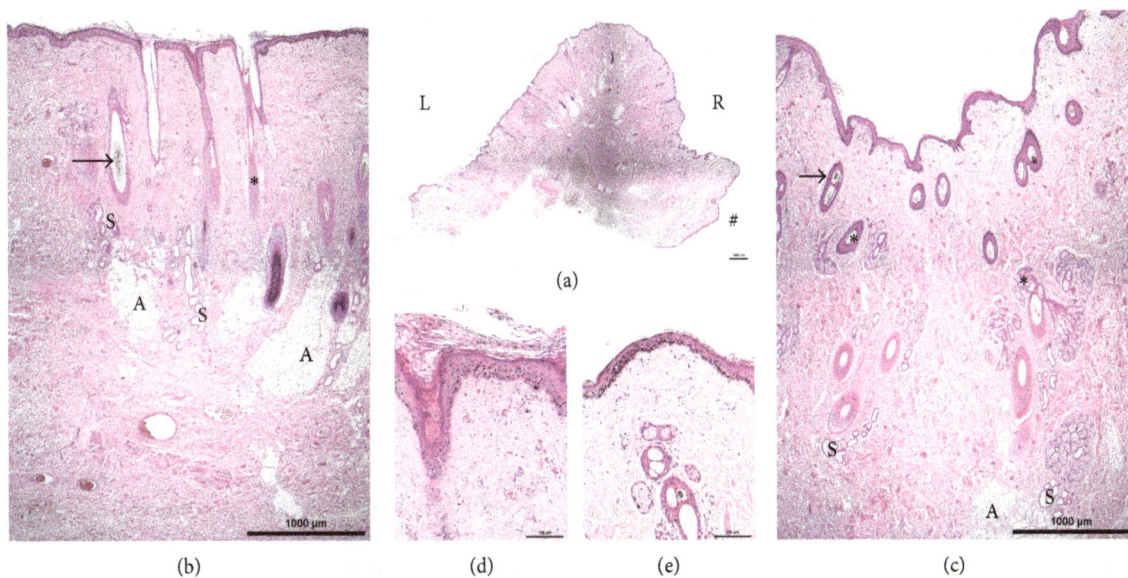

FIGURE 5: Case 2 histopathological image of excised lesion of OD, showing characteristics of normal skin. (a) At low magnification, it is impossible to differentiate the sample from another skin sample. Note the anatomical continuum from the left (eyelid hamartoma, L) to the right (conjunctival dermoid, R) and the conjunctival margin of the sample (#). Medium magnification shows pilosebaceous structures (∗) with hair shafts ( → ), sweat glands (S), and adipose lobules (A) on the cutaneous side (b) and conjunctival side (c) of the dermoid. High power aspect highlights differences between the keratinized epidermis (d) and the smooth, non-, or slight-keratinized thinner epidermis of the conjunctival side (e). Haematoxylin and eosin staining. Original magnification ×10 (a), ×40 (b, c), and ×200 (d, e).

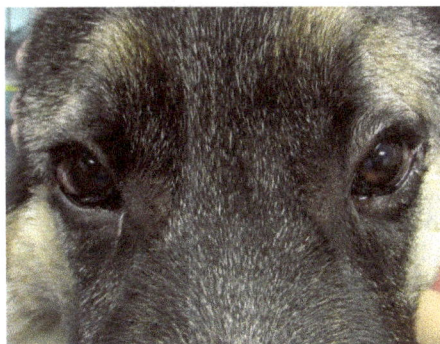

FIGURE 6: Case 1 appearance three month after surgery. No sign of discomfort is observed.

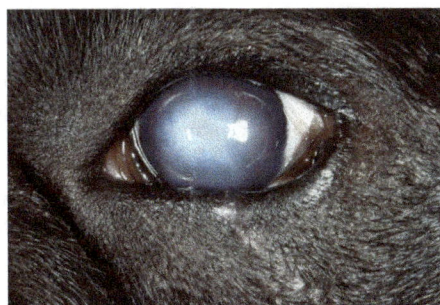

FIGURE 7: Case 2 appearance OS, 1 month after surgery. A discreet oblique scar is still present on the lower eyelid. No sign of discomfort is observed.

## 5. Discussion

The physiopathological mechanism leading to dermoid formation is unknown. The most likely hypothesis is an abnormal differentiation of the surface ectoderm during embryonic development [1]. This tissue then develops into a tegument, with all the histological characteristics of normal skin [1–3]. Although dermoids affecting the eye and its adnexa are mostly unilateral, some authors have reported cases of bilateral disease [6, 12–16, 21]. The hereditary nature of this affliction has been demonstrated in cats [8, 9], cows [14], and horses [11], as well as humans [24].

The conjunctival-palpebral dermoid in dogs is an uncommon form which has previously only been described in veterinary textbooks [1, 3] and not in peer reviewed clinical case reports. The most frequent location is at the external canthus [3], where newly formed tissue interrupts the continuity of the lid margin and continues into the conjunctival fornix [3]. In general, the length of the palpebral opening remains normal, but the presence of this tissue has functional and physical consequences that result from the presence of hairs [3].

In both of these cases, histopathological analysis of the removed modified tissues confirmed the diagnosis of dermoid. In cases of ocular surface dermoids (i.e., conjunctival or corneal dermoids), the skin tissue appears histologically normal but in an abnormal location, corresponding to the definition of choristoma [1]. Embryologically, choristoma results when one or two germ layers form mature tissue that is not normally found in that topographic location [1]. To this definition the notion of mass effect can be added [1]. In our cases, the only difference between the conjunctival portion of the dermoid and normal skin is that the keratinization of the epidermis disappeared or significantly decreased, probably due to the lacrimal fluid that permanently bathed the skin. In cases of cutaneous palpebral dermoids, the location is normal, but the development of the skin is abnormal, with a larger number and size of skin components as compared to normal skin, corresponding to the definition of hamartoma [1, 26]. According to Dubielzig et al., hamartoma is an "excessive amount of mature tissue (hypertrophy and/or hyperplasia) occurring in a location in which tissue is usually found" [1]. The mass effect is also reported as a component of the definition of hamartoma [1].

Both eyes of Case 1 and OD of Case 2 presented with continuous conjunctivo-palpebral dermoid, thus forming composite lesions, whereas OS of Case 2 presented with two distinct lesions affecting the cutaneous portion of the eyelid and the conjunctiva. The abnormal skin island located on the lower eyelid of OS of Case 2 corresponds to the definition of hamartoma. The abnormal skin island located on the conjunctiva of the same eye corresponds to the definition of choristoma. However, we believe that the current accepted terminology inadequately describes the entire composite lesion (OU of Case 1 and OD of Case 2). Indeed, the cutaneous portion of the lesion occurs in a normal location, excluding the term "choristoma." In comparison, the term "hamartoma" does not fit with the conjunctival portion of the lesion, because the anomaly occurs in a location in which skin tissue is usually not found. To the best of our knowledge, there is no specific or accurate term to define the entire cutaneoconjunctival lesion. Both parts of the lesion are probably secondary to the same abnormal event during embryonic development, affecting two adjacent areas of different nature (e.g., the skin and the conjunctival mucosa). The coexistence of distinct separated lesions on OS of Case 2 and continuous cutaneoconjunctival lesion on OD of the same patient make us hypothesize that choristomas and hamartomas may be due to the same developmental process, meaning that the notion of location might be the only difference between the two terms.

The use of the term "dermoid" also seems controversial. For some authors, dermoids are strictly defined as choristomas [1, 2, 4] and cannot be applied for a skin location, whereas for some others [3], by usage and extension, the term "dermoid" can be used for either hamartomas (when occurring on the eyelid) or choristomas (when occurring on the eye surface). In our opinion, as illustrated in these two cases with continuous cutaneoconjunctival lesions, the developmental abnormality and biologic mechanism causing the lesion are probably the same. This is the reason why the term "dermoid" remains accurate for the three possible entities: strictly palpebral lesions, strictly conjunctival (or corneal) lesions, or composite conjunctivo-palpebral lesions with a physical continuum. For this last entity, as the nature of the lesion (dermoid) cannot be associated with "hamartoma" alone or "choristoma" alone, we propose to describe it as a "choristohamartoma."

Independently from the terminology, the clinical presentation of such a lesion is comparable with that observed in cases of conjunctival of corneal dermoid. Hairs chronically traumatize the ocular surface, leading to superficial inflammation characterised by conjunctivitis, corneal neovascularisation, and pigmentation [3]. This abrasion is painful for the patient and provokes a chronic ocular discharge as well as an intense blepharospasm. The patient's abnormal ocular appearance and pain are usually the primary reasons for consultation [3].

The treatment is always surgical and obviously requires resection of the malformed area, sometimes associated with graft procedures [3, 27–29]. During the surgery, particular care must be taken in reconstruction of the palpebral margin in order to conserve palpebral function and remove any risk of iatrogenic ocular irritation. When the palpebral margin deficit is small following resection, a simple edge-to-edge suture can be used, with continuity of the margin being ensured by means of a "figure-of-eight" suture [3]. If the resection leads to a more significant deficit, a more complex oculoplastic procedure is indicated [3]. When the developmental anomaly is severe and has serious consequences (ocular pigmentation or even ulceration and chronic ocular pain), early surgery is recommended [3]. In the case of more discrete conditions having less significant physical and functional consequences, surgery can be carried out at the age of three months [3]. In Case 1, the condition was serious and caused considerable pain as well as intense corneal pigmentation, but surgery was performed at the age of 4 months, following the referring veterinarian's unsuccessful medical treatment. In both cases, the malformation was characteristically located in the outer canthal region except in OS of Case 2. Although it covered a significant portion of the conjunctival fornix, alteration of the palpebral margin was minimal, and so simple resection and classical edge-to-edge reconstruction were sufficient to permanently remove the source of irritation, restore normal palpebral function, and result in the rapid resolution of discomfort and recovery of the dog's normal temperament.

In conclusion, despite the simple but uncommon clinical presentation of these two cases, they illustrate the limitation of the terminology to describe development of abnormalities affecting the ocular surface and adnexa.

## Conflict of Interests

The authors declare that there is no conflict of interests regarding the publication of this paper.

## References

[1] R. R. Dubielzig, K. L. Ketring, G. J. McLellan, and D. M. Albert, "Diseases of eyelids and conjunctiva," in *Veterinary Ocular Pathology: A Comparative Review*, pp. 143–199, Saunders Elsevier, London, UK, 1st edition, 2010.

[2] F. C. Stades and A. van der Woerdt, "Diseases and surgery of the canine eyelid," in *Veterinary Ophthalmology*, K. N. Gelatt, B. C. Gilger, and T. J. Kern, Eds., pp. 832–893, Wiley-Blackwell, Ames, Iowa, USA, 5th edition, 2013.

[3] C. S. Cook, "Ocular embryology and congenital malformations," in *Veterinary Ophthalmology*, K. N. Gelatt, B. C. Gilger, and T. J. Kern, Eds., pp. 3–38, Wiley-Blackwell, Ames, Iowa, USA, 5th edition, 2013.

[4] D. K. Brudenall, M. E. Bernays, and R. L. Peiffer Jr., "Central corneal dermoid in a Labrador retriever puppy," *Journal of Small Animal Practice*, vol. 48, no. 10, pp. 588–590, 2007.

[5] K. Horikiri, K. Ozaki, H. Maeda, and I. Narama, "Corneal dermoid in two laboratory beagle dogs," *Jikken Dobutsu*, vol. 43, no. 3, pp. 417–420, 1994.

[6] K. N. Gelatt, "Bilateral corneal dermoids and distichiasis in a dog," *Veterinary Medicine and Small Animals Clinics*, vol. 66, no. 7, pp. 658–659, 1971.

[7] S. Minamide and K. Suzuki, "Corneal choristoma in a beagle dog," *Australian Veterinary Journal*, vol. 75, no. 2, pp. 93–94, 1997.

[8] M. B. Glaze, "Congenital and hereditary ocular abnormalities in cats," *Clinical Techniques in Small Animal Practice*, vol. 20, no. 2, pp. 74–82, 2005.

[9] P. M. Hendy-Ibbs, "Familial feline epibulbar dermoids," *Veterinary Record*, vol. 116, no. 1, pp. 13–14, 1985.

[10] S. M. Greenberg, C. E. Plummer, D. E. Brooks, S. L. Craft, and J. A. Conway, "Third eyelid dermoid in a horse," *Veterinary Ophthalmology*, vol. 15, no. 5, pp. 351–354, 2012.

[11] J. R. Joyce, J. E. Martin, R. W. Storts, and L. Skow, "Iridial hypoplasia (aniridia) accompanied by limbic dermoids and cataracts in a group of related quarterhorses," *Equine Veterinary Journal Supplement*, no. 10, pp. 26–28, 1990.

[12] S. A. McLaughlin and A. H. Brightman, "Bilateral ocular dermoids in a colt," *Equine Practice*, vol. 5, pp. 10–14, 1983.

[13] K. N. Gelatt, "Corneo-conjunctival dermoid cyst in a calf," *Veterinary Medicine and Small Animals Clinics*, vol. 67, no. 11, article 1217, 1972.

[14] S. D. Barkyoumb and H. W. Leipold, "Nature and cause of bilateral ocular dermoids in Hereford cattle," *Veterinary Pathology*, vol. 21, no. 3, pp. 316–324, 1984.

[15] J. E. Croshaw, "Bilateral corneal dermoid in a calf: a case report," *Journal of the American Veterinary Medical Association*, vol. 135, pp. 216–218, 1959.

[16] D. K. Brudenall, D. A. Ward, L. A. Kerr, and S. J. Newman, "Bilateral corneoconjunctival dermoids and nasal choristomas in a calf," *Veterinary Ophthalmology*, vol. 11, no. 3, pp. 202–206, 2008.

[17] E. E. B. LaDouceur, J. Ernst, and M. K. Keel, "Unilateral corneoscleral choristomas (corneal dermoids) in a white-tailed deer (*Odocoileus virginianus*)," *Journal of Wildlife Diseases*, vol. 48, no. 3, pp. 826–828, 2012.

[18] C. P. Moore, J. B. Shaner, R. M. Halenda, C. S. Rosenfeld, and W. K. Suedmeyer, "Congenital ocular anomalies and ventricular septal defect in a dromedary camel (*Camelus dromedarius*)," *Journal of Zoo and Wildlife Medicine*, vol. 30, no. 3, pp. 423–430, 1999.

[19] C. W. Nichols and M. Yanoff, "Dermoid of a rat cornea," *Pathologia Veterinaria*, vol. 6, no. 3, pp. 214–216, 1969.

[20] D. D. Lawson, "Corneal dermoids in animals," *Veterinary Record*, vol. 97, no. 23, pp. 449–450, 1975.

[21] P. Henkind, G. Marinoff, A. Manas, and A. Friedman, "Bilateral corneal dermoids," *American Journal of Ophthalmology*, vol. 76, no. 6, pp. 972–977, 1973.

[22] A. Mahdavi Fard and L. Pourafkari, "Images in clinical medicine. The hairy eyeball—limbal dermoid," *The New England Journal of Medicine*, vol. 368, no. 1, p. 64, 2013.

[23] M. D. R. A. Gonzalez, A. Navas, A. Haber, T. Ramírez-Luquín, and E. O. Graue-Hernández, "Ocular dermoids: 116 consecutive cases," *Eye and Contact Lens*, vol. 39, no. 2, pp. 188–191, 2013.

[24] J. Zhu, H.-B. Cheng, N. Fan et al., "Studies of a pedigree with limbal dermoid cyst," *International Journal of Ophthalmology*, vol. 5, no. 5, pp. 641–643, 2012.

[25] H. Brandsch and V. Schmidt, "Erbanalytische Untersuchungen zum Dermoid des Auges beim Hund," *Monatshefte für Veterinärmedizin*, vol. 37, pp. 305–306, 1982.

[26] T. L. Gross, P. J. Ihrke, E. J. Walder, and V. K. Affolter, *Skin Diseases of the Dog and Cat. Clinical and Histopathologic Diagnosis*, Blackwell Publishing, Ames, Iowa, USA, 2nd edition, 2005.

[27] M. Kalpravidh, P. Tuntivanich, S. Vongsakul, and S. Sirivaidyapong, "Canine amniotic membrane transplantation for corneal reconstruction after the excision of dermoids in dogs," *Veterinary Research Communications*, vol. 33, no. 8, pp. 1003–1012, 2009.

[28] J.-I. Lee, M.-J. Kim, I.-H. Kim, Y.-B. Kim, and M.-C. Kim, "Surgical correction of corneal dermoid in a dog," *Journal of Veterinary Science*, vol. 6, no. 4, pp. 369–370, 2005.

[29] A. Pirouzian, "Management of pediatric corneal limbal dermoids," *Clinical Ophthalmology*, vol. 7, pp. 607–614, 2013.

# 32

# Exertional Myopathy in a Juvenile Green Sea Turtle (*Chelonia mydas*) Entangled in a Large Mesh Gillnet

Brianne E. Phillips,[1,2] Sarah A. Cannizzo,[1,2] Matthew H. Godfrey,[1,3] Brian A. Stacy,[4] and Craig A. Harms[1,2]

[1]*Department of Clinical Sciences, College of Veterinary Medicine, North Carolina State University, 1060 William Moore Drive, Raleigh, NC 27607, USA*

[2]*Center for Marine Sciences and Technology, North Carolina State University, 303 College Circle, Morehead City, NC 28557, USA*

[3]*North Carolina Wildlife Resources Commission, 1507 Ann Street, Beaufort, NC 28516, USA*

[4]*National Marine Fisheries Service, National Oceanic and Atmospheric Administration, University of Florida, 2187 Mowry Road, P.O. Box 110885, Gainesville, FL 32611, USA*

Correspondence should be addressed to Craig A. Harms; craig_harms@ncsu.edu

Academic Editor: Luciano Espino López

A juvenile female green sea turtle (*Chelonia mydas*) was found entangled in a large mesh gillnet in Pamlico Sound, NC, and was weak upon presentation for treatment. Blood gas analysis revealed severe metabolic acidosis and hyperlactatemia. Plasma biochemistry analysis showed elevated aspartate aminotransferase and creatine kinase, marked hypercalcemia, hyperphosphatemia, and hyperkalemia. Death occurred within 24 hours of presentation despite treatment with intravenous and subcutaneous fluids and sodium bicarbonate. Necropsy revealed multifocal to diffuse pallor of the superficial and deep pectoral muscles. Mild, multifocal, and acute myofiber necrosis was identified by histopathological examination. While histological changes in the examined muscle were modest, the acid-base, mineral, and electrolyte abnormalities were sufficiently severe to contribute to this animal's mortality. Exertional myopathy in reptiles has not been well characterized. Sea turtle mortality resulting from forced submergence has been attributed to blood gas derangements and seawater aspiration; however, exertional myopathy may also be an important contributing factor. If possible, sea turtles subjected to incidental capture and entanglement that exhibit weakness or dull mentation should be clinically evaluated prior to release to minimize the risk of delayed mortality. Treatment with appropriate fluid therapy and supportive care may mitigate the effects of exertional myopathy in some cases.

## 1. Introduction

The green sea turtle (*Chelonia mydas*) is one of five sea turtle species that frequents the coastal waters of North Carolina, USA [1]. Sea turtle stranding cases in this region are attributed to watercraft-related trauma, hypothermic-stunning, commercial and recreational fishing incidental captures, and disease. Incidental captures in fishing gear comprise a large part of North Carolina sea turtle stranding cases [2]. In 2014, there were 255 green sea turtle stranding cases reported in North Carolina and 22% (57/255) were attributed to fisheries interactions [3]. During the North Carolina gillnet fishing season from 1 June to 30 November 2014, incidental captures in large mesh gillnets resulted in 307 nonlethal and 153 lethal interactions with green sea turtles, based on calculations from observer reports and fishing effort [4, 5].

The effect of fishing gear related capture and entanglement on sea turtles is an important area of study for the purposes of mitigating mortality and injury, as well as improving the medical assessment and treatment of these animals. United States shrimp trawlers are required to use Turtle Excluder Devices (TEDs), a grid installed in the trawl net that allows larger animals, particularly sea turtles, to be ejected from the net and thereby minimize incidental captures. In shrimp trawls without TEDs, longer trawl times result in higher sea turtle mortality rates due to the increased duration of forced submergence [6]. The mandatory implementation and use of TEDs were associated with decreased sea turtle stranding cases and reduced rate of population decline [7].

The physiologic effects of voluntary and forced submergence on sea turtles have been examined in both field and laboratory settings. Voluntary submergence is mostly aerobic, with minimal acid-base changes during short dive periods [8]. Prolonged voluntary dives are associated with respiratory acidosis and anaerobic metabolism [9]. Forced submergence due to fishery gear interactions, most notably trawl nets, may result in prolonged periods of hypoxia, seawater aspiration, pulmonary edema, and airway edema and hemorrhage [10]. Kemp's ridley sea turtles (Lepidochelys kempii) placed in trawl nets exhibited a metabolic acidosis with a 6-fold lactate increase in posttrawl blood samples [11]. Loggerhead sea turtles (Caretta caretta) subjected to forced submergence had a respiratory acidosis with hyperlactatemia [12]. As compared to loggerhead sea turtles captured in pound nets, which allow turtles to surface for respiration, trawl-captured loggerhead sea turtles have greater acid-base and lactate derangements [13]. In addition, forced submergence was recently associated with both intra- and extravascular gas embolism in loggerhead sea turtles [14]. That study utilized a combination of clinical pathology, gross necropsy, advanced imaging, and histopathology to demonstrate this clinical scenario in loggerhead sea turtles.

Gillnets are fixed nets used in shallow waters to entrap target teleost species. Interactions between sea turtles and estuarine large mesh gillnets with extended soak periods resulted in high sea turtle mortality rates in North Carolina in the late 1990s and subsequently led to restricted time and area fishing closures in the state [15]. Large mesh net capture of Kemp's ridley sea turtles resulted in high norepinephrine and epinephrine values in postcapture blood samples, suggesting capture-induced neuroendocrine stress response [16]. Greater duration of gillnet entanglement was associated with significant increases in plasma lactate, lactate dehydrogenase (LDH), creatine kinase (CK), and phosphorous levels in green sea turtles [17]. These clinical pathology changes were suspected to be due to the exertion and muscle damage associated with entanglement, but the study lacked supporting evidence from blood gas analysis, gross postmortem examination, and histopathology.

Exertional myopathy, or capture myopathy, is a multifactorial, noninfectious metabolic disease that is well described in mammalian and avian species. This disease is characterized by metabolic acidosis, muscle necrosis, and myoglobinuria [22]. Exertional myopathy can manifest in various clinical presentations and result in a range of clinical pathology changes and histopathologic lesions. While skeletal muscle and renal tissue are predominantly affected, exertional myopathy can also lead to widespread tissue necrosis throughout many organ systems [23]. Severe cases are associated with a poor prognosis. Exertional myopathy in reptile species and other poikilotherms is poorly characterized [24]. Here we present a case of exertional myopathy in a green sea turtle resulting from entanglement in a large mesh gillnet. Diagnostics included blood gas analysis, plasma biochemistry, gross necropsy, and histopathologic examination, which

collectively are not typically available or presented in instances of sea turtle forced submergence and fishery interaction.

## 2. Case Presentation

A 4.65 kg juvenile female green sea turtle (straight carapace length 33.2 cm, curved carapace length 35.1 cm) was found entangled in a large mesh gillnet (stretched mesh length greater than 12.7 cm) on 3 October 2014 in Pamlico Sound, NC (latitude 35° 04.480' and longitude 76° 04.897'). Marine Patrol officers observed the entanglement and reported the severely weak animal to the North Carolina Wildlife Resources Commission. The turtle arrived within approximately 1-2 hours at the North Carolina State University Center for Marine Science and Technology (NCSU CMAST, Morehead City, NC) for further evaluation and care.

On presentation the turtle was dull but responsive to tactile stimulation. It was quadriparetic and did not attempt to move its flippers when handled. A small amount of frank blood was present at the medial canthus of the right eye and sand adhered to both corneas. The turtle was in adequate body condition with no prominent skeletal features. Live barnacles were present, occupying less than 10% of the carapace and plastron. Approximately 10–15 leeches were present on the ventral cervical region and ventral plastron. Superficial abrasions were present on the trailing edge of the right front flipper and ventral aspect of the mandible.

Initial heart rate was 30/min (Pocket-Dop 3 Doppler flow probe, CareFusion, Middleton, WI) and cloacal temperature was 20°C (Barnant Thermocouple Thermometer, Barnant Company, Barrington, IL). Respiratory rate was 2–4/min and no abnormal respiratory sounds were heard. Venipuncture was performed at the left dorsal cervical sinus and the blood sample was evaluated for packed cell volume (PCV) by centrifugation, total solids (TS) by refractometry, and blood gas analysis using an iSTAT point of care analyzer with a CG4+ cartridge (Abaxis, Union City, CA) (Tables 1 and 2). Results revealed a PCV/TS of 40%/4.0 g/dL, a severe metabolic acidosis, and severe hyperlactatemia. Based on history, physical examination, and severity of blood gas derangements, exertional myopathy was suspected. The turtle was treated with intravenous fluids (5 mL/kg of 50% LRS and 50% 0.9% NaCl; Abbott Laboratories, North Chicago, IL) injected over 3 minutes in the left dorsal cervical sinus and subcutaneous fluids (10 mL/kg 0.9% NaCl, 5 mL/kg lactated Ringer's solution) administered over the left and right shoulders. Ceftazidime 20 mg/kg IM (Covis Pharmaceuticals, Inc., Cary, NC) was also administered to the turtle in the right pectoral muscle, in case of aspiration.

Recheck examination was performed approximately 4 hours after initial presentation. The turtle remained weak and heart rate was 4–12/min. Venipuncture was repeated and the blood sample was evaluated using iSTAT CG4+ and CG8+ cartridges and the VetScan VS2 point of care analyzer with an Avian Reptilian Profile Plus reagent rotor (Abaxis, Union City, CA). Clinical pathology results revealed a persistent but slightly improved severe metabolic acidosis (Tables 1 and 2).

TABLE 1: Blood gas results from a large mesh gillnet entangled green sea turtle (*Chelonia mydas*). Values marked with "—" were not obtained. Initial sample was obtained at presentation and the recheck sample was performed approximately 4 hours later. Blood gas analysis performed using iSTAT CG4+ and CG8+ cartridges. Range values based on published iSTAT results of free-ranging juvenile green sea turtles [18, 19]. Temperature correction (TC) was performed at the turtle's cloacal temperature (20.0°C) for pH, $pCO_2$, $pO_2$, and ionized calcium based on formulas presented in Anderson et al. 2011 [18].

| Analyte | Initial (CG4+) | Recheck (CG4+; CG8+) | Range |
|---|---|---|---|
| pH at 37°C | 6.703 | 6.751 | 7.187–7.516[a] |
| pH TC | 6.896 | 6.944 | 7.187–7.516[a] 7.273–7.626[b] |
| Partial pressure carbon dioxide (mmHg) at 37°C | 52.2 | 69.7 | 59.1–84.3[c] |
| Partial pressure carbon dioxide (mmHg) TC | 24.4 | 33.1 | 32.4–65.4[b] |
| Partial pressure oxygen (mmHg) at 37°C | 73 | 28 | 38–53[a] |
| Partial pressure oxygen (mmHg) TC | 58 | 22 | 38–53[a] 14–32[b] |
| Bicarbonate (mmol/L) | 6.5 | 9.7 | 35.6–58.2[b] |
| Total carbon dioxide (mmol/L) | 8 | 12 | 24–43[c] |
| Lactate (mmol/L) | >20.0 | >20.0 | 0.8–8.73[b] |
| Sodium (mmol/L) | — | 137 | 143–153[b] |
| Potassium (mmol/L) | — | >9.0 | 2.7–4.3[b] |
| Ionized calcium (mmol/L) | — | 1.15 | 0.87–1.24[a] 0.57–1.06[b] |
| Glucose (mg/dL) | — | 137 | 97–244[a] |

[a]Anderson et al. 2011 [18], juvenile free-ranging green sea turtles; $n = 8$.
[b]Lewbart et al. 2014 [19], free-ranging green sea turtles; $n = 12$.
[c]CAH unpublished data, study animals in Anderson et al. 2011 [18].

Also noted were a moderately elevated aspartate aminotransferase (AST) and severe hypercalcemia, hyperkalemia, hyperphosphatemia, and hyperlactatemia. The CK and potassium did not read on the VetScan but were suspected to be elevated out of instrument range, and hyperkalemia was confirmed with the iSTAT analyzer. The VetScan Avian Reptile Profile Plus CK and potassium instrument ranges are 5–14,000 U/L and 1.5–8.5 mmol/L, respectively [21]. The iSTAT sodium value was decreased but was suspected to be a spurious result because the VetScan sodium value was within reported green sea turtle sodium ranges [18, 20]. The turtle was treated with additional subcutaneous fluids (10 mL/kg 0.9% NaCl) combined with sodium bicarbonate 0.5 mEq/kg (Hospira, Inc., Lake Forest, IL) split between the shoulders and prefemoral regions.

The turtle was found dead at 08:00 on 4 October 2014 and death was confirmed via Doppler flow probe. A necropsy was performed and tissue samples were saved for histopathology in 10% neutral buffered formalin. The turtle had adequate musculature and fat stores. Multifocal to diffuse regions of muscle pallor were observed in the superficial and deep pectoral muscles (Figure 1). A small amount of foam was found in the distal main stem bronchi. No fluid or foreign material was present in the respiratory tract. The liver appeared mottled and the spleen bulged on cut section. The entire gastrointestinal tract was filled with digesta, mostly sea grass. The mesenteric vessels and serosal vessels on the liver were prominent. The urinary bladder was devoid of urine. There were no gross lesions to either kidney.

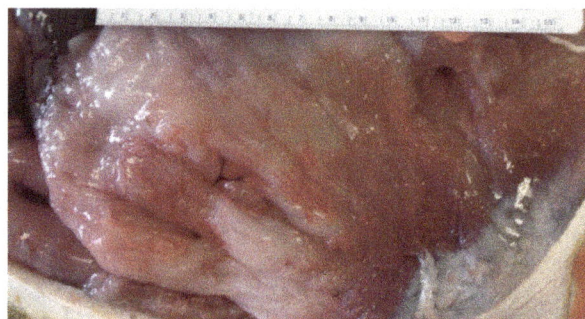

FIGURE 1: The left superficial and deep pectoral muscles of a green sea turtle (*Chelonia mydas*). Multifocal regions of pallor are present.

Histopathology of the pectoral muscles revealed mild, multifocal, acute myofiber necrosis characterized by loss of cross striations, hypercontraction, and segmental disruption of the sarcoplasm. Density of affected myofibers was variable within sections. Some muscle fascicles had rare or no affected myofibers and a few were more diffusely affected (Figure 2). There were no histopathological changes observed in the kidneys. All additional findings were relatively minor and considered incidental, including endarteritis with medial hypertrophy affecting small pulmonary arteries and minimal, chronic endocarditis. These cardiovascular lesions were consistent with response to spirorchiid trematode infection,

TABLE 2: Plasma chemistry and hematology results from a large mesh gillnet entangled green sea turtle (*Chelonia mydas*). PCV/TS was performed at initial presentation. Plasma chemistry performed using the VetScan Avian Reptilian Profile Plus reagent rotor at 4 hours after presentation. Range values based on published free-ranging juvenile green sea turtles from North Carolina caught via pound nets [18] and from the Bahamas during diving [20]. Both studies utilized a benchtop chemistry analyzer at diagnostic laboratories for plasma chemistry analysis. Analytes marked with an * were outside the instrument range. The VetScan Avian Reptile Profile Plus CK and potassium instrument ranges are 5–14,000 U/L and 1.5–8.5 mmol/L, respectively [21]. The CK range reported by Anderson et al. 2011 [18] was likely affected by the capture technique, which included pound net capture for undetermined time and transport on boat prior to blood sample collection.

| Analyte | Value | Range |
|---|---|---|
| Packed cell volume (%) | 40 | 30–39[a]; 26.4–42.0[b] |
| Total solids (g/dL) | 4.0 | 2.5–4.4[a] |
| Total protein (g/dL) | 3.8 | 2.6–3.5[a]; 2.6–6.9[b] |
| Albumin (g/dL) | 1.3 | 1.1–1.6[a]; 0.6–2.1[b] |
| Globulin (g/dL) | 2.5 | 1.3–2.1[a]; 1.9–5.2[b] |
| Aspartate aminotransferase (U/L) | 865 | 134–497[a]; 31–389[b] |
| Bile acids ($\mu$mol/L) | 47 | (No reference available) |
| Creatine kinase (U/L) | * | 841–42,586[a] |
| Uric acid (mg/dL) | 5.7 | 0.7–2.7[a]; 0.5–3.5[b] |
| Glucose (mg/dL) | 163 | 97–244[a]; 87–167[b] |
| Calcium (mg/dL) | 17.0 | 6.3–8.8[a]; 1.6–12.2[b] |
| Phosphorous (mg/dL) | 18.0 | 4.4–9.0[a]; 3.8–10.9[b] |
| Sodium (mmol/L) | 152 | 152–159[a]; 157–183[b] |
| Potassium (mmol/L) | * | 3.6–6.4[a]; 4.1–6.9[b] |

[a]Anderson et al. 2011 [18], juvenile free-ranging green sea turtles; $n$ = 12.
[b]Bolten and Bjorndal 1992 [20], juvenile free-ranging green sea turtles; $n$ = 100.

although spirorchiidiasis was not confirmed by gross or histologic examination [25, 26]. Minimal eosinophilic gastritis and enteric granulocytic infiltrates were also noted and attributed to alimentary endoparasites.

## 3. Discussion

This case documents histopathology and severe clinical pathology abnormalities in a gillnet-entangled juvenile green sea turtle consistent with exertional myopathy. Exertional myopathy is characterized by various degrees of myocyte necrosis on histopathology, which occurs secondary to increased anaerobic metabolism and lactic acid production [22]. In this case, only mild myofiber necrosis was documented, but the severity of muscle lesions was variable within sections examined by histology. Additional affected areas and more severe lesions are possible in other muscles that were not evaluated. It also suggests that the skeletal muscle lesions do not necessarily correlate with the severity of the clinical pathologic changes or, alternatively, that mild necrosis of a large amount of muscle tissue may have similar effects as severe necrosis in a small muscle mass.

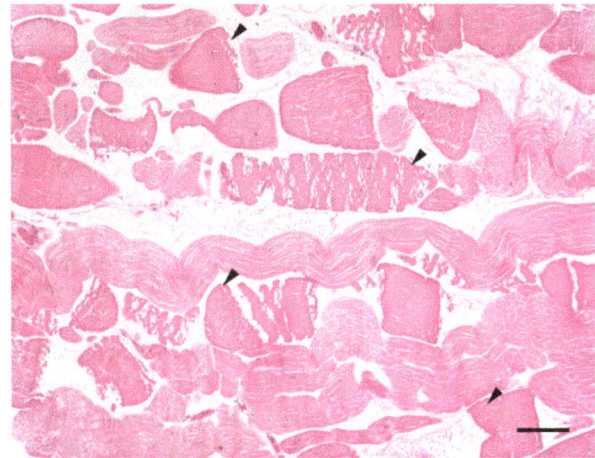

FIGURE 2: Pectoral muscle of a green turtle (*Chelonia mydas*) incidentally captured in a large mesh gillnet. There is multifocal necrosis of individual myofibers that is characterized by hypercontraction, loss of cross striations, and segmental disruption of the sarcoplasm (black arrowheads). Hematoxylin and eosin. Scale = 100 $\mu$m.

Metabolic acidosis is one of the predominant clinical pathology findings associated with exertional myopathy. Acidosis occurs as a result of decreased mitochondrial activity in skeletal muscle and initiation of anaerobic glycolysis that leads to lactic acid production [23]. Capture-related lactic acidosis has previously been documented in several capture effects and forced submergence studies in sea turtles. The severity of acidosis in this case (pH$_{at 37°C}$ 6.703; pH$_{TC}$ 6.896) exceeded the acidosis reported in forced submergence, trawl- and pound net-capture studies (pH range of 6.9–7.3) [11–13]. The decreased bicarbonate ion and total carbon dioxide are further consistent with metabolic acidosis. The lactate in this case exceeded the instrument range (>20 mmol/L). The hyperlactatemia documented here was comparable to or in excess of the lactate concentrations reported in sea turtle forced submergence and capture effects studies, and the blood gas values suggest that exertional myopathy in the green sea turtle can result in extreme acidosis.

Exertional myopathy is often associated with increased plasma AST, CK, and LDH activities in mammals due to myocyte injury [23]. This case included elevations in both AST and CK, and LDH was not evaluated. Multiple tissues express AST activity in loggerhead sea turtles, including cardiac and skeletal muscle [27]. Skeletal muscle damage likely resulted in the moderate elevation in AST and the suspected CK increase seen in this case. Similar enzyme elevations were documented in the evaluation of incidental capture effects on Kemp's ridley and green sea turtles. A positive association with gillnet entanglement time and elevations in plasma LDH and CK was reported in both species [17]. Other capture effects studies have lacked tissue enzyme evaluation as well as histological confirmation of muscle injury, which were documented in the green turtle of this report [17, 28].

The cellular degradation that occurs during exertional myopathy leads to decreased sodium-potassium transport across cell membranes as well as cell rupture [23]. Subsequent increases in extracellular potassium concentrations result, as was seen in the current green sea turtle case. Significant increases in potassium values have been associated with capture stress and forced submergence in sea turtles. Elevated potassium occurred in a single gillnet-associated mortality following release, but insufficient data were available to correlate electrolyte disturbances with mortality, and fresh postmortem examination was not possible [28]. The degree of hyperkalemia was higher in the current case (>9.0 mEq/L) with demonstrated exertional myopathy as compared to reported hyperkalemia secondary to forced submergence and capture effects studies in sea turtles [12, 16, 17]. There was also a marked elevation in phosphorus in this case as compared to values reported in free-ranging green sea turtles [18, 20]. Elevations in phosphorous have been associated with severe tissue trauma secondary to cell leakage in reptiles as well as renal dysfunction [29]. The hyperphosphatemia demonstrated in this exertional myopathy case in combination with elevations of muscle specific enzymes was also documented in gillnet-captured green and Kemp's ridley sea turtles with similar enzyme elevations [17].

This case identified elevations in total calcium and uric acid, which were suspected to be due to acutely decreased renal perfusion. Prolonged sympathetic stimulation, which occurs during exertional myopathy, leads to systemic hypotension and results in decreased cardiac output and blood flow to vital organs including the kidneys [23]. While there were no gross or histopathologic renal lesions and a urine sample was not available postmortem for evaluation, a prolonged decrease in renal perfusion likely decreased renal function and manifested clinically by marked elevations in total calcium and uric acid. Other causes of increased total calcium and uric acid in reptiles including vitellogenesis in reproductively mature females, osteolytic bone disease, granulomatous disease, hyperparathyroidism, gout, and postprandial high protein meal were excluded based on plasma chemistry, gross, and histopathologic examination [29]. Statistically insignificant trends in plasma calcium elevations in comparison to reference ranges were reported following gillnet capture in both green and Kemp's ridley sea turtles [17].

Decompression sickness has recently been documented in gillnet- and trawl-captured loggerhead sea turtles [14]. In these cases, turtles exhibited progressive neurologic signs and positive buoyancy, and widespread intravascular gas embolism was documented using radiography, ultrasonography, and computed tomography. Postmortem and histologic examination typically revealed gas bubbles in the right atrium, lungs, and vasculature. Both duration and depth of capture were associated with gas embolism formation and clinical signs manifested at a minimum capture depth of 10.5 m [14]. Depths in the region of the Pamlico Sound gillnet fishery range between 0 and 2 m. In the case described herein, there were no gas bubbles observed during necropsy or by histology; therefore, there was no evidence that decompression sickness contributed to mortality.

Treatment of exertional myopathy requires aggressive fluid therapy and supportive care. Successful rehabilitation of a rhea with exertional myopathy included fluid therapy, supplemental feedings, methocarbamol, and anxiolytics [30].

Three wild greater sandhill cranes (*Grus canadensis tabida*) with exertional myopathy were successfully released following intensive treatment with fluids, nutritional support, and physical therapy [31]. The empirical treatments, dexamethasone, vitamin E, and selenium, have been administered in cases of exertional myopathy, but therapeutic efficacy has not been evaluated in a controlled manner. Extensive treatment lasting several weeks may be required. Sea turtles markedly affected by exertional myopathy may require housing in a rehabilitation center that could provide daily care and observation. Mammalian and avian cases of exertional myopathy are typically associated with a poor prognosis [22].

Mortality following capture in fishing gear has been attributed to blood gas derangements and seawater aspiration resulting from forced submergence, associated trauma, and decompression sickness. As demonstrated in this case, exertional myopathy is an additional consideration. It may be distinguished by the occurrence of a more severe acidosis, hyperlactatemia, severe elevations in potassium, phosphorous, and CK, as well as concurrent myocyte necrosis on histopathology. Blood chemistry derangements can be severe despite seemingly minor histological lesions in the skeletal muscle, the significance of which may be underappreciated in suspected bycatch animals that are found dead as stranding cases and lack clinical assessment or circumstantial information. Prompt and thorough evaluation of sea turtle entanglement cases exhibiting weakness and dull mentation is recommended if possible. Cases exhibiting these clinical signs and with clinical pathology abnormalities consistent with exertional myopathy should be treated aggressively with fluid therapy and supportive care. Immediate release of sea turtles involved in fishery gear entanglements that exhibit overt clinical signs may result in delayed, unobserved mortality due to the physiologic effects, including those related to exertional myopathy.

## Conflict of Interests

The authors declare that there is no conflict of interests regarding the publication of this paper.

## Acknowledgments

The authors thank Heather Broadhurst and Emily Christiansen for their technical assistance during this case.

## References

[1] S. P. Epperly, J. Braun, and A. Veishlow, "Sea turtles in North Carolina waters," *Conservation Biology*, vol. 9, no. 2, pp. 384–394, 1995.

[2] C. M. McClellan, A. J. Read, W. M. Cluse, and M. H. Godfrey, "Conservation in a complex management environment: the bycatch of sea turtles in North Carolina's commercial fisheries," *Marine Policy*, vol. 35, no. 2, pp. 241–248, 2011.

[3] North Carolina Wildlife Resources Commissions, Seaturtle.org, 2015, http://www.seaturtle.org/strand/summary/.

[4] J. Boyd, "Fall 2014 seasonal progress report," Incidental Take Permit 16230, North Carolina Division of Marine Fisheries, Morehead City, NC, USA, 2014.

[5] J. Boyd, "Summer 2014 seasonal progress report," Incidental Take Permit 16230, North Carolina Division of Marine Fisheries, 2014.

[6] C. R. Sasso and S. P. Epperly, "Seasonal sea turtle mortality risk from forced submergence in bottom trawls," *Fisheries Research*, vol. 81, no. 1, pp. 86–88, 2006.

[7] L. B. Crowder, S. R. Hopkins-Murphy, and J. A. Royle, "Effects of turtle excluder devices (TEDs) on loggerhead sea turtle strandings with implications for conservation," *Copeia*, no. 4, pp. 773–779, 1995.

[8] M. E. Lutcavage and P. L. Lutz, "Voluntary diving metabolism and ventilation in the loggerhead sea turtle," *Journal of Experimental Marine Biology and Ecology*, vol. 147, no. 2, pp. 287–296, 1991.

[9] P. L. Lutz and T. B. Bentley, "Respiratory physiology of diving in the sea turtle," *Copeia*, vol. 1985, no. 3, pp. 671–679, 1985.

[10] T. M. Work and G. H. Balazs, "Pathology and distribution of sea turtles landed as bycatch in the hawaii-based north pacific pelagic longline fishery," *Journal of Wildlife Diseases*, vol. 46, no. 2, pp. 422–432, 2010.

[11] E. K. Stabenau, T. A. Heming, and J. F. Mitchell, "Respiratory, acid-base and ionic status of kemp's ridley sea turtles (*Lepidochelys kempi*) subjected to trawling," *Comparative Biochemistry and Physiology A*, vol. 99, no. 1-2, pp. 107–111, 1991.

[12] E. K. Stabenau and K. R. N. Vietti, "The physiological effects of multiple forced submergences in loggerhead sea turtles (*Caretta caretta*)," *Fishery Bulletin*, vol. 101, no. 4, pp. 889–899, 2003.

[13] C. A. Harms, K. M. Mallo, P. M. Ross, and A. Segars, "Venous blood gases and lactates of wild loggerhead sea turtles (*Caretta caretta*) following two capture techniques," *Journal of Wildlife Diseases*, vol. 39, no. 2, pp. 366–374, 2003.

[14] D. García-Párraga, J. L. Crespo-Picazo, Y. Bernaldo de Quirós et al., "Decompression sickness ('the bends') in sea turtles," *Diseases of Aquatic Organisms*, vol. 111, no. 3, pp. 191–205, 2014.

[15] B. L. Byrd, A. A. Hohn, and M. H. Godfrey, "Emerging fisheries, emerging fishery interactions with sea turtles: a case study of the large-mesh gillnet fishery for flounder in Pamlico Sound, North Carolina, USA," *Marine Policy*, vol. 35, no. 3, pp. 271–285, 2011.

[16] L. A. Hoopes, A. M. Landry Jr., and E. K. Stabenau, "Physiological effects of capturing Kemp's ridley sea turtles, *Lepidochelys kempii*, in entanglement nets," *Canadian Journal of Zoology*, vol. 78, no. 11, pp. 1941–1947, 2000.

[17] J. E. Snoddy, M. Landon, G. Blanvillain, and A. Southwood, "Blood biochemistry of sea turtles captured in gillnets in the lower cape fear river, North Carolina, USA," *Journal of Wildlife Management*, vol. 73, no. 8, pp. 1394–1401, 2009.

[18] E. T. Anderson, C. A. Harms, E. M. Stringer, and W. M. Cluse, "Evaluation of hematology and serum biochemistry of cold-stunned green sea turtles (*Chelonia mydas*) in North Carolina, USA," *Journal of Zoo and Wildlife Medicine*, vol. 42, no. 2, pp. 247–255, 2011.

[19] G. A. Lewbart, M. Hirschfeld, J. Denkinger et al., "Blood gases, biochemistry, and hematology of galapagos green turtles (*Chelonia mydas*)," *PLoS ONE*, vol. 9, no. 5, Article ID e96487, 2014.

[20] A. B. Bolten and K. A. Bjorndal, "Blood profiles for a wild population of green turtles (*Chelonia mydas*) in the southern Bahamas: size-specific and sex-specific relationships," *Journal of Wildlife Diseases*, vol. 28, no. 3, pp. 407–413, 1992.

[21] Abaxis, "VetScan Avian Reptilian Profile Plus package insert," 2007, http://www.abaxis.com/pdf/Avian-Reptilian%20Profile%20Plus.pdf.

[22] J. Patterson, "Capture myopathy," in *Zoo Animal and Wildlife Immobilization*, G. West, D. Heard, and N. Chalkett, Eds., pp. 171–179, Wiley-Blackwell, 2nd edition, 2014.

[23] T. R. Spraker, "Stress and capture myopathy in artiodactyls," in *Zoo and Wild Animal Medicine, Current Therapy*, M. E. Fowler, Ed., pp. 481–488, W.B. Saunders Company, Philadelphia, Pa, USA, 3rd edition, 1993.

[24] E. S. Williams and E. T. Thorne, "Exertional myopathy (capture myopathy)," in *Noninfectious Diseases of Wildlife*, A. Fairbrother, L. N. Locke, and G. L. Hoff, Eds., pp. 181–193, Iowa State University Press, Ames, Iowa, USA, 2nd edition, 1996.

[25] A. N. Gordon, W. R. Kelly, and T. H. Cribb, "Lesions caused by cardiovascular flukes (Digenea: Spirorchidae) in stranded green turtles (*Chelonia mydas*)," *Veterinary Pathology*, vol. 35, no. 1, pp. 21–30, 1998.

[26] M. Santoro, J. A. Morales, and B. Rodríguez-Ortíz, "Spirorchiidiosis (Digenea: Spirorchiidae) and lesions associated with parasites in Caribbean green turtles (*Chelonia mydas*)," *Veterinary Record*, vol. 161, no. 14, pp. 482–486, 2007.

[27] E. T. Anderson, V. L. Socha, J. Gardner, L. Byrd, and C. A. Manire, "Tissue enzyme activities in the loggerhead sea turtle (*Caretta caretta*)," *Journal of Zoo and Wildlife Medicine*, vol. 44, no. 1, pp. 62–69, 2013.

[28] J. E. Snoddy and A. S. Williard, "Movements and post-release mortality of juvenile sea turtles released from gillnets in the lower Cape Fear River, North Carolina, USA," *Endangered Species Research*, vol. 12, no. 3, pp. 235–247, 2010.

[29] T. W. Campbell, "Clinical pathology," in *Current Therapy in Reptile Medicine and Surgery*, D. R. Mader and S. J. Divers, Eds., pp. 70–92, Saunders, St. Louis, Mo, USA, 2014.

[30] K. M. Smith, S. Murray, and C. Sanchez, "Successful treatment of suspected exertional myopathy in a rhea (*Rhea americana*)," *Journal of Zoo and Wildlife Medicine*, vol. 36, no. 2, pp. 316–320, 2005.

[31] N. K. Businga, J. Langenberg, and L. Carlson, "Successful treatment of capture myopathy in three wild greater sandhill cranes (*Grus canadensis tabida*)," *Journal of Avian Medicine and Surgery*, vol. 21, no. 4, pp. 294–298, 2007.

# 33

# Clinical, Bacteriological, and Histopathological Findings of a Testicular Fibrosis in a 6-Year-Old Lusitano Stallion

**A. Rocha,**[1, 2] **T. Guimarães,**[1, 2] **J. C. Duarte,**[3] **C. Cosinha,**[3] **V. T. A. Lopes,**[4] **F. Faria,**[1] **I. Amorim,**[1, 5] **and F. Gärtner**[1, 5]

[1] *Department of Immuno-Physiology and Farmacology (AR), Department of Veterinary Clinics (TG) and Department of Pathology and Molecular Immunology (FF, IA and FG) of the Institute of Biomedical Sciences Abel Salazar (ICBAS), University of Porto, Campus Agrário de Vairão, Rua Jorge Viterbo Ferreira no. 228, 4050-313 Porto, Portugal*
[2] *Center for the Study of Animal Sciences (CECA), ICETA, University of Porto, Campus Agrário de Vairão, Rua Padre Armando Quintas 7, 4485-661 Vairão, Portugal*
[3] *LusoPecus, Rua da Fábrica-Azinhaga do Catalão, Loja 2-A-Porto Alto, 2135-000 Samora Correia, Portugal*
[4] *EVP Lda, Rua Luís Derouet 27, Esquerdo 1, 1250-151 Lisbon, Portugal*
[5] *Institute of Molecular Pathology and Immunology of the University of Porto (IPATIMUP), Rua Dr. Roberto Frias s/n, 4200-465 Porto, Portugal*

Correspondence should be addressed to F. Gärtner, fgartner@ipatimup.pt

Academic Editors: G. Sironi and D. M. Wong

A 6-year-old Lusitano stallion was referred to our centre due to an enlarged left testicle. Anamnesis indicated that the stallion had a chronic hypertrophy of the left testicle, with no apparent ill effect on work (dressage training) or semen production. Prolonged use of anti-inflammatory drugs (NSAIDs) and antibiotics were probable. Upon examination of the animal, it was found that clinical signs were compatible with chronic testicular degeneration or fibrosis. Ultrasound scanning did not evidence the exuberant macroscopic lesions seen upon hemicastration of the left testicle, but it showed in the left spermatic cord a conspicuous absence of the typical hypoechogenic areas representing the pampiniform plexus. Swabbing of the penis, prepuce, and distal urethra resulted in the isolation of *Rhodococcus equi* and *Corynebacterium* spp. However, histopathological examination did not support infectious orchitis as cause of the lesions and no bacterial growth was obtained from swabbing of the parenchyma in the excised testicle. Histopathological findings were compatible with chronic orchitis with fibrosis and necrosis, probably secondary to ischemia of the testicular parenchyma. After hemi-castration, the stallion resumed semen production at acceptable levels.

## 1. Introduction

Testicular hypertrophy may have multiple causes, namely, testicular trauma, infectious orchitis, hydrocele, hematocele, neoplasia, or be secondary to torsion of the spermatic cord [1]. Publications on testicular pathology of the stallion in conjunction with clinical findings, ultrasound imaging, microbiological isolations, histopathological exams, and semen evaluation are scarce. In the present paper we describe the clinical, microbiological, and histopathological findings in a 6-year-old Lusitano stallion with an enlarged left testicle. Semen evaluation was assessed before and after hemi-castration, and possible etiology of the pathology is discussed.

## 2. Case Presentation

A 6-year-old Lusitano stallion was referred to our centre, due to an enlarged left testicle. When referred to us by a colleague, the stallion had been medicated with enrofloxacin, meloxicam and dexamethasone for the last 24 hrs. A previous use of anti-inflamatory drugs (NSAIDs) and antibiotics was probable. No colic-like signs had been noted in the stallion, but the owner referred to a transient "locomotion problem", several months before, during a horse show. The stallion was under dressage training and had been used intensively for semen collection and was reported as having very good libido, producing large volume ejaculates with a low concentration.

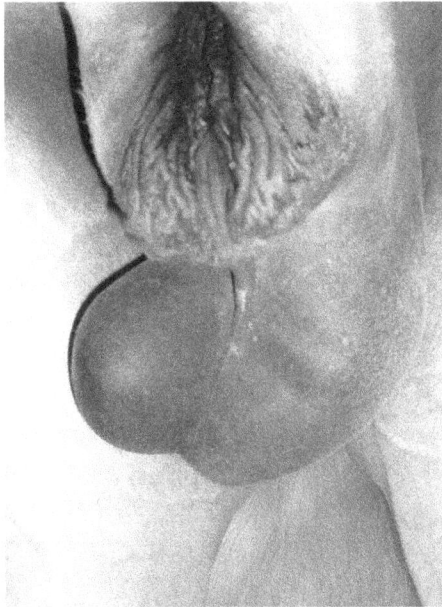

FIGURE 1: View of the testicles of the affected stallion with a greatly enlarged left testicle.

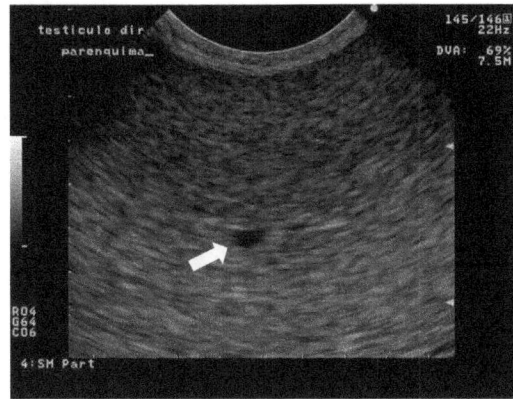

FIGURE 2: Ultrasonogram of the right testicle, showing homogenous parenchyma. White arrow indicates the central vein.

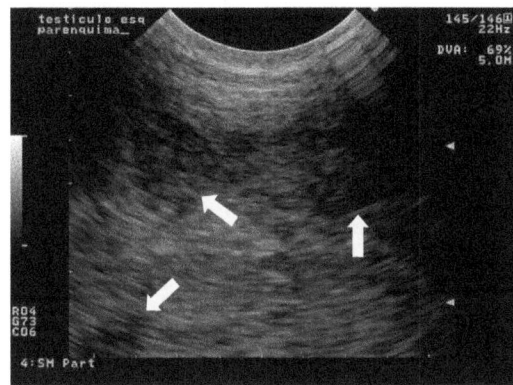

FIGURE 3: Ultrasonogram of the left testicle with several hypoechoic areas (white arrows).

On arrival at our centre after a 4 hr road trip, the stallion was eating normally (hay), did not limp, and at visual inspection displayed an obviously enlarged left scrotum, about two to three times the volume of the right normal-sized testicle (Figure 1). The rectal temperature was 37.6°C. No other alterations were detected on physical exam. On hearing the mares vocalizing, the stallion immediately got a full erection. Semen was collected utilizing an artificial vagina (Missouri model) and a phantom as a mount. The stallion displayed very good libido and mounted and ejaculated with no signs of pain. Volume of the gel-free fraction of the ejaculate was 100 mL, with a concentration of 85 million sperm cells/mL, a subjective motility of 30% (optical microscopy, 200x), and linear motility assessed by computer-assisted sperm analysis (Integrated Sperm Analysis System, ISAS) of 20%. Sperm cell morphology was assessed by optical microscopy ($\times$1000) in a Diff-Quik stained slide, counting 333 sperm cells. A total of 20.1% total abnormal forms were found, namely, 10.2% of the head (including acrosome), 8.1% of the middle piece, and 1.8% of the tail. A few round, epithelial cells were seen as well as 3 monocytes.

Swabbing of the penis, prepuce, and distal urethra of the stallion was performed, and samples were sent for bacterial culture. A blood sample was collected by venipuncture of the jugular and sent for a complete blood analysis.

After semen collection the stallion was restrained in a stock and subjected to genital examination. At palpation, the skin of scrotum and spermatic cord was elastic and pliable without evidence of edema or dermal bruising. No edema was present in the prepuce either. The right scrotal contents felt normal, as well as the right spermatic cord, that measured 5 cm in its largest width. The head, body, and tail of the right epididymis were easily palpated and had a normal consistency. The left testicle felt very hard and tense and

had reduced mobility inside the scrotum. The animal did not display any sign of pain or discomfort at palpation, and scrotal temperature was not increased. The head and body of the left epididymis were difficult to individualize, but the tail was palpable in a normal position and location, attached to the caudal pole of the testicle. The left spermatic cord was very hard, with a width of 10 cm in the largest section.

Testicles, epididymides, and spermatic cord were scanned utilizing an Aloka ultrasound scanner model Prosound 2 with a 7.5 MHz sector transducer. An abundant amount of ultrasound gel was used, but no stand-off pad was utilized. The parenchyma of the right testicle (Figure 2) presented a uniformly echogenic homogenous image, and the central vein could be visualized. No deviation from the expected ultrasound images was seen for the right head and cauda epididymis. The right spermatic cord presented the typical hypoechoic areas of the pampiniform plexus. No changes of echogenicity were seen in the left testicle and no scrotal edema was noticed, but the general texture of the testicular parenchyma was more granulose and coarse than the right testicle, with several anechoic, round areas with small (50 mm) diameter (Figure 3). The central vein could not be visualized. The tail of the epididymis had normal echogenicity. The left spermatic cord did not show the typical

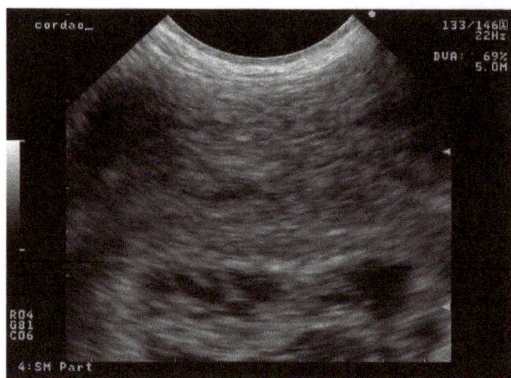

FIGURE 4: Ultrasonogram of the left spermatic cord without evidence of hypoechoic areas characteristic of the pampiniform plexus.

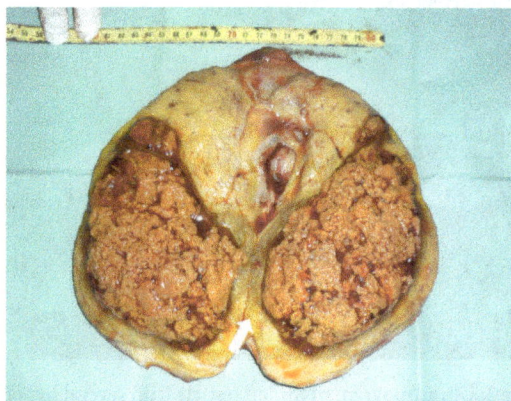

FIGURE 6: A view of the left epididymal head and body, appearing as a fibrotic dense tissues.

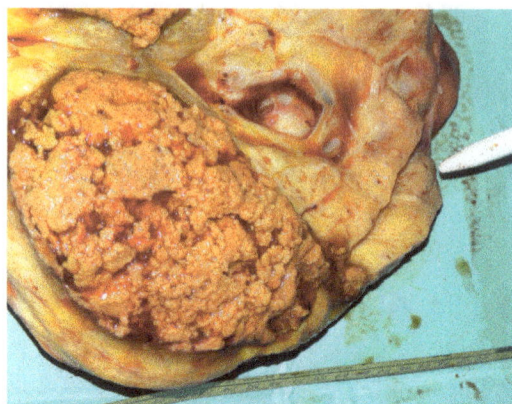

FIGURE 5: View of the excised testicle with the testicular parenchyma appearing as a soft mass. Note the increased thickness of the tunics (arrow).

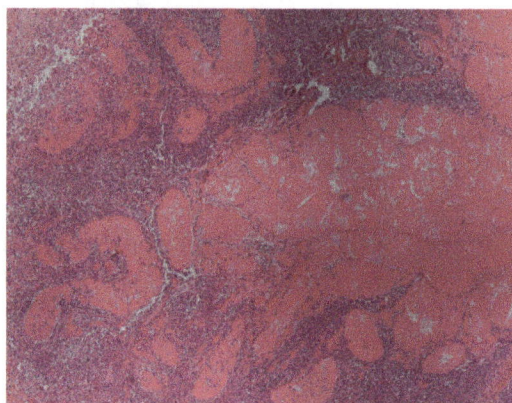

FIGURE 7: H&E, 40x. Histologically, the lesion was composed of an extensive and central area of necrosis surrounded by large amount of diffuse mononuclear inflammatory infiltration.

hypoechoic areas characteristic of the pampiniform plexus. Instead, it seemed a rather solid, hyperechogenic area without much irrigation (Figure 4). Ultrasound scanning of the accessory sex glands, with the same ultrasound scanner using a linear 5.0 MHz probe, did not evidence any alterations. A presumptive diagnosis of testicular degeneration or fibrosis of the left testicle was made, based on the findings of palpation and ultrasound examination. It was speculated that the testicular pathology could have been due to ischemia of the testicular parenchyma, possibly secondary to spermatic cord torsion. Given the possibility of formation of anti-sperm antibodies [2] that could be deleterious to the right, healthy testicle, immediate hemicastration was advised. The owner was renitent to that solution. Thus, the stallion was kept under NSAID and antibiotic therapy, without corticosteroids, and subjected to 15-minute cold showers every 3 hrs, in the affected testicle. As no improvements were seen in 48 hrs, the stallion was subjected to hemicastration of the left testicle, under general anesthesia. As soon as the excised testicle was opened, samples of four different areas of the parenchyma were collected aseptically, for bacterial isolation.

The excised testicle was enlarged, with increased thickness of the tunics. The testicular parenchyma consisted of soft pink tissues forming cordons which string with easiness and presented a red liquefied appearance (Figure 5). The epididymis was hard at palpation and looked like a fibrotic dense tissue (Figure 6). Samples of the testicle were placed in formaldehyde and sent to the pathology lab for processing and histological analysis.

The microbiological isolation from the genital yielded pure cultures of *Rhodococcus equi* and *Corynebacterium* spp.. As no separated cultures were performed for the penis, prepuce, and distal urethra, it was not possible to precisely indicate where the growth of *R. equi* and *Corynebacterium* spp. occurred. No microbial growth was obtained from the testicular parenchyma samples.

At the histopathological exam, the testicular architecture was deeply modified, due to an extensive and central area of coagulation necrosis, with some neutrophils and cellular debris (Figure 7). At the periphery, moderate to severe amount of diffuse mononuclear inflammatory infiltration (rich in macrophages showing intense phagocytic activity, plasma cells, and lymphocytes) associated with

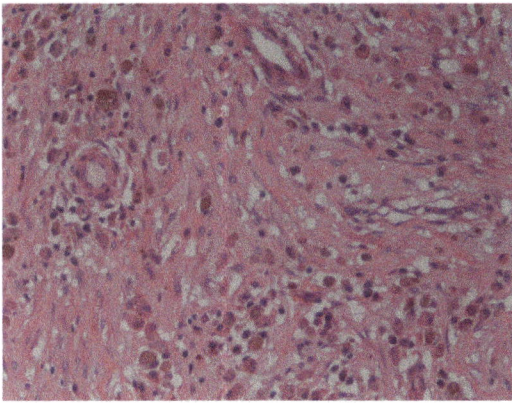

FIGURE 8: H&E, 200x. The inflammatory infiltrate constited of macrophages showing intense phagocytic activity, plasma cells, and lymphocytes, with formation of an exuberant granulation tissue.

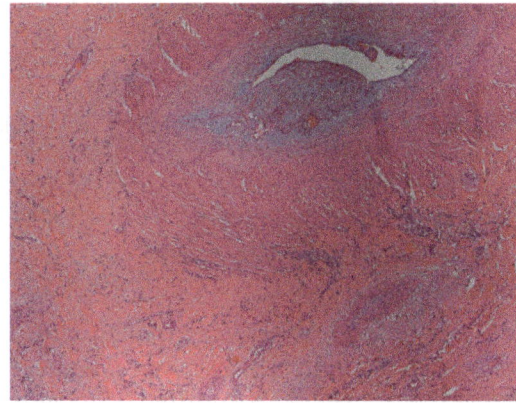

FIGURE 9: H&E, 40x. Most vessels evidenced degeneration of the walls, with accumulation of mucin-like material and cellular vacuolization.

exuberant granulation tissue, rich in active fibroblasts and blood vessels, was noted (Figure 8). Also, multiple foci of lymphoplasmocitary infiltrate were observed. Most vessels evidenced degeneration of the walls, with accumulation of mucine-like material and cellular vacuolization (Figure 9). The epididymis was atrophic with very few sperm cells. Vital stains (periodic acid-Schiff and Gram) did not reveal any microorganisms. The histopathological findings were compatible with chronic orchitis, with severe fibrosis and necrosis. These findings, associated with the clinical signs, were compatible with lesions due to ischemia, possibly secondary to torsion of the spermatic cord > 180 degrees.

All blood parameters were within normal range, including creatinine, aspartate aminotransferase (AST), gamma-glutamyl transferase (GGT), and creatine kinase (CK).

Records from the semen collection centre (LusoPecus), just before the hemi-castration, showed that the progressive motility of the fresh semen in the 2 collected ejaculates was 60%; a total of 60 straws with $100 \times 10^6$ sperm cells/mL were frozen, with progressive motility at thawing of 40% and 30% for the first and second ejaculates, respectively. Four months after the hemi-castration, the stallion was collected 14 times during a period of 42 days, producing ejaculates with a subjective progressive motility ranging from 60% to 70%, which resulted in the freezing of 20 to 60 straws with $100 \times 10^6$ sperm cells/mL per ejaculate, with a postthaw progressive motility varying from 35% to 40%.

## 3. Discussion

Visual examination and palpation of the testicles were enough to clearly evidence a serious pathology of the left testicle, in this stallion. The use of ultrasonic imaging added some additional information that was not enough to establish a definitive diagnosis or to clearly show the existing total destruction of testicular parenchyma. However, ultrasonic images of the affected spermatic cord were useful to highlight the absence of images compatible with a functional pampiniform plexus. Extensive (>180°) torsion of the spermatic cord results in occlusion of the testicular

vasculature [2] and even 180° torsions may cause retrograde blood flow and affect testicular function [3]. Thrombosis of the testicular artery may mimic the effects of testicular torsion, but is a rare condition [2]. Thus, we speculated that the lesions seen in the affected testicle could have been due to ischemia secondary to torsion of the spermatic cord, as no evidence of trauma was detected in the skin of the scrotum or of the spermatic cord.

Virulent strains Rhodococcus equi cause diseases in horses [4] including pyogranulomatous pneumonia in foals [5] and sporadically other lesions in several organs [2, 6]. Rhodococcus equi has been isolated from the genital tract of mares [7, 8] and can cause abortion [7]. Upon receiving the microbiology results and considering the macroscopic aspect of the testicular parenchyma, the possibility of an ascending infection by Rhodococcus equi was considered. Together with the stallion of this case report, we collected during the reproductive season genital samples of 61 additional stallions, and the only positive result for R. equi was the reported case. Such a low prevalence is in agreement with results from Althouse et al. [9] that isolated R. equi only in 1 of 31 samples but differs from the findings of Spergser et al. [10] that isolated R. equi in 56 out of 116 stallions. The lack of isolation of bacteria from the parenchyma, associated with the histopathological findings, rules out an infectious origin of the testicular lesions observed.

In conclusion, visual inspection and testicular palpation of the scrotal contents were the best approach to reach a presumptive diagnosis, with ultrasonographic examination, particularly of the spermatic cord, adding some useful information. The real extent of the pathology was only seen after excision of the affected testicle. The most probable cause of the testicular pathology was ischemia of the testicular parenchyma, possibly after torsion of the spermatic cord. The isolation of pure colonies of Rhodococcus equi and Corynebacterium spp. from the genitalia may be due to opportunistic growth of these bacteria after prolonged use of antibiotics. Hemicastration of the affected testicle did not decrease the quality of the ejaculate or the freezability of the semen, compared to precastration levels.

## Acknowledgments

This work was partially financed by Projects PTDC/CVT/ 108456/2008 (FCT) and COMPETE: FCOMP-01-0124- FEDER-009565. The authors appreciatively acknowledge Carla Mendonça, Luis Atayde, and Tiago Pereira for the castration of the stallion and Carla Miranda, Eliane Silva, and Gertrude Thompson for the microbiological isolations.

## References

[1] W. Beard, "Abnormalities of the testicles," in *Equine Reproduction*, A. O. McKinnon, E. L. Squires, W. E. Vaala, and D. D. Varner, Eds., pp. 1161–1165, Wiley-Blackwell, 2nd edition, 2011.

[2] J. Schumacher and D. D. Varner, "Abnormalities of the spermatic cord," in *Equine Reproduction*, A. O. McKinnon, E. L. Squires, W. E. Vaala, and D. D. Varner, Eds., pp. 1145–1155, Wiley-Blackwell, 2nd edition, 2011.

[3] M. A. Pozor and S. M. McDonnell, "Color Doppler ultrasound evaluation of testicular blood flow in stallions," *Theriogenology*, vol. 61, no. 5, pp. 799–810, 2004.

[4] R. Wada, M. Kamada, T. Anzai et al., "Pathogenicity and virulence of *Rhodococcus equi* in foals following intratracheal challenge," *Veterinary Microbiology*, vol. 56, no. 3-4, pp. 301–312, 1997.

[5] D. L. Dungworth, "*Rhodococcus (Corynebacterium) equi* infection," in *Pathology of Domestic Animals*, K. V. F. Jubb, P. C. Kennedy, and N. Palmer, Eds., vol. 2, pp. 652–655, Academic Press, 4th edition, 1993.

[6] M. C. Zink, J. A. Yager, and N. L. Smart, "*Corynebacterium equi* infections in horses, 1958–1984: a review of 131 cases," *Canadian Veterinary Journal*, vol. 27, pp. 213–217, 1986.

[7] L. Szeredi, T. Molnár, R. Glávits et al., "Two cases of equine abortion caused by *Rhodococcus equi*," *Veterinary Pathology*, vol. 43, no. 2, pp. 208–211, 2006.

[8] A. M. Bain, "*Corynebacterium equi* infections in the equine," *Australian Veterinary Journal*, vol. 39, pp. 116–121, 1963.

[9] G. C. Althouse, J. Skaife, and P. Loomis, "Prevalence and types of contaminant bacteria in extended, chilled equine semen," *Animal Reproduction Science*, vol. 121, pp. S224–S225, 2010.

[10] J. Spergser, C. Aurich, J. E. Aurich, and R. Rosengarten, "High prevalence of mycoplasmas in the genital tract of asymptomatic stallions in Austria," *Veterinary Microbiology*, vol. 87, no. 2, pp. 119–129, 2002.

# 34

# *Mycobacterium tuberculosis* and Dual *M. tuberculosis*/*M. bovis* Infection as the Cause of Tuberculosis in a Gorilla and a Lioness, Respectively, in Ibadan Zoo, Nigeria

**Aina Adeogun,[1] Olutayo Omobowale,[2] Chiaka Owuamanam,[3] Olugbenga Alaka,[4] Victor Taiwo,[4] Dick van Soolingen,[5,6] and Simeon Cadmus[7]**

[1]*Department of Zoology, University of Ibadan, Ibadan 200005, Nigeria*

[2]*Department of Veterinary Medicine, University of Ibadan, Ibadan 200005, Nigeria*

[3]*Zoological Garden, University of Ibadan, Ibadan 200005, Nigeria*

[4]*Department of Veterinary Pathology, University of Ibadan, Ibadan 200005, Nigeria*

[5]*Department of Pulmonary Diseases and Department of Clinical Microbiology, Radboud University, Nijmegen Medical Centre, Nijmegen, Netherlands*

[6]*Diagnostic Laboratory for Bacteriology and Parasitology (BPD), Center for Infectious Disease Research, Diagnostics and Perinatal Screening (IDS), National Institute for Public Health and the Environment (RIVM), P.O. Box 1, 3720 BA Bilthoven, Netherlands*

[7]*Tuberculosis and Brucellosis Research Laboratories, Department of Veterinary Public Health & Preventive Medicine, University of Ibadan, Ibadan 200005, Nigeria*

Correspondence should be addressed to Simeon Cadmus; simeonc5@gmail.com

Academic Editor: Isabel Pires

Tuberculosis (TB) in zoo animals is an important public health problem in places where it occurs. This is even very important in countries where there is little public health awareness about the disease; thus confined animals in the zoo can be infected directly or indirectly by infected humans and vice versa. In Nigeria, the problem of TB is a major concern among both humans and cattle. Here, we present cases of *Mycobacterium tuberculosis* and *M. tuberculosis*/*M. bovis* infections in a female gorilla and a lioness, respectively, in a zoo in Ibadan, Nigeria. These cases were confirmed after bacteriological examinations and DNA from granulomatous lesions of the animals' carcasses were subjected to the Hain and spoligotyping techniques. Our findings reveal the first documented report of TB infections in a gorilla and a lioness in zoo animals in Nigeria. The public health risks of tuberculosis in zoological settings are therefore reemphasized.

## 1. Introduction

Tuberculosis (TB) remains a major public health problem globally [1]. The disease affects humans and other wide range species of nonhuman primates, elephants, carnivores, marine mammals, giraffes, rhinoceroses, buffaloes, and psittacine birds in different countries of the world including USA, Thailand, Sweden [2–6]. Globally, TB is mainly caused by *Mycobacterium tuberculosis* in humans and *M. tuberculosis* is one of the seven species constituting the *M. tuberculosis* complex (MTC) which includes *M. bovis,* a major pathogen of cattle causing bovine tuberculosis (BTB). Reports of TB infections in gorillas and members of the lion family are scarce in Nigeria despite the huge burden of the disease in the human population [1] and the endemicity of BTB in cattle [7, 8].

## 2. Case Report

Between 2009 and 2010, we investigated the death of a female gorilla and a lioness due to TB in Zoological Garden in Ibadan, Ibadan, southwestern Nigeria.

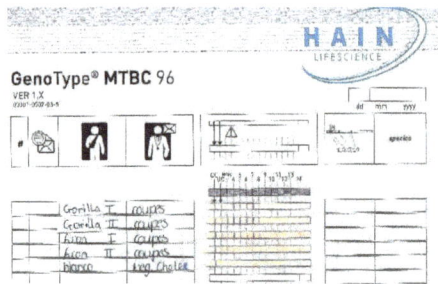

FIGURE 1: The result of the Hain test for the gorilla and the lioness.

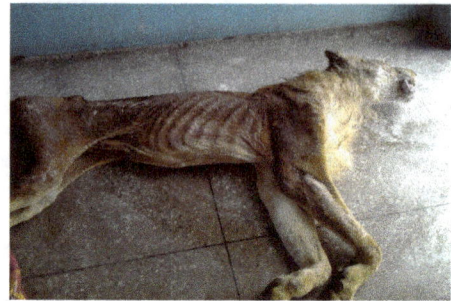

FIGURE 2: Emaciated lioness.

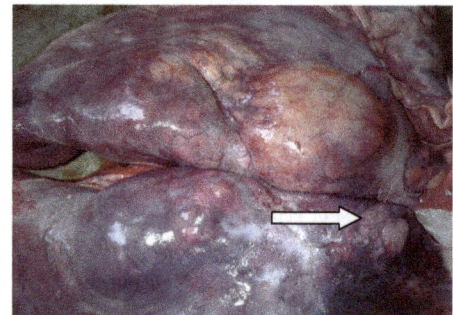

FIGURE 3: Photograph of lioness lungs showing multiple solitary and coalescing nodules of varying sizes (arrow).

*2.1. Case 1.* A female lowland gorilla (*Gorilla gorilla*) of about 47 years of age was presented dead at the postmortem unit of the Department of Veterinary Pathology, University of Ibadan. The carcass was markedly emaciated with bony projections of the rib. The ocular and oral mucous membranes were moderately pale. There were several cream coloured firm nodules of varying sizes (5 mm–2 cm) in multiple organs including the lungs, liver, spleen, and the serosa. Microscopic examination of these nodules revealed typical granulomatous inflammation in affected organs characterised by caseous necrosis surrounded by zone of inflammation comprising macrophages, lymphocytes, plasma cells, and occasional giant cells. Based on the above, tentative diagnoses of generalized TB and uterine leiomyoma (fibroid) were made at the Department of Veterinary Pathology, University of Ibadan, Nigeria.

Specimens from the lungs and other affected tissues and organs with miliary nodules were decontaminated and digested as previously described by Cadmus et al. [9] using NALC- (N-acetyl-L-cysteine-) NaOH and followed by DNA extraction. Briefly, decontaminated samples were centrifuged for 10 minutes at 5 000 rmp and the supernatant was removed. 200 $\mu$L of InstaGene matrix was added to the pellet and incubated and mixed in a thermomixer at 56°C for 30 min and later vortexed for 10 seconds. The product was again incubated and mixed at 99°C for 30 minutes and spun down for 3 minutes at 12 000 rmp. Finally, 20 $\mu$L of supernatant from the resulting supernatant was aliquotted to carry out PCR reaction for spoligotyping and the Hain test as previously described [10, 11].

Our result showed that only the Hain test confirmed *M. tuberculosis* (Figure 1) as the incriminating agent of the infection in the gorilla while the spoligotyping failed.

*2.2. Case 2.* A female lion (*Panthera leo*) of about 15 years of age was presented at the postmortem unit of the Department of Veterinary Pathology, University of Ibadan. Postmortem examination revealed a markedly emaciated carcass with sunken eyes and pale mucous membrabes (Figure 2). The trachea and bronchi contained thick brownish mucopurulent froth. The lungs were diffusedly hyperemic with some localized foci of ecchymotic heamorrhages on the ventral surfaces of the left caudal and right middle lobes. Both lungs were consolidated and firm in consistency with nodules ranging from 0.5 to 2 cm in diameter spread throughout

the parenchyma. Many of the nodules were solitary, while a few were confluent (Figure 3). Upon incision, the large nodules were observed to have abscesses in the caudal lobe of the right lung, while others were firm to hard with cheesy core. Some of the associated lymph nodes, particularly the pharyngeal and mediastinal, were edematous and enlarged. The liver, spleen, and kidneys were markedly congested and enlarged. Tentative morphological diagnoses were marked dehydration and emaciation; pneumonia; granulomatous, chronic active, and severe lymphadenopathy. Histopathology results revealed alveolar spaces containing infiltration of neutrophils and macrophages mixed with fibrin and extensive alveolar collapse with multiple foci of granulomatous reactions (Figure 4).

Specimens from the lungs and pharyngeal and mediastinal lymph nodes with miliary nodules were decontaminated and digested and DNA extraction was carried out as described for the gorilla above.

The results of the Hain test (Figure 1) and spoligotyping technique (Figure 5) revealed the presence of *M. tuberculosis* and *M. bovis* from the lungs and mediastinal lymph nodes, respectively.

## 3. Discussion

We report the isolation of *M. tuberculosis* and *M. tuberculosis*/*M. bovis* in a gorilla and a lioness, respectively, in a private zoo in Ibadan, southwestern Nigeria. Tuberculosis caused by *M. tuberculosis* and *M. bovis* has been identified in a wide range of species, including nonhuman primates,

(a)        (b)

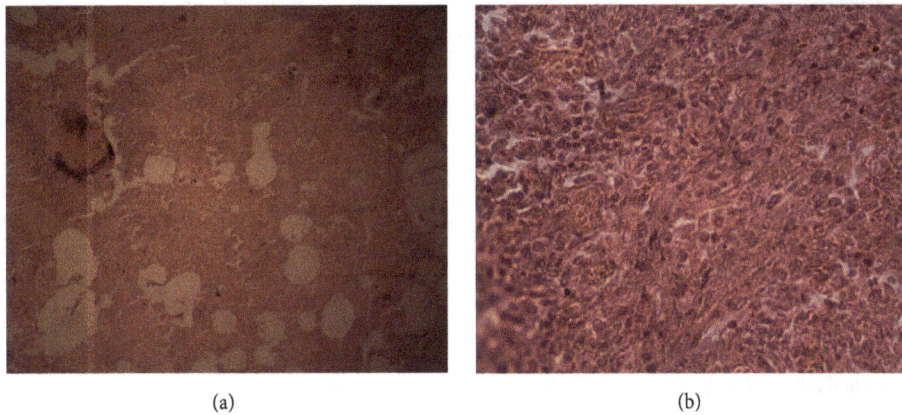

FIGURE 4: The micrograph in section (a) shows the lioness lungs with extensive alveolar collapse and multiple foci of granulomatous reactions in the lungs, ×100 H&E. (b) Higher magnification of section (a) showing extensive fibrosis, marked alveolar collapse, and mononuclear cellular infiltrations.

FIGURE 5: *M. bovis* spoligotype recovered from a lioness in a zoo in Ibadan, Nigeria.

elephants, and other exotic ungulates, carnivores, marine mammals, and psittacine birds [2, 3]. Disease associated with *M. tuberculosis* has occurred mostly within captive settings and does not appear to occur naturally in free-living mammals. *Mycobacterium tuberculosis* associated disease mostly occurs within captive settings and rarely appears naturally in free-living mammals [3]. In Nigeria, several reports have been made concerning human and bovine TB [7, 9, 12–15]. Globally, Nigeria ranks 4th among the TB burdened nations [1]; coupled with this, BTB is endemic among farm and slaughtered animals [7–9, 14]. Due to the high prevalence of human pulmonary TB in Nigeria and observed poor hygienic habits of zookeepers as well as visitors, animals within the private zoo in Ibadan are therefore exposed to possible risk of TB infections from humans.

The gorilla at this zoo was particularly at grave risk of exposure to TB, given the multitude of people who went visiting her, since she was a center of attraction in the zoo. The fact that she also lived in the zoo for about 42 years (brought into the zoo in 1962 when she was about 5 years) also meant that old age and confinement might have contributed to her vulnerability and death to TB.

The lioness had dual infection resulting from *M. tuberculosis* and *M. bovis*. The *M. tuberculosis* infection could be due to similar scenario presented for the gorilla (particularly as it relates to occasional confinement during which the human contact is close and highest) and her relatively old age. The most likely source of her *M. bovis* infection could be due to contaminated raw meat she was fed, mainly from the abattoir where 4.3% prevalence of BTB has been reported in slaughtered cattle [16] and with reports of *M. bovis* infection in slaughtered goats [14]. The fact that the animals fed to the lions in the zoo are not subjected to prior postmortem checks makes them vulnerable to *M. bovis* infection.

From the public health perspective, since the zoo environment is mostly congested with human population at festive seasons, it becomes easy for animals and zookeepers to become infected by TB patients who in most instances may be unaware of their illnesses despite obvious symptoms due to limited public health awareness about the disease [17, 18]. Similar scenario has accounted for zoo animal infection in other settings in Sweden, Thailand, and USA, [3, 5, 6, 19].

In conclusion, this study confirms cases of TB due to *M. tuberculosis* and *M. tuberculosis/M. bovis* in a gorilla and a lioness, respectively, in a zoo in Nigeria. Due to the high prevalence of human and BTB in Nigeria, we advocate that more public health precautions be taken by zookeepers in the country and most TB endemic countries with high contact between humans and wildlife. In addition, efforts should be put in place to routinely screen zookeepers who can indirectly transmit infections from the visiting public to the animals. In the same vein, public contacts with the animals must be reduced to the barest minimum. More importantly, raw meat/animals fed to zoo animals should go through routine meat inspection checks in order to control infection with *M. bovis*. Finally, we advocate continuous public health awareness to zoo visitors as a way of stepping up TB enlightenment and control in disease endemic countries.

## Competing Interests

The authors declare that they have no competing interests.

## Acknowledgments

The authors sincerely thank the entire team of the National Tuberculosis Reference Laboratory, National Institute for Public Health and the Environment, Bilthoven, Netherlands, for assisting with part of the laboratory analysis.

# References

[1] World Health Organization, *Global Tuberculosis Report 2015*, 20th edition, 2015, http://apps.who.int/iris/bitstream/10665/191102/1/9789241565059_eng.pdf?ua=1.

[2] M.-F. Thorel, C. Karoui, A. Varnerot, C. Fleury, and V. Vincent, "Isolation of *Mycobacterium bovis* from baboons, leopards and a sea-lion," *Veterinary Research*, vol. 29, no. 2, pp. 207–212, 1998.

[3] R. J. Montali, S. K. Mikota, and L. I. Cheng, "*Mycobacterium tuberculosis* in zoo and wildlife species," *Scientific and Technical Review*, vol. 20, no. 1, pp. 291–303, 2001.

[4] S. S. Lewerin, S.-L. Olsson, K. Eld et al., "Outbreak of *Mycobacterium tuberculosis* infection among captive Asian elephants in a Swedish zoo," *Veterinary Record*, vol. 156, no. 6, pp. 171–175, 2005.

[5] T. Angkawanish, W. Wajjwalku, A. Sirimalaisuwan et al., "*Mycobacterium tuberculosis* infection of domesticated Asian elephants, Thailand," *Emerging Infectious Diseases*, vol. 16, no. 12, pp. 1949–1951, 2010.

[6] A. Zlot, J. Vines, L. Nystrom et al., "Diagnosis of tuberculosis in three zoo elephants and a human contact—oregon, 2013," *Morbidity and Mortality Weekly Report (MMWR)*, vol. 64, no. 52, pp. 1398–1402, 2016, Erratum: vol. 64, no. 52. Morbidity and Mortality Weekly Report (MMWR), vol. 65, article 131, 2016.

[7] S. I. B. Cadmus, A. A. Atsanda, S. O. Oni, and E. E. U. Akang, "Bovine tuberculosis in one cattle herd in Ibadan in Nigeria," *Veterinary Medicine—Czech*, vol. 49, no. 11, pp. 406–412, 2004.

[8] S. Ibrahim, C. A. Agada, J. U. Umoh, I. Ajogi, U. M. Farouk, and S. I. B. Cadmus, "Prevalence of bovine tuberculosis in Jigawa State, northwestern Nigeria," *Tropical Animal Health and Production*, vol. 42, no. 7, pp. 1333–1335, 2010.

[9] S. Cadmus, S. Palmer, M. Okker et al., "Molecular analysis of human and bovine tubercle bacilli from a local setting in Nigeria," *Journal of Clinical Microbiology*, vol. 44, no. 1, pp. 29–34, 2006.

[10] M. P. Romero Gómez, L. Herrera-León, M. S. Jiménez, and J. García Rodríguez, "Comparison of GenoType® MTBC with RFLP-PCR and multiplex PCR to identify *Mycobacterium tuberculosis* complex species," *European Journal of Clinical Microbiology & Infectious Diseases*, vol. 26, pp. 63–66, 2007.

[11] J. Kamerbeek, L. Schouls, A. Kolk et al., "Simultaneous detection and strain differentiation of *Mycobacterium tuberculosis* for diagnosis and epidemiology," *Journal of Clinical Microbiology*, vol. 35, no. 4, pp. 907–914, 1997.

[12] B. P. Thumamo, A. E. Asuquo, L. N. Abia-Bassey et al., "Molecular epidemiology and genetic diversity of Mycobacterium tuberculosis complex in the Cross River State, Nigeria," *Infection, Genetics and Evolution*, vol. 12, no. 4, pp. 671–677, 2012.

[13] A. Ani, T. Bruvik, Y. Okoh et al., "Genetic diversity of *Mycobacterium tuberculosis* Complex in Jos, Nigeria," *BMC Infectious Diseases*, vol. 10, article 189, 2010.

[14] S. I. Cadmus, H. K. Adesokan, A. O. Jenkins, and D. Van Soolingen, "*Mycobacterium bovis* and *M. tuberculosis* in Goats, Nigeria," *Emerging Infectious Diseases*, vol. 15, no. 12, pp. 2066–2067, 2009.

[15] A. O. Jenkins, S. I. B. Cadmus, E. H. Venter et al., "Molecular epidemiology of human and animal tuberculosis in Ibadan, Southwestern Nigeria," *Veterinary Microbiology*, vol. 151, no. 1-2, pp. 139–147, 2011.

[16] S. I. B. Cadmus, H. K. Adesokan, A. F. Adepoju, and E. B. Otesile, "Zoonotic risks and transmission of *Mycobacteria* species from cows' milk and slaughtered cattle to man in Ibadan: role of butchers," *Nigerian Veterinary Journal*, vol. 29, no. 1, pp. 30–39, 2008.

[17] O. O. Odusanya and J. O. Babafemi, "Patterns of delays amongst pulmonary tuberculosis patients in Lagos, Nigeria," *BMC Public Health*, vol. 4, article 18, 2004.

[18] A. A. Fatiregun and C. C. Ejeckam, "Determinants of patient delay in seeking treatment among pulmonary tuberculosis cases in a government specialist hospital in Ibadan, Nigeria," *Tanzania Journal of Health Research*, vol. 12, no. 2, pp. 1–9, 2010.

[19] K. Michalak, C. Austin, S. Diesel, J. M. Bacon, P. Zimmerman, and J. N. Maslow, "*Mycobacterium tuberculosis* infection as a zoonotic disease: transmission between humans and elephants," *Emerging Infectious Diseases*, vol. 4, no. 2, pp. 283–287, 1998.

# 35

# Oestrus ovis L. (Diptera: Oestridae) Induced Nasal Myiasis in a Dog from Northern Italy

Sergio A. Zanzani,[1] Luigi Cozzi,[1] Emanuela Olivieri,[2]
Alessia L. Gazzonis,[1] and Maria Teresa Manfredi[1]

[1]Dipartimento di Medicina Veterinaria, Università degli Studi di Milano, Via Celoria 10, 20133 Milano, Italy
[2]Dipartimento di Medicina Veterinaria, Università degli Studi di Perugia, Via S. Costanzo 4, 06126 Perugia, Italy

Correspondence should be addressed to Sergio A. Zanzani; sergio.zanzani@unimi.it

Academic Editor: Sheila C. Rahal

A companion dog from Milan province (northern Italy), presenting with frequent and violent sneezing, underwent rhinoscopy, laryngoscopy, and tracheoscopy procedures. During rhinoscopy, a dipteran larva was isolated from the dog and identified as first instar larval stage of O. ovis by morphological features. Reports of O. ovis in domestic carnivores are sporadic and nevertheless this infestion should be considered as a possible differential diagnosis of rhinitis in domestic carnivores living in contaminated areas by the fly as consequence of the presence of sheep and goats. This report described a case of autochthonous infestion in a dog from an area where O. ovis was not historically present but it could be affected by a possible expansion of the fly as a consequence of climate change. This is the first record of Oestrus ovis infestion in a dog in Italy and, at the same time, the most northerly finding of larvae of sheep bot fly in the country.

## 1. Introduction

Oestrus ovis L. (Diptera: Oestridae), a sheep nasal bot fly, affects sheep and goats worldwide and, particularly, in areas where adult flies can be active all the year round thanks to favourable climatic conditions [1]. In central and southern Italy prevalence of infestion in sheep is high: 55.8%, 72.8%, and 91% of infected sheep were observed during necropsies in Sicily [2], Tuscany [3], and Sardinia [4], respectively. Zoonotic infestions sustained by O. ovis are numerous and diffused all over the world. In Italy, O. ovis infestions in humans were first described in Sicily in the 19th century [5] and several infestions have been reported even in more recent years, mostly in southern rural areas [6]. Sporadic descriptions of zoonotic infestions by O. ovis are reported also in central [7] and northern Italy [8, 9] as well as in an urban area [10]. O. ovis infestions in ovine and humans in the most northerly parts of Italy are reported below 45 degrees north latitude: in Liguria, Emilia-Romagna, and northern Tuscany. Reports of O. ovis infestions in domestic carnivores are sporadic [11–16] and have not been yet described in Italy.

The aim of the present study is to describe an autochthonous case of O. ovis infestion in a companion dog bred in northern Italy.

## 2. Case Presentation

In July 2015, an 8-month-old female of Staffordshire Bull Terrier, housed in Milan province (northern Italy) and purchased from an Italian dog breeder, was taken to a veterinary clinic on account of her frequent and violent sneezing that lasts for two days. During anamnestic data collection, the owner reported that sneezing occurred after the dog had been taken for a walk in a rural area close to his house. At clinical examination the bitch also presented stertorous and reversal sneezing. Anamnesis, dog breed, and symptoms made clinicians suspect a nasal foreign body and/or a brachycephalic airway obstructive syndrome (BAOS). No antimicrobial or anti-inflammatory therapies were being administered to the dog. The bitch was then anesthetized for laryngoscopy, tracheoscopy, and anterior and posterior rhinoscopy. Laryngeal

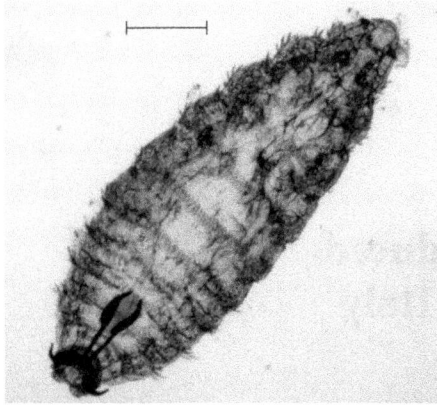

FIGURE 1: *O. ovis* L1 collected from the dog after nasal lavage (40x). Black bar indicates 200 μm length.

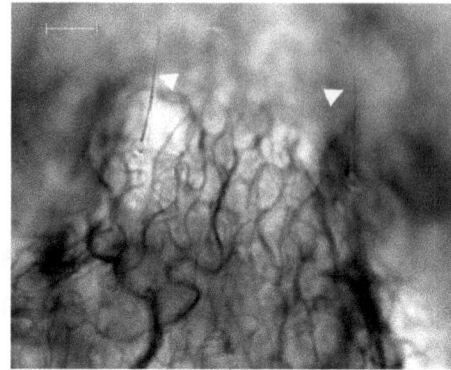

FIGURE 2: *O. ovis* L1 surface (630x). White arrows indicate cuticular sensilla and white bar indicates 10 μm length.

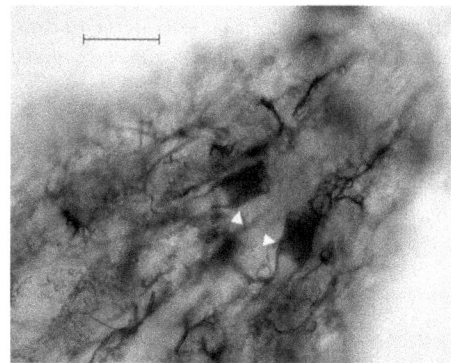

FIGURE 3: Terminal segments of *O. ovis* L1 (200x). White arrows indicate tracheal trunks and black bar indicates 50 μm length.

inspection revealed everted laryngeal saccules, whereas tracheoscopy did not show any remarkable alteration. Posterior rhinoscopy evidenced few small mucosal erosions (diameter < 2 mm) surrounded by mildly thickened and oedematous mucosae in the rhinopharynx; a small quantity of mucus-like material was also present. The anterior rhinoscopy highlighted two and three whitish fusiform organisms in the right and in the left nasal cavities, respectively; all the observed organisms appeared to be vital, presenting high mobility on the nasal mucosal surface. Attempts to catch them using endoscopic forceps failed and only after nasal lavage was one of them isolated and collected. Noticeably, following nasal lavage, the acute and violent sneezing improved considerably which might be due to removal of most of the observed organisms. The collected organism resembled a larva of Diptera and while waiting for further investigations after rhinoscopy the dog was also treated for three times every 7 days (days 0, 7, and 14) with subcutaneous administration of 300 μg/kg of ivermectin. After treatment, sneezing disappeared completely, and only moderate reversal sneezing, probably due to everted laryngeal saccules, remained present. The larva was sent to the Department of Veterinary Medicine of Milan for identification; it was studied under the light microscope and identified according to morphological keys [17–21]. The specimen was identified as a first instar larval stage (L1) of *O. ovis* L. (Diptera: Oestridae). The fusiform and dorsoventrally flattened L1, about 1.18 mm long and 0.44 mm wide, was divided into 11 segments (Figure 1). On its surface, these segments presented trichoid cuticular sensilla (Figure 2). Such structures are thermosensitive; they allow L1 to both locate and, in association with its quick mobility, rapidly reach the nasal cavities to find a suitable niche for its development. Ventral and lateral clusters of spines were also evident on the larva surface. They measured about 20 μm and 30 μm in length, respectively, and their distribution resembled the typical pattern described in *Oestrus* larvae. In subfamily Oestrinae, lateral and ventral spines can help a larva attach to and move on the host's mucosal surface without being expelled by its sneezing. The larva under investigation showed a distinctive cluster of spines on the terminal abdominal segment, though its bilobated shape was not perfectly preserved. Cranially, a pair of prominent, dark brown oral hooks, connected to the internal cephalopharyngeal skeleton, as well as defined antennal lobes, measuring about 18 × 22 μm could be noticed. Broad tracheal trunks, about 20 μm wide, ended between the tenth and eleventh body segments (Figure 3).

## 3. Discussion

*O. ovis* is an agent of myiasis in sheep and goats. Members of Oestridae family tend to be highly host-specific, with preference for herbivores. We described the first record of *O. ovis* infestation in a dog in Italy and, at the same time, the most northerly finding of larvae of sheep bot fly in our country. The infected dog we examined lives in a village near Milan and might have come down with the infestation in an area located about 60 km north of the 45th parallel north. Reasonably, it is a case of autochthonous infestation. In fact, contacts between sheep parasites and companion dogs are likely to occur because even though Milan with its territory is highly urbanized rural areas crossed by transhumant flocks from the PreAlpine areas are still present. Furthermore, unlike other regions such as Tuscany, Liguria, and Emilia Romagna, Lombardy is not characterised by immigration of shepherds and flocks from Sardinia or southern Italy; thus, it can be hypothesised that the presence of sheep nasal bot fly in the studied area is a consequence of temperature increase as observed in several surveys conducted in northern Italy [22–24]. Climate change there might have favoured a habitat more suitable to adult flies survival, as emphasized by some authors [25]. This hypothesis is also supported by the findings (after the record of the infestation in the dog) of other cases of O. ovis infestation in small ruminants bred in three provinces (Bergamo, Varese, and Brescia) located to the north of Milan and referred to our laboratories.

As to dogs, it should be noted that in domestic carnivores (dogs and cats) O. ovis infestations are less common than in humans, having been sporadically described in dogs from India [11], Spain [12, 13], New Zealand [14], and UK [16] and in a cat from Australia [15]. Low occurrence of O. ovis infestations in domestic carnivores might be due to peculiar sheep bot fly preferences and, in general, due to the strong relationship between oestrids and herbivores. In fact, the only species belonging to Oestridae family that naturally infects carnivores is Dermatobia hominis, although it mainly parasitizes herbivores [19]. Moreover, in rural areas and in developing countries, infestations in dogs and cats could go unnoticed or undetected most likely because an in vivo diagnosis of nasal myiasis in carnivores is possible only if larvae and/or puparia are collected by pet owners or clinicians and correctly identified. It is a fact that no serological tests are available for dogs and cats and the described symptoms of infestation are nonspecific (i.e., sneezing, stertor, nasal discharge, excitation, loss of appetite, coughing fits, unilateral epistaxis, and fever). Then, collection of larvae and/or puparia in vivo can be performed only if spontaneous expulsion from nasal cavities through nostrils is noticed by pet owners or occurs during a diagnostic procedure such as a rhinoscopy.

Thus, in case of rhinitis in domestic carnivores, nasal myiasis due to O. ovis should be considered as a possible differential diagnosis, especially when proximity to small ruminant farms is reported in the anamnesis and usual antimicrobial and/or anti-inflammatory treatments result to be ineffective.

## Competing Interests

The authors declare that there are no competing interests regarding the publication of this paper.

## References

[1] S. Sotiraki and M. J. R. Hall, "A review of comparative aspects of myiasis in goats and sheep in Europe," Small Ruminant Research, vol. 103, no. 1, pp. 75–83, 2012.

[2] S. Caracappa, S. Riili, P. Zanghi, V. di Marco, and P. Dorchies, "Epidemiology of ovine oestrosis (Oestrus ovis Linné 1761, Diptera: Oestridae) in Sicily," Veterinary Parasitology, vol. 92, pp. 233–237, 2000.

[3] A. Marconcini and C. Ercolani, "Ovine oestrosis in Tuscany," Annali della Facoltà di Medicina Veterinaria di Pisa, vol. 42, pp. 159–165, 1989.

[4] A. Scala, G. Solinas, C. V. Citterio, L. H. Kramer, and C. Genchi, "Sheep oestrosis (Oestrus ovis Linné 1761, Diptera: Oestridae) in Sardinia, Italy," Veterinary Parasitology, vol. 102, no. 1-2, pp. 133–141, 2001.

[5] G. A. Galvani, "Storia naturale fisiologica e medica del villagese dell'Etna," Atti della Accademia Gioenia di Scienze Naturali in Catania, vol. 15, pp. 123–185, 1839.

[6] S. Pampiglione, S. Giannetto, and A. Virga, "Persistence of human myiasis by Oestrus ovis L. (Diptera: Oestridae) among shepherds of the Etnean area (Sicily) for over 150 years," Parassitologia, vol. 39, no. 4, pp. 415–418, 1997.

[7] D. Crotti, M. L. D'Annibale, and A. Ricci, "A case of ophthalmomyiasis: description and diagnosis," Infezioni in Medicina, vol. 13, no. 2, pp. 120–122, 2005.

[8] M. Dono, M. R. Bertonati, R. Poggi et al., "Three cases of ophthalmomyiasis externa by sheep botfly Oestrus ovis in Italy," New Microbiologica, vol. 28, no. 4, pp. 365–368, 2005.

[9] F. Rivasi, L. Campi, G. M. Cavallini, and S. Pampiglione, "External ophthalmomyiasis by Oestrus ovis larvae diagnosed in a Papanicolaou-stained conjunctival smear," Cytopathology, vol. 20, no. 5, pp. 340–342, 2009.

[10] D. Otranto, C. Cantacessi, M. Santantonio, and G. Rizzo, "Oestrus ovis causing human ocular myiasis: from countryside to town centre," Journal of Clinical and Experimental Ophthalmology, vol. 37, no. 3, pp. 327–328, 2009.

[11] S. K. Tanwani and P. C. Jain, "Oestrus ovis larva in the nasal cavity of a dog," Haryana Veterinarian, vol. 25, pp. 37–38, 1986.

[12] J. Lucientes, M. Ferrer-Dufol, M. J. Andres, M. A. Peribañez, M. J. Gracia-Salinas, and J. A. Castillo, "Canine myiasis by sheep bot fly (Diptera: Oestridae)," Journal of Medical Entomology, vol. 34, no. 2, pp. 242–243, 1997.

[13] L. Luján, J. Vázquez, J. Lucientes, J. A. Pañero, and R. Varea, "Nasal myiasis due to Oestrus ovis infestation in a dog," Veterinary Record, vol. 142, no. 11, pp. 282–283, 1998.

[14] A. C. G. Heath and C. Johnson, "Nasal myiasis in a dog due to Oestrus ovis (Diptera: Oestridae)," New Zealand Veterinary Journal, vol. 49, no. 4, p. 164, 2001.

[15] S. M. Webb and V. L. Grillo, "Nasal myiasis in a cat caused by larvae of the nasal bot fly, Oestrus ovis," Australian Veterinary Journal, vol. 88, no. 11, pp. 455–457, 2010.

[16] J. McGarry, F. Penrose, and C. Collins, "Oestrus ovis infestation of a dog in the UK," Journal of Small Animal Practice, vol. 53, no. 3, pp. 192–193, 2012.

[17] F. Zumpt, Myiasis in Man and Animals in the Old World, Butterworths, London, UK, 1965.

[18] D. D. Colwell and P. J. Scholl, "Cuticular sensilla on newly hatched larvae of Gasterophilus intestinalis and Oestrus ovis," Medical and Veterinary Entomology, vol. 9, no. 1, pp. 85–93, 1995.

[19] D. D. Colwell, "Larval morphology," in The Oestrid Flies: Biology, Host-parasite Relationship, Impact and Management, D. D. Colwell, M. J. R. Hall, and P. J. Sholl, Eds., pp. 98–122, CABI, Cambridge, Mass, USA, 2006.

[20] C. E. Angulo-Valadez, P. J. Scholl, R. Cepeda-Palacios, P. Jacquiet, and P. Dorchies, "Nasal bots... a fascinating world!," Veterinary Parasitology, vol. 174, no. 1-2, pp. 19–25, 2010.

[21] R. Cepeda-Palacios, C. E. A. Valadez, J. P. Scholl, R. Ramírez-Orduña, P. H. Jacquiet, and P. H. Dorchies, "Ecobiology of the sheep nose bot fly (Oestrus ovis L.): a review," Revue de Médecine Vétérinaire, vol. 162, no. 11, pp. 503–507, 2011.

[22] M. Pisetta, L. Montecchio, C. M. O. Longa, C. Salvadori, F. Zottele, and G. Maresi, "Green alder decline in Italian Alps," Forest Ecology and Management, vol. 281, pp. 75–83, 2012.

[23]  A. M. Mercuri, P. Torri, E. Casini, and L. Olmi, "Climate
      warming and the decline of *Taxus airborne* pollen in urban
      pollen rain (Emilia Romagna, northern Italy)," *Plant Biology*,
      vol. 15, no. 1, pp. 70–82, 2013.

[24]  G. Bertini, T. Amoriello, G. Fabbio, and M. Piovosi, "Forest
      growth and climate change: evidences from the ICP-Forests
      intensive monitoring in Italy," *iForest*, vol. 4, pp. 262–267, 2011.

[25]  M. A. Taylor, "Emerging parasitic diseases of sheep," *Veterinary
      Parasitology*, vol. 189, no. 1, pp. 2–7, 2012.

# 36

# Case Report of Bilateral 3-4 Metatarsal Syndactyly in a Pet Rabbit

**M. Gallego[1] and L. Avedillo[2]**

[1]*Centro Veterinario Madrid Exóticos, Calle Meléndez Valdés 17, 28015 Madrid, Spain*
[2]*Centro Veterinario Salud Animal, Calle de la Iglesia 10, Griñón, 28971 Madrid, Spain*

Correspondence should be addressed to M. Gallego; miguel.galego@gmail.com

Academic Editor: Renato L. Santos

We report the first case of spontaneous syndactyly reported in a pet rabbit. Syndactyly only caused an atypical gait in the rabbit. The radiological study revealed bilateral 3rd and 4th metatarsal bones fused in its entire length preserving normal joint surfaces resembling syndactyly type Ia. The cause of this congenital malformation was unknown.

## 1. Introduction

Syndactyly is a congenital malformation in which two or more fingers are joined because they fail to separate or fuse during limb development. The fusion of carpal, tarsal, metacarpal, and metatarsal bones is included in the term syndactyly, as they often occur together [1]. In human and veterinary medicine syndactyly has been classified into several types: simple, which affects only soft tissue; complex, involving synostosis; complete, involving entire length synostosis of the fused bones; incomplete, when synostosis does not comprise the entire bone length; complicated, when syndactyly appears with other malformations in the same individual; and uncomplicated if there are no more malformations [1–3].

Congenital syndactyly has been observed in dogs, cats, sheep, pigs, and cows [3–8]. Although in dogs and cats are cited isolated cases in the literature, it has been considered by some authors that syndactyly is hereditary in these species [2, 3]. Syndactyly in dogs can be complicated: in a family of Australian Shepherd dogs a multiple inherited teratologic syndrome that was lethal to males has been reported [7]. Although in sheep heritability has been suggested, it is in cows in the species in which hereditary syndactyly, in autosomal recessive form, is best described [4, 6, 8].

In humans syndactyly is associated with a mutation in the HoxD-13 gene in a syndrome called synpolydactyly, where bone fusions and duplications in hands and feet occur [9]. There are other causes of syndactyly in people; in fact, in more than 90 multiple malformation syndromes syndactyly is present [1, 10].

Mice genetically modified for experimental embryology have been employed to investigate the embryonic development of the limbs. In these studies syndactyly appeared in the offspring occasionally. Syndactyly was found both in mice lacking laminin alpha-5 chain gene and in mice null for fibrillin-2 gene. Retinoic acid receptor gene mutation in mouse also caused syndactyly. Inhibition of interdigital cell death was observed in functional cell proteins TGF Beta-2/TGF Beta-3 double knockout mice. Mice null for both Apaf1 and bax/bak, respectively, gene, and cell proteins implicated in apoptosis developed soft tissue syndactyly [11, 12].

In reference texts of pet rabbit medicine the following congenital conditions are cited: cryptorchidism, incisor malocclusion, spinal deformities, incomplete tracheal rings, splay leg, uterine malformations, renal agenesis, congenital cardiac disease, polycystic kidney disease, hereditary ataxia, glaucoma, cataracts, lymphoma, and cutaneous asthenia [13–15]. However there are few congenital diseases described in pet rabbits; in the other conditions literature refers to laboratory rabbits or to observations in daily clinical practice. Except for the congenital incisor malocclusion, which is best described [16], there are only sparse case reports: two reports

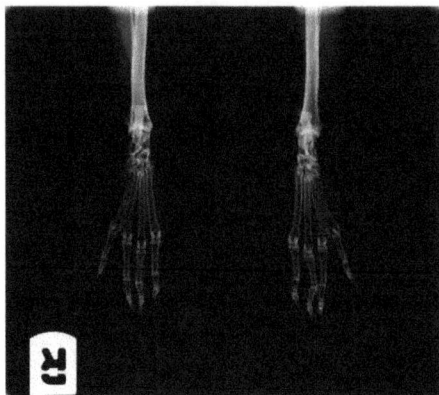

FIGURE 1: Dorsoplantar view of bilateral syndactyly in a pet rabbit.

TABLE 1: Relevant laboratory findings in a syndactyly rabbit.

| | Value | Reference interval |
| --- | --- | --- |
| Hematology | | (a) |
| Biochemistry | | |
| Globulins (g/dL) | 3,7* | 1,5–2,7 (b) |
| Calcium, total (mg/dL) | 14,4* | 11–14 (b) |
| Calcium, ionized (mmol/L) | 1,83 | 1,67–1,85 (c) |
| Urinalysis | | |
| Sediment | Triple phosphate | Triple phosphate, calcium oxalate, calcium carbonate (d) |
| Proteins (mg/dL) | 45,96 | 7,64–70,37 (e) |
| Creatinine (mg/dL) | 67,45 | — |
| GGT (U/L) | 38,25 | 2,7–96,5 (f) |
| Ratio PU : CrU | 0,68* | 0,11–0,4 (e)/<0,6 (b) |
| Ratio GGT : CrU | 0,57 | 0,043–1,034 (f) |

*Value out of the reference interval.
(a) RBC, WBC, hemoglobin, and hematocrit value were within the reference interval for rabbits by Graham and Mader [47].
(b) Melillo 2007 [39]. ALT, ALP, total protein, albumin, BUN, creatinine, and phosphorus were within the reference interval for rabbits by Melillo [39].
(c) Ardiaca et al. 2013 [42]. Gasometry and electrolyte values (pH, $HCO_{3-}$, BEecf, AnGap, Na, K, and Cl) were within the reference interval for rabbits by Ardiaca et al. [42].
(d) Urine strip values were within the reference interval by Hoefer [43].
(e) Reusch et al. 2009 [34].
(f) Mancinelli et al. 2012 [35].

of congenital ventricular septal defects, one case of incomplete tracheal rings, various cases of cutaneous asthenia, one case of bilateral tibial agenesis, two cases of congenital uterine malformations, congenital cataracts, and one corneal dermoid [17–26]. Syndactyly has not been reported in pet rabbits.

Previously, syndactyly has only been observed in laboratory rabbits on studies to assess the teratogenic effects in fetuses of different compounds administered to pregnant does. Vitamin A, 6-aminonicotinamide, hydroxyurea, thalidomide, and cyclophosphamide resulted in offspring syndactyly, in addition to other malformations [27–30]. Syndactyly was induced in rabbits as a result of aberrant scarring after causing traumatic injury on fetuses in utero or caused by uterine puncture to obtain amniotic fluid [31, 32]. After an exhaustive literature review, the authors founded only a citation of spontaneous syndactyly in a laboratory rabbit, a fetus of New Zealand white rabbit that was part of one of the 33 malformed individuals from a total of 2821 control rabbits from a breeding laboratory colony [33].

## 2. Case Histories

A three-year-old mixed breed pet male rabbit weighing 1.6 kg was admitted in a veterinary surgeon for routine sterilization. During the consultation, the owner referred an unusual walking since he bought it in a store when it was 6 weeks old. A detailed physical examination revealed no abnormalities. A radiological study of the hindlimbs was accepted by the owner.

The radiological study showed bilateral 3rd and 4th metatarsal bones fused in its entire length preserving normal joint surfaces (Figure 1). The owner was informed of the unusual radiological findings and a comprehensive prechirurgical analytical profile was accepted.

Two blood samples were obtained. The first blood sample was obtained from the right saphenous vein for hematology (MS4 Vet®; Melet Schloesing) and biochemical profile (Chemray 120®; Rayto) and to obtain a serum sample for serology of Encephalitozoon cuniculi by indirect immunofluorescence in an external laboratory. The second blood sample

was obtained from the left saphenous vein with a special heparinized syringe (PICO 50®; Radiometer) for the evaluation of blood gases and electrolytes in a gasometer (ABL80 Basic® FLEX, Radiometer).

A urinalysis was also performed. The urine was collected with a sterile syringe from a clean surface by manual expression of the bladder. Urinalysis consisted in determination of urine specific gravity by refractometry, protein : creatinine (UP/UCr), and gamma-glutamyl transferase : creatinine (GGTU/CrU) ratios as indicated in the literature [34, 35] and urine strip test (10 Combur test UX®; Roche) with an automatic tester (Urisys®; Roche).

The probes revealed the following alterations (Table 1): hyperglobulinemia, hypercalcemia, and increased UP/UCr. The antibody titer against Encephalitozoon cuniculi was positive, 1 : 640 [36].

Orchiectomy and follow-up were uneventful. During anesthesia a complete radiological exam, previously approved by the owner, was performed and no other abnormalities were observed.

## 3. Discussion

The rabbit presented in this case report is the first case of spontaneous syndactyly in a domestic rabbit. Authors have done a comprehensive search in animal dysmorphology databases [37] resulting in the fact that this presented phenotype is not previously reported in rabbits and resembles syndactyly type Ia in humans [37, 38]. Syndactyly was complex, complete, and not complicated and only caused an atypical walking in the rabbit.

Hyperglobulinemia in rabbits has been associated with inflammatory or infectious processes; in this case the encephalitozoonosis can explain this finding [39].

Increased plasma total calcium was not considered relevant because the value of venous ionized calcium (iCa) was within the reference range [40]. Although iCa reference range for domestic rabbits was established in arterial blood it is assumed that there are no significant differences between arterial or venous samples [41, 42].

Raised UP/UCr ratio value (without active sediment) has been associated with renal damage in rabbits [34, 39, 43]. Although positive *Encephalitozoon cuniculi* titer does not always correspond with histological lesions [36] and elevated UP/UCr ratio has not been associated with the parasite in seropositive rabbits by Reusch et al. [34], the parasite can cause kidney damage, whereas it is considered transient and of little relevance [44]. Neither *Encephalitozoon* or other microsporidia have been associated with congenital malformations in animals or people [45].

Due to the absence of symptoms it was decided to evaluate kidney function in later visits, but the owner refused further testing. It is interesting to note that in human medicine syndactyly appears in numerous multiple malformation syndromes, some with renal impairment [10].

The etiology of syndactyly of this rabbit is difficult to assess but is linked to the embryology of the limbs. The development of fingers in rabbits occurs between 14 and 18 days of gestation [28, 46], after the limb bud and the digital rays appear. Although embryology of the limbs is complex and not fully understood, grossly these rays are composed of mesenchymal condensations that will form the digits after separating from each other by cell apoptosis [11, 12]. The authors aim that in that time interval an unknown etiologic agent (e.g., toxic, trauma, or genetic defect) acted. Exposition to environmental toxins or nonprescription products was unlikely in this case. Considering the symmetry of the syndactyly and the suspected etiology in other species a genetic origin is proposed by the authors. Although presented as an isolated malformation, the presence of other malformations in similar cases should be considered by the clinician.

## Additional Points

The source is Centro Veterinario Madrid Exóticos.

## Competing Interests

The authors declare that there is no conflict of interests regarding the publication of this paper.

## References

[1] S. Malik, "Syndactyly: phenotypes, genetics and current classification," *European Journal of Human Genetics*, vol. 20, no. 8, pp. 817–824, 2012.

[2] H. A. M. Towle and G. J. Breur, "Dysostoses of the canine and feline appendicular skeleton," *Journal of the American Veterinary Medical Association*, vol. 225, no. 11, pp. 1685–1692, 2004.

[3] H. A. M. Towle, W. E. Blevins, L. R. Tuer, and G. J. Breur, "Syndactyly in a litter of cats," *Journal of Small Animal Practice*, vol. 48, no. 5, pp. 292–296, 2007.

[4] S. M. Dennis and H. W. Leipold, "Congenital dactylous malformations in sheep," *The Cornell Veterinarian*, vol. 62, no. 2, pp. 322–327, 1972.

[5] H. W. Leipold and S. M. Dennis, "Syndactyly in a pig," *The Cornell Veterinarian*, vol. 62, no. 2, pp. 269–273, 1972.

[6] L. Hart-Elcock, H. W. Leipold, and R. Baker, "Hereditary bovine syndactyly: diagnosis in bovine fetuses," *Veterinary Pathology*, vol. 24, no. 2, pp. 140–147, 1987.

[7] L. E. Freeman, D. P. Sponenberg, and D. G. Schabdach, "Morphologic characterization of a heritable syndrome of cleft lip/palate, polydactyly, and tibial/fibular dysgenesis in Australian Shepherd dogs," *Anatomia Histologia Embryologia*, vol. 17, article 81, 1988.

[8] I. Yeruham, T. Goshen, D. Lahav, and S. Perl, "Simultaneous occurrence of epitheliogenesis imperfecta with syndactyly in a calf and a lamb," *Australian Veterinary Journal*, vol. 83, no. 3, pp. 149–150, 2005.

[9] P. Sharpe, "HOX gene mutations—the wait is over," *Nature Medicine*, vol. 2, no. 7, pp. 748–749, 1996.

[10] D. Smith, K. Jones, M. Jones, and M. Del Campo, *Smith's Recognizable Patterns of Human Malformation*, Saunders, Philadelphia, Pa, USA, 2013.

[11] V. Zuzarte-Luís and J. M. Hurlé, "Programmed cell death in the developing limb," *International Journal of Developmental Biology*, vol. 46, no. 7, pp. 871–876, 2002.

[12] J. J. Sanz-Ezquerro and C. Tickle, "Digital development and morphogenesis," *Journal of Anatomy*, vol. 202, no. 1, pp. 51–58, 2003.

[13] K. Quesenberry and J. Carpenter, *Ferrets, Rabbits, and Rodents*, Elsevier/Saunders, St. Louis, Mo, USA, 2012.

[14] A. Meredith and B. Lord, *BSAVA Manual of Rabbit Medicine*, British Small Animal Veterinary Association, Quedgeley, UK, 2014.

[15] M. Varga, *Textbook of Rabbit Medicine*, Elsevier, Edinburg, UK, 2014.

[16] E. Böhmer, "Diseases of the incisors," in *Dentistry in Rabbits and Rodents*, E. Böhmer, Ed., pp. 118–152, John Wiley & Sons, Chichester, UK, 1st edition, 2015.

[17] K. N. Gelatt, "Congenital cataracts in a litter of rabbits," *Journal of the American Veterinary Medical Association*, vol. 167, no. 7, pp. 598–599, 1975.

[18] R. G. Harvey, P. J. Brown, R. D. Young, and T. J. Whitbread, "A connective tissue defect in two rabbits similar to the Ehlers-Danlos syndrome," *Veterinary Record*, vol. 126, no. 6, pp. 130–132, 1990.

[19] S. Damsch and C. Messow, "Tibial aplasia and agenesis in a rabbit (case report)," *Deutsche Tierärztliche Wochenschrift*, vol. 98, no. 11, pp. 427–429, 1991.

[20] P. J. Brown, R. D. Young, and P. J. Cripps, "Abnormalities of collagen fibrils in a rabbit with a connective tissue defect similar to Ehlers-Danlos syndrome," *Research in Veterinary Science*, vol. 55, no. 3, pp. 346–350, 1993.

[21] J. D. Sinke, J. E. Van Dijk, and T. Willemse, "A case of Ehlers-Danlos-like syndrome in a rabbit with a review of the disease in

other species," *Veterinary Quarterly*, vol. 19, no. 4, pp. 182–185, 1997.

[22] F. Wagner, M. Brügmann, W. Drommer, and M. Fehr, "Corneal dermoid in a dwarf rabbit (*Oryctolagus cuniculi*)," *Contemporary Topics in Laboratory Animal Science*, vol. 39, no. 5, pp. 39–40, 2000.

[23] S. Redrobe, "Imaging techniques in small mammals," *Journal of Exotic Pet Medicine*, vol. 10, no. 4, pp. 187–197, 2001.

[24] B. Deeb, "The dyspneic rabbit," *Exotic DVM*, vol. 7, pp. 39–42, 2005.

[25] H. P. Thode III and M. S Johnston, "Probable congenital uterine developmental abnormalities in two domestic rabbits," *Veterinary Record*, vol. 164, no. 8, pp. 242–244, 2009.

[26] N. Hildebrandt, C. Leuser, D. Miltz, E. Henrich, and M. Schneider, "Restrictive ventricular septal defect in a dwarf rabbit," *Tierärztliche Praxis Ausgabe K: Kleintiere/Heimtiere*, vol. 44, no. 1, pp. 59–64, 2016.

[27] S. Fabro and R. L. Smith, "The teratogenic activity of thalidomide in the rabbit," *The Journal of Pathology and Bacteriology*, vol. 91, no. 2, pp. 511–519, 1966.

[28] H. A. Hartman, "The fetus in experimental technology," in *The Biology of the Laboratory Rabbit*, S. Weisbroth, R. Flatt, and A. Kraus, Eds., p. 117, Academic Press, New York, NY, USA, 1974.

[29] E. Ujházy, T. Balonová, M. Durisová, A. Gajdosík, J. Jansák, and A. Molnárová, "Teratogenicity of cyclophosphamide in New Zealand white rabbits," *Neoplasma*, vol. 40, no. 1, pp. 45–49, 1993.

[30] S. C. Hyoun, S. G. Običan, and A. R. Scialli, "Teratogen update: methotrexate," *Birth Defects Research Part A: Clinical and Molecular Teratology*, vol. 94, no. 4, pp. 187–207, 2012.

[31] J. M. Clavert, A. Clavert, A. Berlizon, and P. Buck, "Abnormalities resulting from intra-adnexal injection of glucose in the rabbit embryo—an experimental model of 'amniotic disease,'" *Progress in Pediatric Surgery*, vol. 12, pp. 143–164, 1978.

[32] A. Galvan, E. Alvarez, S. Parraguirre, M. L. Suarez, and A. Perez, "Development of a fetal rabbit model to study amniotic band syndrome," *Fetal and Pediatric Pathology*, vol. 31, no. 5, pp. 300–308, 2012.

[33] D. D. Cozens, "Abnormalities of the external form and of the skeleton in the New Zealand white rabbit," *Food and Cosmetics Toxicology*, vol. 3, pp. 695–700, 1965.

[34] B. Reusch, J. K. Murray, K. Papasouliotis, and S. P. Redrobe, "Urinary protein:creatinine ratio in rabbits in relation to their serological status to *Encephalitozoon cuniculi*," *Veterinary Record*, vol. 164, no. 10, pp. 293–295, 2009.

[35] E. Mancinelli, D. J. Shaw, and A. L. Meredith, "$\gamma$-Glutamyltransferase (GGT) activity in the urine of clinically healthy domestic rabbits (*Oryctolagus cuniculus*)," *Veterinary Record*, vol. 171, no. 19, p. 475, 2012.

[36] J. Csokai, A. Joachim, A. Gruber, A. Tichy, A. Pakozdy, and F. Künzel, "Diagnostic markers for encephalitozoonosis in pet rabbits," *Veterinary Parasitology*, vol. 163, no. 1-2, pp. 18–26, 2009.

[37] OMIA, Online Mendelian Inheritance in Animals, http://omia.angis.org.au/home/.

[38] OMIM, "Online Mendelian Inheritance in Man," http://www.omim.org/entry/609815.

[39] A. Melillo, "Rabbit clinical pathology," *Journal of Exotic Pet Medicine*, vol. 16, no. 3, pp. 135–145, 2007.

[40] P. A. Schenck, D. J. Chew, L. A. Nagode, and T. J. Rosol, "Disorders of calcium: hypercalcemia and hypocalcemia," in *Fluid,*

*Electrolyte and Acid-Base Disorders in Small Animal Practice*, S. P. DiBartola, Ed., pp. 120–194, Elsevier/Saunders, St. Louis, Mo, USA, 4th edition, 2012.

[41] R. Bilkovski, C. Cannon, S. Adhikari, and I. Nasr, "Arterial and venous ionized calcium measurements: is there a difference?" *Annals of Emergency Medicine*, vol. 44, no. 4, p. S56, 2004.

[42] M. Ardiaca, C. Bonvehí, and A. Montesinos, "Point-of-care blood gas and electrolyte analysis in rabbits," *Veterinary Clinics of North America: Exotic Animal Practice*, vol. 16, no. 1, pp. 175–195, 2013.

[43] L. Hoefer, "Rabbit and ferret renal disease diagnosis," in *Laboratory Medicine: Avian and Exotic Pets*, A. Fudge, Ed., pp. 311–318, Saunders, Philadelphia, Pa, USA, 1st edition, 2000.

[44] F. Künzel and A. Joachim, "Encephalitozoonosis in rabbits," *Parasitology Research*, vol. 106, no. 2, pp. 299–309, 2010.

[45] P. Ramanan and B. S. Pritt, "Extraintestinal microsporidiosis," *Journal of Clinical Microbiology*, vol. 52, no. 11, pp. 3839–3844, 2014.

[46] A. P. Dyban, V. F. Puchkov, N. A. Samoshkina, L. I. Khozhai, N. A. Chebotar, and V. S. Baranov, "Chapter 12: laboratory mammals: mouse (*Mus musculus*), rat (*Rattus norvergicus*), rabbit (*Oryctolagus cuniculus*), and golden hamster (*Cricetus auratus*)," in *Animal Species for Developmental Studies, Volume II: Vertebrates*, T. Dettlaff and F. Billett, Eds., pp. 351–442, Consultants Bureau, New York, NY, USA, 1st edition, 1991.

[47] J. Graham and D. R. Mader, "Basic approach to veterinary care," in *Ferrets, Rabbits, and Rodents*, K. Quesenberry and J. Carpenter, Eds., pp. 174–182, Elsevier/Saunders, St. Louis, Mo, USA, 3rd edition, 2012.

# 37

# Benign Pigmented Dermal Basal Cell Tumor in a Namibian Cheetah (*Acinonyx jubatus*)

**Sonja K. Heinrich,**[1] **Bettina Wachter,**[1] **and Gudrun Wibbelt**[2]

[1]*Leibniz Institute for Zoo and Wildlife Research, Department Evolutionary Ecology, Alfred-Kowalke-Strasse 17, 10315 Berlin, Germany*
[2]*Leibniz Institute for Zoo and Wildlife Research, Department Wildlife Diseases, Alfred-Kowalke-Strasse 17, 10315 Berlin, Germany*

Correspondence should be addressed to Sonja K. Heinrich; heinrich@izw-berlin.de

Academic Editor: Paola Roccabianca

A 3.5-year-old wild born cheetah (*Acinonyx jubatus*), living in a large enclosure on a private Namibian farm, developed a large exophytic nodular neoplasm in its skin at the height of the left shoulder blade. We describe the clinical appearance, the surgical removal, and histological examination of the tumor, which was diagnosed as a moderately pigmented benign basal cell tumor. A three-year follow-up showed no evidence of recurrence after the surgery. Although neoplasia is reported in nondomestic felids, only very few concern cheetahs. So far, no case of basal cell tumor was described in this species.

## 1. Introduction

The number of reports on neoplasms in exotic felids is continuously rising, particularly due to an increase in longevity in captive animals [1]. Several types of neoplasia are published in captive cheetahs, but no basal cell tumor has been described so far [2–6]. Basal cell tumors arise from nonkeratinizing cells that originate in the basal layer of the epidermis and are one of the most common skin tumors in domestic cats [7].

Namibia hosts the worldwide largest free-ranging cheetah population with most of these animals roaming on privately owned commercial farmland [8, 9]. While some farmers regularly eliminate cheetahs to reduce the threat to their livestock and game animals [8], others keep cheetahs in large enclosures on their guest farms as tourist attractions. Such privately kept animals have to go through an annual health check by an authorized veterinarian. The cheetah research project of the Leibniz Institute for Zoo and Wildlife Research has been working on Namibian farmland since 2002 and has examined more than 400 free-ranging as well as more than 100 captive cheetahs. In 2011, we removed a benign basal cell tumor from a wild born captive cheetah living on a Namibian farm. This was the first neoplastic lesion found by the project in about 14 years of cheetah research.

## 2. Case Presentation

We were contacted by a local farmer who kept a cheetah on his farm, which exhibited a slow growing alopecic dermal mass at the height of the left shoulder blade that began to grow approximately 1.5 years earlier (Figure 1). The animal was a castrated 3.5-year-old wild born male cheetah, living since the age of 3 months in a large fenced area surrounding the farmhouse. He had been vaccinated yearly against rabies (Rabisin®), feline calicivirus, feline panleukemia virus, feline viral rhinotracheitis virus (Feligen CRP®, Virbac), and feline leukemia virus (Tricat, Nobivac). The surgical option was made. A fine needle aspirate of the mass was not attempted before surgery, as this would have required an additional anesthesia. During the clinical investigation, the cheetah was found in a good health status with a body weight of 47 kg.

The cheetah was immobilized with a mixture of ketamine (3.2 mg/kg, Ketavet®, Kyron Laboratories, Benrose, RSA) and medetomidine (0.06 mg/kg, Novartis, Spartan, Republic of South Africa) administered with a dart shot from a dartgun (Telinject, Dudenhofen, Germany). The skin around the mass was shaved and the surgical field was washed and disinfected with 70% ethanol. The mass and covering skin were excised from the adjacent tissue. The neoplasia was well encapsulated and no infiltrative growth into the surrounding

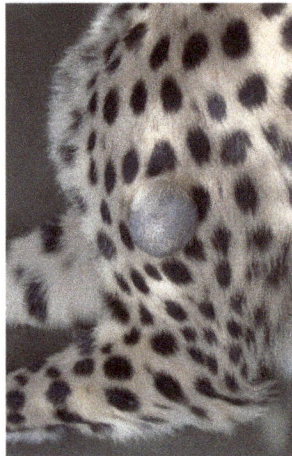

FIGURE 1: Exophytic solid basal cell tumor of a Namibian cheetah located on the left shoulder.

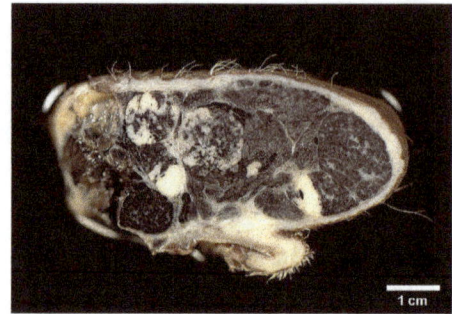

FIGURE 2: Cut surface of the solid basal cell tumor in a Namibian cheetah (5.5 cm in diameter).

tissue was visible, but it had one large supportive blood vessel, which was ligated and cut. The wound was closed with a subcutaneous consecutive suture and several cutaneous suture stiches both with absorbable material. The animal was treated prophylactically with 2 mg/kg ketoprofen (Ketofen®, Merial) as anti-inflammatory and pain medication and with a combination of 15.000 IU/kg procaine benzyl penicillin and 15.000 IU/kg benzathine benzyl penicillin (Peni-LA Phenix®, Virbac) to prevent a wound infection. To keep the wound clean from dust and dirt, we dressed the animal with children's shirt, which was removed by the farmer seven days after surgery. The immobilization was reversed with Atipamezole (0.11 mg/kg, Antisedan®, Pfizer, RSA). The wound remained uninfected and was nearly invisible at the annual medical check-up one year after the surgery and the cheetah was still alive 3.5 years after removal of the tumor without any signs of recurrence.

The excised neoplasia was fixed in 10% buffered formalin and shipped to Germany in full compliance with the Convention on International Trade in Endangered Species (CITES) for histological examination at the Leibniz Institute for Zoo and Wildlife Research in Berlin.

The tumor presented itself as an exophytic firm encapsulated broad based nodular dermal to subcutaneous mass measuring 5.5 cm × 4.5 cm × 2.5 cm, covered by intact sparsely haired dark pigmented skin. Cut surfaces revealed multiple small lobules separated by fine white strands of connective tissue (Figure 2). Lobules were mottled light to dark grey or whitish with multinodular solid growth pattern and they did not exceed the surgical excision margins. Microscopically, some lobules were populated by high numbers of heavily dark brown, pigmented cells, while others contained lightly pigmented cells, which were mostly distributed in the periphery of each lobule (Figures 3(a) and 3(b)). Within the lobules, cells were oriented in cords and trabeculae or small islands separated by thin collagen, while distinct sheets of collagen-rich connective tissue surrounded the entire lobules (Figure 3(c)). Rarely, small assemblies of dark pigmented cells (melanophages) were found in the separating connective

tissue septa. The neoplastic cells were cuboidal to polygonal with uniformly large round to ovoid central nuclei with stippled chromatin and 1-2 nucleoli (Figure 3(d)). Cytoplasm was scant to moderate, pale eosinophilic, sparsely stained and finely granular. The majority of the tumor cells had indistinct cell borders (Figures 3(c) and 3(d)). Occasionally, single mitotic figures were found (one per 10 high power fields). The overlying epidermis was made of five to six even layers of unremarkable keratinocytes containing some melanosomes in the basal cells as well as some cells of the stratum germinativum. There was mild orthokeratosis and a few remaining hair follicles. The superficial dermis contained mild nodular perivascular neutrophilic infiltrates and dermal collagen was markedly thickened as a response to the expanding tumor, but no other pathological changes were apparent.

A panel of immunohistochemistry stains was applied and revealed tumor cells being positive for pancytokeratin but negative for MelanA, S100, and vimentin. Although the dark pigmentation and nests and islands of polygonal cells prompted the differential diagnosis of a melanocytoma, the immunohistochemistry results lead to the final diagnosis of a moderately pigmented basal cell tumor.

## 3. Discussion

Basal cell tumors are common cutaneous epithelial neoplasms in domestic dogs and cats [10] originating from cells of the basal layer of the epidermis but without epidermal or adnexal differentiation [11, 12]. Two distinct growth forms, cystic and solid basal cell tumors, are found with the former representing the majority of cases in cats [7]. Their microscopic appearance is notoriously pleomorphic with many pattern variations [13], but some features are commonly described such as the dermal position or the singularity in occurrence of these nodular masses. In solid basal cell tumors the cell morphology often varies, whereas the nuclei are usually uniformly ovoid and surrounded by scant cytoplasm [13]. While this holds true for the solid tumor described here in the Namibian cheetah, the majority of its lobules featured a slightly different cellular growth pattern than expected for a basal cell tumor. The nests and clusters of neoplastic cells as well as the sometimes high amount of dark brown pigmentation lead to the first assumption of a melanocytoma.

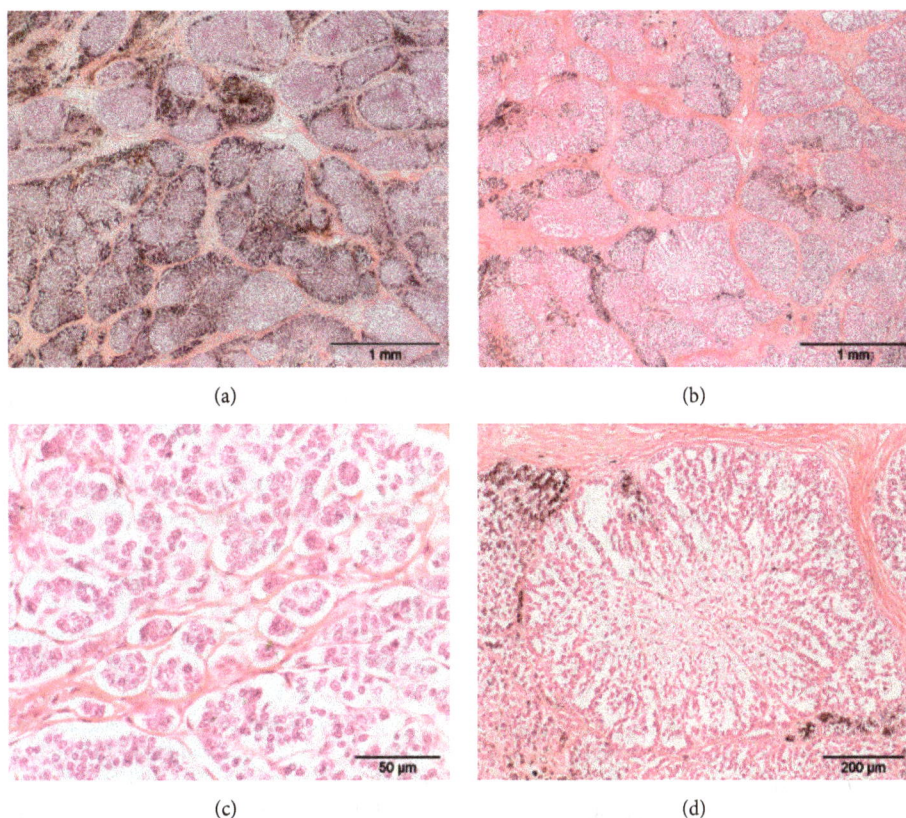

FIGURE 3: Basal cell tumor in a Namibian cheetah. (a) Area of heavily pigmented dark brown tumor lobules and (b) tumor lobules sparsely pigmented. (c) Tumor cells oriented in cords and nests separated by thin collagen. (d) Tumor nodule with cells with indistinct cell borders delineated by fine connective tissue. HE stain.

However, basal cell tumors often also contain pigment [14]. One survey on basal cell tumors in cats described 25% of 46 tumors as black or grey masses [10], while another review of 56 of cystic and solid feline basal cell tumors in cats found almost 50% pigmented [7]. Thus, confusion between melanocytoma and basal cell tumors is a recognized obstacle [15]. The application of immunohistochemistry stains including epithelial as well as melanocytic markers [16, 17] was necessary to lead to the diagnosis of a basal cell tumor. An additional differential diagnosis is the trichoblastoma. This benign neoplasia is derived from the trichoblastic epithelium, the primitive hair germ of embryonic follicular development, and occurs in four different variants: ribbon, trabecular, granular, and spindle cell trichoblastoma [18]. Their distinct growth pattern differentiates these entities from the tumor described here, as they usually comprise one to two layers of cells oriented in long and narrow winding cords of cells as well as adnexal differentiation. The trabecular trichoblastoma would appear as the closest resemblance of the tumor in the cheetah. But the characteristic peripheral palisading growth of trabecular trichoblastoma cells is not a feature in the tumor of the animal described here. Currently, there are ongoing discussions whether basal cell tumors should still be recognized as an own entity or whether they should be integrated into trichoblastomas together with all neoplasms

deriving from cells of the hair follicle [19, 20]. But until this debate is resolved, we will use the term basal cell tumor.

The most common location of this neoplasia in domestic cats is the head or the trunk [11], while the tumor found in the cheetah was removed at the height of the left shoulder blade. Basal cell tumors are considered benign neoplasms which is also reflected in this case because, although the tumor was of rather large size, three years after removal no sign of recurrence on the skin of the cheetah was visible.

In nondomestic felids, a similar solid basal cell tumor was described in a captive Indian leopard (*Panthera pardus fusca*) [21] and a basal cell epithelioma was found in a captive African lion (*P. leo*) [22]. However, also malignant dermal melanomas have been described in exotic cat species. One was detected in a lion, located at the upper lip and successfully treated with a combination of radio- and immunotherapy [23], and the other was reported in a white tiger (*P. tigris tigris*), which had metastasized to most lymph nodes and the lung [24].

In cheetahs, the most common neoplasia is myelolipoma, which was first described in 1968 [5]. It occurs only in captive cheetahs and is reported with an unusually high frequency [4, 25–27]. It is mostly located in the liver and spleen and it has been suggested as an indicator for chronic disease or stress [26]. Other reports on neoplasia in captive cheetahs include three cases of fibroleiomyoma [3, 4], a mesothelioma [28], and a T-cell lymphoma associated with feline leukemia virus [2]. This is the first description of a solid basal cell tumor in a cheetah. After approximately 14 years of cheetah research in Namibia and no other cases published in the literature, it seems that the described neoplasm occurs, unlike to domestic cats, very rarely in this animal species.

## Competing Interests

The authors declare that they have no competing interests.

## Acknowledgments

The authors thank the Namibian Ministry of Environment and Tourism for permission to conduct the study and the owner of the cheetah for cooperation. The authors are grateful to D. Krumnow for her technical assistance in the histology lab. This work was supported by the Messerli Foundation, Switzerland.

## References

[1] M. A. Owston, E. C. Ramsay, and D. S. Rotstein, "Neoplasia in felids at the Knoxville Zoological gardens, 1979–2003," *Journal of Zoo and Wildlife Medicine*, vol. 39, no. 4, pp. 608–613, 2008.

[2] L. Marker, L. Munson, P. A. Basson, and S. Quackenbush, "Multicentric T-cell lymphoma associated with feline leukemia virus infection in a captive Namibian cheetah (*Acinonyx jubatus*)," *Journal of Wildlife Diseases*, vol. 39, no. 3, pp. 690–695, 2003.

[3] C. Walzer, A. Kübber-Heiss, and B. Bauder, "Spontaneous uterine fibroleiomyoma in a captive cheetah," *Journal of Veterinary Medicine Series A: Physiology Pathology Clinical Medicine*, vol. 50, no. 7, pp. 363–365, 2003.

[4] L. Munson, "Diseases of captive cheetahs (*Acinonyx jubatus*): results of the cheetah research council pathology survey, 1989–1992," *Zoo Biology*, vol. 12, no. 1, pp. 105–124, 1993.

[5] L. S. Lombard, H. M. Fortna, F. M. Garner, and G. Brynjolfsson, "Myelolipomas of the liver in captive wild felidae," *Pathologia Veterinaria*, vol. 5, no. 2, pp. 127–134, 1968.

[6] M. J. Hartman, R. M. Kirberger, A. S. Tordiffe, S. Boy, and J. P. Schoeman, "Laparoscopic removal of a large abdominal foreign body granuloma using single incision laparoscopic surgery (SILS) and extraction bag in a cheetah (*Acinonyx jubatus*)," *Veterinary Record Case Reports*, vol. 3, no. 1, Article ID e000162, 2015.

[7] M. A. Miller, S. L. Nelson, J. R. Turk et al., "Cutaneous neoplasia in 340 cats," *Veterinary Pathology*, vol. 28, no. 5, pp. 389–395, 1991.

[8] L. L. Marker, M. G. L. Mills, and D. W. Macdonald, "Factors influencing perceptions of conflict and tolerance toward cheetahs on Namibian farmlands," *Conservation Biology*, vol. 17, no. 5, pp. 1290–1298, 2003.

[9] L. Marker, "Current Status of the cheetah (*Acinonyx jubatus*)," in *Proceedings of the Symposium on Cheetahs as Game Ranch Animals*, pp. 1–17, 1998.

[10] R. W. Diters and K. M. Walsh, "Feline basal cell tumors: a review of 124 cases," *Veterinary Pathology*, vol. 21, no. 1, pp. 51–56, 1984.

[11] M. Goldschmidt and M. Hendrick, "Tumors of the skin and soft tissues," in *Tumors in Domestic Animals*, D. J. Meuten, Ed., pp. 45–118, Blackwell, London, UK; Iowa State Press, Ames, Iowa, USA, 2002.

[12] M. H. Goldschmidt, R. Dunstan, A. Stannard, C. von Tscharner, E. J. Walder, and J. Yager, *Histological Classification of Epithelial and Melanocytic Tumors of the Skin of Domestic Animals*, Armed Forces Institute of Pathology: American Registry of Pathology: World Health Organization Collaborating Center for Comparative Oncology, Washington, DC, USA, 1998.

[13] J. A. Yager and B. P. Wilcock, "Basal cell and appendage tumours," in *Color Atlas and Text of Surgical Pathology of the Dog and Cat, Volume 1: Dermatopathology and Skin Tumors*, J. A. Yager and B. P. Wilcock, Eds., pp. 259–260, Wolfe Publishing, 1994.

[14] M. Goldschmidt and M. Hendrick, "Tumors of the skin and soft tissues," in *Tumors in Domestic Animals*, D. J. Meuten, Ed., pp. 45–117, John Wiley & Sons, 4th edition, 2008.

[15] D. W. Scott, "Feline dermatology 1900–1978: a monograph," *Journal of the American Animal Hospital Association*, vol. 16, no. 3, pp. 331–459, 1980.

[16] J. A. Ramos-Vara, M. A. Miller, G. C. Johnson, S. E. Turnquist, J. M. Kreeger, and G. L. Watson, "Melan A and S100 protein immunohistochemistry in feline melanomas: 48 cases," *Veterinary Pathology*, vol. 39, no. 1, pp. 127–132, 2002.

[17] J. S. van der Linde-Sipman, M. M. L. de Wit, E. van Garderen, R. F. Molenbeek, D. van der Velde-Zimmermann, and R. A. de Weger, "Cutaneous malignant melanomas in 57 cats: identification of (amelanotic) signet-ring and balloon cell types and verification of their origin by immunohistochemistry, electron microscopy, and in situ hybridization," *Veterinary Pathology*, vol. 34, no. 1, pp. 31–38, 1997.

[18] E. A. Mauldin and J. Peter-Kennedy, "Integumentary system; tumors arising from hair follicles," in *Jubb, Kennedy & Palmer's Pathology of Domestic Animal*, M. Maxie, Ed., chapter 6, pp. 714–715, Saunders Elservier, Philadelphia, Pa, USA, 2007.

[19] A. R. Kiehl and M. B. C. Mays, "Selected lesions of skin and subcutis of the trunk," in *Atlas for the Diagnosis of Tumors in the Dog and Cat*, pp. 80–82, John Wiley & Sons, 2016.

[20] T. L. Gross, P. J. Ihrke, E. J. Walder, and V. K. Affolter, *Skin Diseases of the Dog and Cat: Clinical and Histopathologic Diagnosis*, Blackwell Science, 2nd edition, 2005.

[21] R. J. Brown, R. D. Davis, W. P. Trevethan, and N. L. Johnson, "Basal cell tumor in an Indian leopard," *Journal of Wildlife Diseases*, vol. 8, no. 3, pp. 237–238, 1972.

[22] G. White, "A basal cell epithelioma in an African lion," *Veterinary Medicine and Small Animal Clinician*, vol. 70, no. 9, p. 1096, 1975.

[23] J. C. Steeil, J. Schumacher, K. Baine et al., "Diagnosis and treatment of a dermal malignant melanoma in an African lion (*Panthera leo*)," *Journal of Zoo and Wildlife Medicine*, vol. 44, no. 3, pp. 721–727, 2013.

[24] A. Rao, L. Acharjyo, and A. Mohanty, "Malignant melanoma in a white tiger," *Indian Journal of Veterinary Pathology*, vol. 15, pp. 113–114, 1991.

[25] R. H. Cardy and R. E. Bostrom, "Multiple splenic myelolipomas in a cheetah (*Acinonyx jubatus*)," *Veterinary Pathology*, vol. 15, no. 4, pp. 556–558, 1978.

[26] C. Walzer, K. Hittmair, and C. Walzer-Wagner, "Ultrasonographic identification and characterization of splenic nodular lipomatosis or myelolipomas in cheetahs (*Acinonyx jubatus*)," *Veterinary Radiology & Ultrasound*, vol. 37, no. 4, pp. 289–292, 1996.

[27] P. Wadsworth and D. Jones, "Myelolipoma in the liver of a cheetah (*Acinonyx jubatus*)," *The Journal of Zoo Animal Medicine*, vol. 11, no. 3, pp. 75–76, 1980.

[28] A. Whiton, J. Schumacher, E. E. Evans et al., "Mesothelioma in two nondomestic felids: North American cougar (*Felis concolor*) and cheetah (*Acinonyx jubatus*)," *Case Reports in Veterinary Medicine*, vol. 2013, Article ID 286793, 6 pages, 2013.

# 38

# Common Arterial Trunk in a 3-Day-Old Alpaca Cria

**Tsumugi Anne Kurosawa,**[1] **Tamilselvam Gunasekaran,**[2]
**Robert Sanders,**[3] **and Elizabeth Carr**[4]

[1]*Royal Veterinary College, Clinical Science and Services, Royal Veterinary College, Hawkshead Ln, Hatfield AL9 7TA, UK*
[2]*BluePearl Veterinary Partners, 4126 Packard Road, Ann Arbor, MI 48187, USA*
[3]*Veterinary Medical Center, Small Animal Clinical Sciences, College of Veterinary Medicine, Michigan State University, 736 Wilson Road, East Lansing, MI 48187, USA*
[4]*Veterinary Medical Center, Large Animal Clinical Sciences, College of Veterinary Medicine, Michigan State University, 736 Wilson Road, East Lansing, MI, USA*

Correspondence should be addressed to Robert Sanders; ras@cvm.msu.edu

Academic Editor: Luciano Espino López

A 3-day-old alpaca cria presented for progressive weakness and dyspnea since birth. Complete bloodwork, thoracic radiographs, and endoscopic examination of the nasal passages and distal trachea revealed no significant findings. Echocardiogram and contrast study revealed a single artery overriding a large ventricular septal defect (VSD). A small atrial septal defect or patent foramen ovale was also noted. Color flow Doppler and an agitated saline contrast study revealed bidirectional but primarily right to left flow through the VSD and bidirectional shunting through the atrial defect. Differential diagnosis based on echocardiographic findings included common arterial trunk, Tetralogy of Fallot, and pulmonary atresia with a VSD. Postmortem examination revealed a large common arterial trunk with a quadricuspid valve overriding a VSD. Additionally, defect in the atrial septum was determined to be a patent foramen ovale. A single pulmonary trunk arose from the common arterial trunk and bifurcated to the left and right pulmonary artery, consistent with a Collet and Edwards' type I common arterial trunk with aortic predominance. Although uncommon, congenital cardiac defects should be considered in animals presenting with clinical signs of hypoxemia, dyspnea, or failure to thrive.

## 1. Introduction

South American camelids have been reported to have a predisposition to be born with complex congenital heart diseases and it has been hypothesized that this may be associated with the relatively small genetic pool available for breeding outside South America [1]. As such it is important to be aware of the clinical presentation of congenital heart disease in llamas and alpacas. This case report describes the clinical presentation and the physical examination findings of a young cria with complex congenital heart disease. The diagnostic methods used to identify are described and a discussion of the embryologic origins is presented.

## 2. Case Presentation

A 3-day-old, 9.5 kg female alpaca cria was presented for progressive weakness and dyspnea of a few hours' duration. The cria had an uneventful birth, stood, nursed, and passed urine and feces normally, but was less active than normal. The cria nursed regularly but only for very short periods. On presentation, the patient was tachycardic (heart rate 148) and appeared to be dyspneic (respiratory rate 28) with cyanosis of the oral mucous membranes and had a capillary refill time of 3 seconds. Cardiac auscultation revealed no significant abnormalities (excluding the tachycardia) and pulse pressure was considered normal. During examination, the cria intermittently lowered its head, became ataxic, and

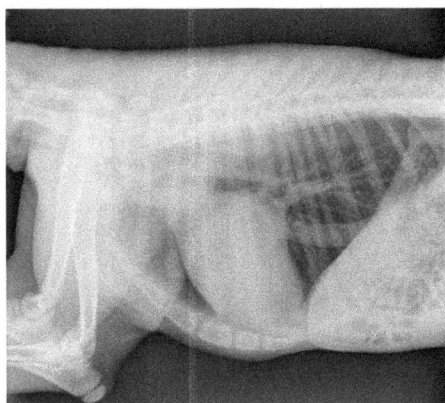

FIGURE 1: Thoracic radiograph: left lateral thoracic view of the skeletally immature alpaca cria demonstrating mild loss of the cranial waist, distention of the caudal vena cava, and a mild diffuse unstructured interstitial pattern in the lungs warranting cardiac evaluation. A reduced cervical tracheal diameter is also evident.

collapsed. These episodes were precipitated by handling or when nursing. After a few moments the cria sat sternal and then stood, appearing normal. Behavior and neurologic exam between episodes were normal. Differential diagnosis included septicemia, pneumonia, choanal atresia, meningitis, persistent fetal circulation, and cardiac abnormalities. No significant abnormalities were noted on complete blood cell count and blood chemistry. Standard lateral thoracic radiographs (evaluated by a board certified veterinary radiologist) revealed slight loss of cranial cardiac waist, distention of the caudal vena cava, and a mild diffuse interstitial lung pattern (Figure 1) without significant evidence of pulmonary venous congestion or overcirculation. A dorsoventral or ventrodorsal view may have provided additional information regarding the heart, but it is not routinely obtained in an unsedated or unanesthetized cria [1]. An attempt was made to perform upper airway endoscopy to assess for suspected choanal atresia; however, the procedure was aborted as the cria became progressively more distressed. The cria was subsequently anesthetized and placed on 100% oxygen. An endoscopic examination of the nasal passages and distal trachea revealed no significant abnormalities. An arterial blood gas was performed while on oxygen supplementation which revealed a marked hypoxemia ($PaO_2$ 19 mmHg, $PaCO_2$ 29.6 mmHg, and $SaO_2$% 31.7) making cardiac disease with right to left shunting of blood more likely. As such, with no evidence of respiratory diseases or septicemia as the cause of the clinical signs, a congenital cardiac malformation was highly suspected and a cardiac evaluation was performed.

Two-dimensional (2D) echocardiography, color flow, and spectral Doppler examinations were performed under general anesthesia with an ultrasound unit (Vivid 7, General Electric Medical System, Waukesha, WI, USA) equipped with 1.5–3.6, 2.2–5, and 4.4–10 MHz phased-array transducers. Two-dimensional images revealed severe dilation of the right atrium and ventricle. Thickening of the right ventricle free wall was also identified. No significant dilation of the left atrium or thickening of the left ventricle was noted. The

interventricular septum (IVS) was flattened and there was paradoxical motion of the IVS. At the base of the IVS a large ventricular septal defect (VSD) was detected (Figure 2(a)). Additionally, a patent foramen ovale (PFO) was noted in the atrial septum (Figure 2(b)) and a single large artery overriding the VSD was also identified. The right ventricular outflow tract, origins of the pulmonary arteries, and a patent ductus arteriosus could not be visualized during the echocardiographic examination. Systolic function appeared normal as estimated by 27% fractional shortening (normal 32.8 ± 7.6) [1]. Color flow Doppler evaluation revealed bidirectional but primarily right to left shunting across both the defect in the atrial septum and VSD. Mild regurgitation across mitral, tricuspid, and the valve of the single large artery was noted. A contrast study was performed by injecting agitated heparinized saline into the external jugular vein while viewing the heart from the right parasternal view. Presence of bubbles from the right heart crossing the VSD into the left heart and main artery during systole confirmed the presence of a right to left shunting VSD (Figure 3; Supplementary Information: Video 1 and Video 2 in Supplementary Material available online at http://dx.doi.org/10.1155/2016/4609126). Differential diagnosis based on the echocardiographic findings included Tetralogy of Fallot, severe pulmonic stenosis or pulmonary atresia with a VSD, and common arterial trunk (CAT). Surgical implantation of a vascular shunt and open-heart surgical correction of the malformation was discussed with the owners but due to the poor prognosis and limited treatment options, the owner elected humane euthanasia and postmortem examination.

On macroscopic examination, there was evidence of both right sided (liver congestion and pleural, pericardial, and peritoneal effusion) and left sided (marked pulmonary edema) congestive heart failure. Examination of the heart revealed marked dilation of the right atrium, a small PFO, a large VSD, and a single large vessel overriding the IVS. The vessel had a mildly thickened quadricuspid valve and appeared to be the only outflow tract for both the right and left ventricles consistent with a CAT. A separate pulmonary artery originating from the right ventricular outflow tract could not be identified despite careful dissection. However, a single pulmonary trunk arose from the common trunk prior to the arch and branched to the right and left pulmonary arteries. A patent ductus arteriosus was not identified. Coronary artery structure appeared to be normal. Histological examination identified the presence of pulmonary edema and hepatic congestion consistent with left and right sided congestive heart failure. There was an incidental finding of a cerebellar pseudocyst. Based on the postmortem examination, a diagnosis of a type I CAT (according to Collett and Edwards' classification) and PFO was made.

## 3. Discussion

Common arterial trunk is described as the presence of a single vessel with a semilunar valve, originating from the base of the heart serving as an outlet for both ventricles supplying blood to the systemic, pulmonary, and coronary circulations together with a VSD [2]. In people, CAT is

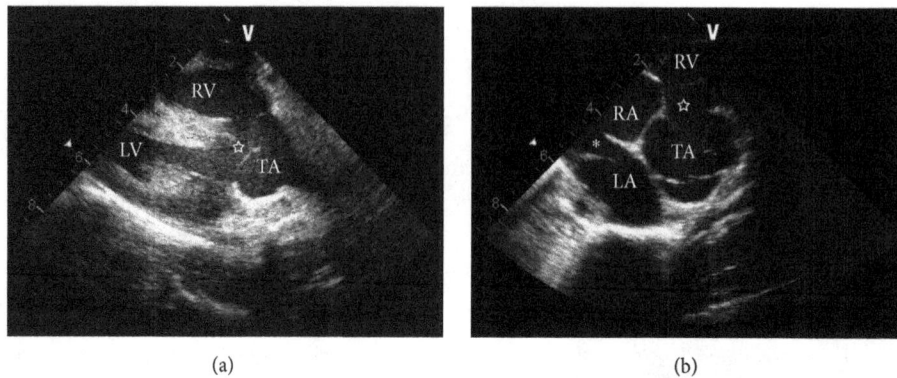

(a)                                                        (b)

FIGURE 2: Two-dimensional echocardiographic images. (a) Right parasternal long axis view. Note the truncus arteriosus overriding the ventricular septal defect (star). (b) Right parasternal short axis view at the level of the heart base. Note the ventricular septal defect (star), atrial septal defect (asterisk), and lack of an obvious right ventricular outflow tract. LA, left atrium; RA, right atrium; RV, right ventricle; TA, truncus arteriosus.

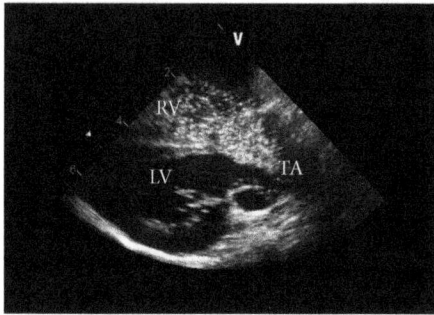

FIGURE 3: Two-dimensional echocardiographic images of agitated saline contrast study. Two-dimensional echocardiographic right parasternal image of an agitated saline contrast study demonstrating primarily right to left flow of bubbles across the large ventricular septal defect. LV, left ventricle; RV, right ventricle; TA, truncus arteriosus.

uncommon representing 1-2% of all congenital heart defects with no gender predilection [3, 4]. There have been various associated cardiac anomalies with a right aortic arch (28%) and interrupted aortic arch (18%) as the most frequently reported concurrent defects [4, 5]. In veterinary patients, CAT is rare with a few reported cases in a llama, cats, dogs, cattle, monkey, and a horse [6–14]. The incidence of congenital cardiac diseases in alpacas is currently unknown. However, in a large retrospective of 663 llamas, VSD was the most common congenital cardiac abnormality reported (14/24 cases) [15]. Reports of cardiac defects in camelid species include VSD, patent ductus arteriosus, transposition of the great vessels, persistent right aortic arch, pulmonary atresia with a VSD, and CAT in a llama [1, 6, 15–17]. To the best of authors' knowledge, this is the first report detailing echocardiographic findings of a CAT and PFO in an alpaca. It is not uncommon for the foramen ovale to remain patent for up to 2 weeks in a llama cria and once the left atrial pressure exceeds the right atrial pressure, the embryologic structure closes [15].

Common arterial trunk is widely described as a conotruncal malformation occurring during fetal development. This categorization arose mainly from the use of two outflow tract components: "conus" and "truncus" by the early investigators to classify congenital outflow tract abnormalities [18]. However, recent studies using electron micrsopy and episcopy on human and mice embryos recognized three outflow tract components, namely, the proximal, intermediate, and distal components in the developing primary heart tube [19]. With ongoing contributions of nonmyocardial tissues from the second heart field and from neural crest cells these outflow tract components transform to form intrapericardial trunks, arterial roots, and subvalvular ventricular outflow tracts, respectively, in the postnatal heart. During development, the common lumen of the distal outflow tract is initially divided into separate intrapericardial arteries by the aortopulmonary septum derived from the dorsal wall of the aortic arch [20]. This is followed by the progressive fusion of the outflow tract cushions that spiral through the intermediate and proximal components. But these septal structures disappear later as the intrapericardial aorta and pulmonary trunks form their own discrete walls. The proximal cushions then fuse with the muscular crest of the right ventricle to form the septal component of the subpulmonary infundibulum [21]. In the left ventricle the posterior wall of the outflow tract is formed by the fibrous extension of the aortic and mitral valve leaflets followed by the closure of the interventricular communications by formation of membranous septum [20].

In normal fetal development the spiral septum separates the common trunk into the pulmonary trunk and proximal ascending aorta, allowing proper delivery of deoxygenated and oxygenated blood, respectively. Failure of fusion of the outflow tract cushions results in formation of a single large trunk with a common ventriculoarterial junction and a single semilunar valve, overriding a VSD [22]. The common trunk supplies a mixture of oxygenated and deoxygenated blood into the systemic, pulmonary, and coronary circulations [2]. The VSD associated with CAT is typically large, extending from the truncal valve to the pars membranacea septi [3].

There is usually a fibrous tissue connecting the septal leaflet of the mitral valve to the noncoronary leaflet of the truncal valve which distinguishes CAT from a form of transposition of the great arteries [3]. The CAT more often originates from both either ventricles or the right ventricle and less frequently the left ventricle [4, 5]. The truncal valve is most commonly tricuspid but can be bicuspid, quadricuspid, or pentacuspid [2]. The valves can have marked changes such as abnormal thickening that can lead to truncal insufficiency or stenosis [2].

Common arterial trunk is often categorized according to a classification system based on the origins of the pulmonary arteries [23]. In type I, the most common type in humans, a single pulmonary trunk arises from the CAT, which subsequently bifurcates into the right and left pulmonary arteries [4]. In types II and III, separate right and left pulmonary arteries arise directly from the CAT [23]. In type II the arteries originate from the dorsal wall of the CAT while in type III they are more laterally oriented [23]. The pulmonary artery is absent in type IV (absence of the 6th aortic arches) and blood supply to the lungs is via the bronchial arteries and is now considered to be pulmonary atresia with a VSD [4, 23]. A second classification system was later described primarily based on the presence (type A) or absence (type B) of a VSD and development of the aorticopulmonary septum [2]. Most cases of type B were actually aortopulmonary window defects, and as such type B classification is no longer used [4]. Type A is subdivided into 4 categories with type A1 corresponding to Collett and Edwards type 1 and type A2 to Collett and Edwards type II and type III. Type A3 describes an absence of one pulmonary artery with a presence of a ductus arteriosus or collateral vessels to provide blood flow to the lungs [3]. Finally, type A4 includes hypoplasia, coarctation, and atresia or absence of the aortic arch [3]. Recently, a simplified categorization that classifies CAT based on the presence of systemic or pulmonary predominance was proposed [24, 25]. In pulmonary dominance, the common trunk trifurcates into right and left branch pulmonary arteries and ductal continuation to descending aorta. The ascending aorta emerges from common trunk as a side branch and is typically hypoplastic [24]. In aortic dominance, the common trunk resembles the ascending aorta continuing to have normal aortic arch. The pulmonary arteries originate from the left posterior aspect of the trunk [24]. This simplified approach helps in surgical risk stratification since the number one risk factor defining surgical mortality is the presence of hypoplastic or interrupted aortic arch [25]. For the cria of this report, a single pulmonary trunk arose from the common trunk before bifurcating into right and left pulmonary arteries prior to the aortic arch consistent with the type aortic predominance.

Clinical presentation of veterinary patients with CAT can be variable. As with this case, newborn patients can present with severe clinical signs shortly after birth while others may be asymptomatic or develop clinical signs later in life and go undetected for several years [8, 10]. In humans, CAT is usually detected early in infancy (or in utero), and early intervention can improve long-term survival [26]. Patients usually present with symptoms of congestive heart failure soon after birth and survival to adulthood is rare without correction [27–29]. Accurate echocardiographic diagnosis of CAT is challenging. Differential diagnosis based on echocardiographic findings included CAT, Tetralogy of Fallot, and severe pulmonic stenosis or pulmonary atresia with a VSD. In Tetralogy of Fallot, a large VSD with an overriding vessel is identified, but unlike CAT, a separate pulmonary artery is present. In pulmonary atresia there is an overriding aorta with atresia of the pulmonary artery which can appear very similar to a CAT on echocardiographic examination. Pulmonary circulation in pulmonary atresia can be supplied by a concurrent patent ductus arteriosus or bronchial arteries whereas in CAT, distinct pulmonary arteries arise from the trunk as previously described [4, 29]. As such, a diagnosis of CAT must identify a single arterial vessel giving rise to systemic, pulmonary, and coronary arteries. Cardiac catheterization and angiography or magnetic resonance imaging may be required to obtain an accurate antemortem diagnosis [2]. Contrast studies such as one performed in this case can provide additional information regarding the hemodynamics of the anomaly.

The classification of CAT and origin of the trunk are important factors when evaluating patients before corrective surgery. For example, patients with only one pulmonary artery often develop severe pulmonary vascular disease even with correction during the neonatal period [30]. In people, surgical correction involves separating the pulmonary arteries from the CAT and creating a connection to the right ventricle via a valved conduit and the CAT is then connected to the left ventricle and the VSD is closed [26]. Complete surgical repair early during infancy is preferred as progression of pulmonary vascular obstructive disease can increase mortality postoperatively [2]. In the last 30 years, the improvements in surgical techniques and postoperative management have contributed to a favorable prognosis in people after surgical repair of CAT with over 90% survival for one year postoperatively [26]. Without surgical repair, 80% of human patients do not live past one year of age [29]. Factors impacting long-term survival include age at diagnosis, conduit stenosis, truncal valve insufficiency, truncal valve stenosis, myocardial failure, pulmonary hypertension, and concurrent interrupted aortic arch [26]. The prognosis in veterinary patients is currently unknown as reported cases are lacking but is presumed to be poor. At this time surgical repair has not yet been described in the veterinary literature.

This case describes an unusual complex cardiac anomaly in a camelid species. The alpaca cria described in this report presented with severe clinical signs that were associated with right to left shunting of blood due to a type I CAT with PFO. The radiographic evaluation of the lung fields did not match the finding noted on necropsy. This may have been due to progression of the patient's condition to severe respiratory distress after the radiographs were taken. To the best of authors' knowledge, this is the first case report detailing the echocardiographic findings associated with CAT in an alpaca cria. Although uncommon, congenital cardiac defects should be considered in animals presenting with clinical signs of hypoxemia, dyspnea, or failure to thrive.

## Competing Interests

The authors declare that there is no conflict of interests regarding the publication of this paper.

## References

[1] M. L. Margiocco, B. A. Scansen, and J. D. Bonagura, "Camelid cardiology," *Veterinary Clinics of North America—Food Animal Practice*, vol. 25, no. 2, pp. 423–454, 2009.

[2] A. K. Cabalka, W. D. Edwards, and J. A. Dearani, "Truncus arteriosus," in *Moss and Adam's Heart Disease in Infants, Children and Adolescents*, H. D. Allen, D. J. Driscoll, R. E. Shaddy, and T. F. Feltes, Eds., pp. 911–922, Lippincott Williams & Wilkins, Philadelphia, Pa, USA, 7th edition, 2008.

[3] R. Van Praagh and S. Van Praagh, "The anatomy of common aorticopulmonary trunk (truncus arteriosus communis) and its embryologic implications. A study of 57 necropsy cases," *The American Journal of Cardiology*, vol. 16, no. 3, pp. 406–425, 1965.

[4] J. Deshpande, M. Desai, and S. Kinare, "Persistent truncus arteriosus—an autopsy study of 16 cases," *International Journal of Cardiology*, vol. 37, no. 3, pp. 395–399, 1992.

[5] F. Butto, R. V. Lucas Jr., and J. E. Edwards, "Persistent truncus arteriosus: pathologic anatomy in 54 cases," *Pediatric Cardiology*, vol. 7, no. 2, pp. 95–101, 1986.

[6] M. Godynicka and S. Godynicki, "A case of persistent arterial trunk in a guanaco llama," *Folia Morphologica*, vol. 2, pp. 212–215, 1971.

[7] C. D. Buergelt, P. F. Suter, and W. J. Kay, "Persistent truncus arteriosus in a cat," *Journal of the American Veterinary Medical Association*, vol. 153, pp. 548–552, 1968.

[8] A. P. Nicolle, D. Tessier-Vetzel, E. Begon, C. C. Sampedrano, J.-L. Pouchelon, and V. Chetboul, "Persistent truncus arteriosus in a 6-year-old cat," *Journal of Veterinary Medicine Series A: Physiology Pathology Clinical Medicine*, vol. 52, no. 7, pp. 350–353, 2005.

[9] T. Chuzel, I. Bublot, L. Couturier et al., "Persistent truncus arteriosus in a cat," *Journal of Veterinary Cardiology*, vol. 9, no. 1, pp. 43–46, 2007.

[10] F. Serres, V. Chetboul, C. C. Sampedrano, V. Gouni, and J.-L. Pouchelon, "Ante-mortem diagnosis of persistent truncus arteriosus in an 8-year-old asymptomatic dog," *Journal of Veterinary Cardiology*, vol. 11, no. 1, pp. 59–65, 2009.

[11] R. S. Downey and R. M. Liptrap, "An unusual congenital cardiac defect in a dog," *Canadian Veterinary Journal*, vol. 7, no. 10, pp. 233–238, 1966.

[12] E. Heath and J. P. Kukreti, "Persistent truncus arteriosus communis in a two-year-old steer," *Veterinary Record*, vol. 105, no. 23, pp. 527–530, 1979.

[13] D. J. Brandt, D. R. Canfield, P. E. Peterson, and A. G. Hendrickx, "Persistent truncus arteriosus in a rhesus monkey," *Comparative Medicine*, vol. 52, no. 3, pp. 269–272, 2002.

[14] J. E. Sojka, "Persistent truncus arteriosus in a foal," *Equine Practice*, vol. 9, pp. 19–26, 1987.

[15] J. A. Boon, A. P. Knight, and D. H. Moore, "Llama cardiology," *The Veterinary Clinics of North America. Food Animal Practice*, vol. 10, no. 2, pp. 353–370, 1994.

[16] M. L. Cebra, C. K. Cebra, F. B. Garry, J. A. Boon, and E. C. Orton, "Atrioventricular septal defects in three llamas (*Lama glama*)," *Journal of Zoo and Wildlife Medicine*, vol. 29, no. 2, pp. 225–227, 1998.

[17] J. Slack, I. Johns, A. Van Eps, and V. B. Reef, "Imaging diagnosis—tricuspid atresia in an alpaca," *Veterinary Radiology & Ultrasound*, vol. 49, no. 3, pp. 309–312, 2008.

[18] T. C. Kramer, "The partitioning of the truncus and conus and the formation of the membranous portion of the interventricular septum in the human heart," *American Journal of Anatomy*, vol. 71, no. 3, pp. 343–370, 1942.

[19] R. H. Anderson, S. Mori, D. E. Spicer, N. A. Brown, and T. J. Mohun, "Development and morphology of the ventricular outflow tracts," *World Journal for Pediatric and Congenital Heart Surgery*, vol. 7, no. 5, pp. 561–577, 2016.

[20] R. H. Anderson, B. Chaudhry, T. J. Mohun et al., "Normal and abnormal development of the intrapericardial arterial trunks in humans and mice," *Cardiovascular Research*, vol. 95, no. 1, pp. 108–115, 2012.

[21] M. J. B. van den Hoff, A. F. M. Moorman, J. M. Ruijter et al., "Myocardialization of the cardiac outflow tract," *Developmental Biology*, vol. 212, no. 2, pp. 477–490, 1999.

[22] L. H. S. Van Mierop, D. F. Patterson, and W. R. Schnarr, "Pathogenesis of persistent truncus arteriosus in light of observations made in a dog embryo with the anomaly," *The American Journal of Cardiology*, vol. 41, no. 4, pp. 755–762, 1978.

[23] R. W. Collett and J. E. Edwards, "Persistent truncus arteriosus: a classification according to anatomic types," *Surgical Clinics of North America*, vol. 29, no. 4, pp. 1245–1270, 1949.

[24] M. L. Jacobs, "Congenital Heart Surgery Nomenclature and Database Project: truncus arteriosus," *Annals of Thoracic Surgery*, vol. 69, no. 4, pp. S50–S55, 2000.

[25] H. M. Russell, J. L. Marshal, A. H. Robert et al., "A simplified categorization for common arterial trunk," *The Journal of Thoracic and Cardiovascular Surgery*, vol. 141, no. 3, pp. 645–653, 2011.

[26] L. D. Thompson, D. B. McElhinney, V. M. Reddy, E. Petrossian, N. H. Silverman, and F. L. Hanley, "Neonatal repair of truncus arteriosus: continuing improvement in outcomes," *Annals of Thoracic Surgery*, vol. 72, no. 2, pp. 391–395, 2001.

[27] V. Bodí, L. Insa, J. Sanchis, M. Ibáez, A. Losada, and F. J. Chorro, "Persistent truncus arteriosus type 4 with survival to the age of 54 years," *International Journal of Cardiology*, vol. 82, no. 1, pp. 75–77, 2002.

[28] G. Carvalho, A. A. Silva, R. B. Bestetti, and A. C. Leme-Neto, "Long-term survival in truncus arteriosus communis type A1 associated with Ehlers-Danlos syndrome—a case report," *Angiology*, vol. 53, no. 3, pp. 363–365, 2002.

[29] P. Hicken, D. Evans, and D. Heath, "Persistent truncus arteriosus with survival to the age of 38 years," *British Heart Journal*, vol. 28, no. 2, pp. 284–286, 1966.

[30] D. A. Fyfe, D. J. Driscoll, R. M. Di Donato et al., "Truncus arteriosus with single pulmonary artery: influence of pulmonary vascular obstructive disease on early and late operative results," *Journal of the American College of Cardiology*, vol. 5, no. 5, pp. 1168–1172, 1985.

# Permissions

# List of Contributors

**E. J. Ehrhart, G. Mason and T. Spraker**
CSU Veterinary Diagnostic Medicine Center, Fort Collins, CO, USA

**G. Krafsur**
CSU Veterinary Diagnostic Medicine Center, Fort Collins, CO, USA
North Slope Borough Department ofWildlife Management, Barrow, AK, USA

**J. Ramos-Vara**
Indiana Animal Disease Diagnostic Laboratory and Department of Comparative Pathobiology, Purdue University, West Lafayette, IN, USA

**F. Sarren, B. Adams and C. Hanns**
North Slope Borough Department ofWildlife Management, Barrow, AK, USA

**C. Duncan**
CSU Veterinary Diagnostic Medicine Center, Fort Collins, CO, USA
Colorado State University Veterinary Diagnostic Laboratory, 300West Drake Avenue, Fort Collins, CO 80526, USA

**Sonia E. Kuhn and Diane V. H. Hendrix**
Department of Small Animal Clinical Sciences, College of Veterinary Medicine, University of Tennessee, 2407 River Drive, Knoxville, TN 37996, USA

**J. Riggs and S. J. Langley-Hobbs**
The Queen's Veterinary School Hospital, Department of Veterinary Medicine, University of Cambridge, Madingley Road, Cambridge CB3 0ES, UK

**Keiichi Ueda, Hirokazu Miyahara and Senzo Uchida**
General Research Center, Okinawa Churaumi Aquarium, Aza Ishikawa 888, Motobu-Cho, Kunigami-Gun, Okinawa 905-0206, Japan

**Ayako Sano**
Department of Animal Sciences, Faculty of Agriculture, University of the Ryukyus, Sembaru 1, Nishihara-Cho, Nakagusuku-Gun, Okinawa 903-0213, Japan

**Jyoji Yamate, Mitsuru Kuwamura, Takeshi Izawa, Miyuu Tanaka and Yuko Hasegawa**
Laboratory of Veterinary Pathology, Division of Veterinary Sciences, Rinku-Campus, Osaka Prefecture University, Rinku Ohrai Kita 1-58, Izumisano, Osaka 598-8531, Japan

**Eiko Itano Nakagawa**
Department of Pathological Science, CCB, State University of Londrina, P.O. Box 6001, 86051-970 Londrina, PR, Brazil

**Hiroji Chibana**
Medical Mycology Research Center, Chiba University, Inohana 1-8-1, Chiba 260-8673, Japan

**Yasuharu Izumisawa**
Department of Veterinary Medicine, Rakuno Gakuen University, Bunkyodai Midorimachi 582, Ebetu, Hokkaido 069-0836, Japan

**Judit Viu, Lara Armengou, Carla Cesarini and Eduard Jose-Cunilleras**
Servei de Medicina Interna Equina, Departament de Medicina i Cirugia Animals, Facultat de Veterinària, Universitat Autònoma de Barcelona, Bellaterra, 08193 Barcelona, Spain

**Cristian de la Fuente and Sònia Añor**
Servei de Neurologia i Neurocirurgia, Departament de Medicina i Cirugia Animals, Facultat de Veterinària, Universitat Autònoma de Barcelona, Bellaterra, 08193 Barcelona, Spain

**Lora R. Ballweber**
Veterinary Diagnostic Laboratory, College of Veterinary Medicine and Biomedical Sciences, Colorado State University, Fort Collins, CO 80523-1644, USA

**Deanna Dailey**
Cell and Molecular Biology Graduate Program, College of Veterinary Medicine and Biomedical Sciences, Colorado State University, Fort Collins, CO 80523-1005, USA

**Gabriele Landolt**
Department of Clinical Sciences, College of Veterinary Medicine and Biomedical Sciences, Colorado State University, 300 West Drake Road, Fort Collins, CO 80523-1678, USA

**Claudia Cruz Villagrán, Nicholas Frank and James Schumacher**
Department of Large Animal Clinical Sciences, University of Tennessee College of Veterinary Medicine, 2407 River Drive, Knoxville, TN 37996, USA

**Danielle Reel**
Department of Biomedical and Diagnostic Sciences, University of Tennessee College of Veterinary Medicine, 2407 River Drive, Knoxville, TN 37996, USA

**Natalia Azevedo Philadelpho, Marta B. Guimarães and Antonio J. Piantino Ferreira**
Department of Pathology, School of Veterinary Medicine, University of São Paulo, Avenida Prof. Orlando Marques de Paiva 87, 05508-900 São Paulo, SP, Brazil

**Alexander E. Gallagher and Andrew J. Specht**
Department of Small Animal Clinical Sciences, College of Veterinary Medicine, University of Florida, Gainesville, FL 32608, USA

**S. Stephan and M. Hilbe**
Institute of Veterinary Pathology, Vetsuisse Faculty, University of Zurich, 8057 Zurich, Switzerland

**S. Hug**
Department of Equine Medicine, Vetsuisse Faculty, University of Zurich, 8057 Zurich, Switzerland

**Terry M. Jacobs, Bruce R. Hoppe and Cathy E. Poehlmann**
Park Pet Hospital, 7378 N. Teutonia Avenue, Milwaukee,WI 53209, USA

**Marie E. Pinkerton**
Department of Pathobiological Sciences, School of Veterinary Medicine, University ofWisconsin, 2015 Linden Drive, Madison, WI 53706, USA

**Milan Milovancev**
Wisconsin Veterinary Referral Center,Waukesha,WI 53188, USA
Department of Small Animal Surgery, College of Veterinary Medicine, Oregon State University, 267 Magruder Hall, Corvallis, OR 97331, USA

**Alberto Alberti and Gessica Tore**
Department of Veterinary Medicine, University of Sassari, Via Vienna 2, 07100 Sassari, Italy

**Alessandra Scagliarini, Laura Gallina and Federica Savini**
Department of Veterinary Medical Sciences, University of Bologna, Via Zamboni 33, 40126 Bologna, Italy

**Chiara Caporali**
Private Practitioner, Via Giovanni da Verrazzano 19, 52100 Arezzo, Italy

**Francesca Abramo**
Department of Veterinary Sciences, University of Pisa, Viale delle Piagge 2, 56124 Pisa, Italy

**Carl Adagra**
Tropical Queensland Cat Clinic, Townsville City, QLD 4810, Australia

**Susan Amanda Piripi**
University of Sydney, Sydney, NSW2006, Australia

**M. Argano and C. Adami**
Anesthesiology and PainTherapy Division, Department of Veterinary Clinical Science, Vetsuisse Faculty, University of Berne, Switzerland

**K. Gendron**
Radiology Division, Department of Veterinary Clinical Science, Vetsuisse Faculty, University of Berne, Switzerland

**U. Rytz**
Surgery Division, Department of Veterinary Clinical Science, Vetsuisse Faculty, University of Berne, Switzerland

**Gustavo L. G. Almeida**
Department of Internal Medicine, Faculty of Medicine, Gama Filho University, 20740-900 Rio de Janeiro, RJ, Brazil
Cardiology Division, Centro Veterinário Colina, Rua Colina 60 Lj-09, Ilha do Governador, 21931-380 Rio de Janeiro, RJ, Brazil

**Marcelo B. Almeida, Ana Carolina M. Santos and Ângela V. Mattos**
Cardiology Division, Centro Veterinário Colina, Rua Colina 60 Lj-09, Ilha do Governador, 21931-380 Rio de Janeiro, RJ, Brazil

**Ludmila S. C. Oliveira**
Clinical Division, Pet-Gávea, Marquês de São Vicente 07, Gávea, 22451-041 Rio de Janeiro, RJ, Brazil

**Rômulo C. Braga**
Radiology Department, CRV Imagem, Avenida das Américas 595, Barra da Tijuca, 22631-000 Rio de Janeiro, RJ, Brazil

**Katherine Baine**
Department of Small Animal Clinical Sciences, College of Veterinary Medicine, University of Tennessee, 2407 River Drive, Knoxville, TN 37996, USA

**Kim Newkirk, Kellie A. Fecteau and Marcy J. Souza**
Department of Biomedical and Diagnostic Sciences, College of Veterinary Medicine, University of Tennessee, 2407 River Drive, Knoxville, TN 37996, USA

**Alexandre Le Roux, Nathalie Rademacher and Lorrie Gaschen**
Department of Veterinary Clinical Sciences, Section of Diagnostic Imaging, School of Veterinary Medicine, Louisiana State University, Skip Bertman Drive, Baton Rouge, LA 70803, USA

**Sanjeev Gumber and Rudy W. Bauer**
Department of Pathobiological Sciences, School of Veterinary Medicine, Louisiana State University, Baton Rouge, LA 70803, USA

**Emiko Van Wie**
Texas A&M University College of Veterinary Medicine, 422 Raymond Stotzer Parkway, College Station, TX 77843, USA

**Annie V. Chen, Stephanie A. Thomovsky and Russell L. Tucker**
Washington State University College of Veterinary Medicine, P.O. Box 647010, Pullman, WA 99164, USA

**Karen A. McCormick**
Large Animal Clinical Sciences, University of Tennessee, College of Veterinary Medicine, 2407 River Drive, Knoxville, TN 37996, USA

**Daniel Ward**
Small Animal Clinical Sciences, University of Tennessee, College of Veterinary Medicine, 2407 River Drive, Knoxville, TN 37996, USA

**Kimberly M. Newkirk**
Diagnostic and Biomedical Sciences, University of Tennessee, College of Veterinary Medicine, 2407 River Drive, Knoxville, TN 37996, USA

**Joseph Smith**
William R. Pritchard Veterinary Medical Teaching Hospital, University of California Davis, Davis, CA 95616, USA

**David Kovalik**
Union Veterinary Clinic, 609 2nd Street NE, Washington, DC 20002, USA

**Anita Varga**
Department of Medicine and Epidemiology, School of Veterinary Medicine, University of California, Davis, TupperHall, Davis, CA 95616, USA

**Suresh Gonde, L. D. Singla and B. K. Bansal**
College of Veterinary Science, Guru Angad Dev Veterinary and Animal Sciences University, Ludhiana, Punjab 141004, India

**Sushma Chhabra**
Department of Veterinary Medicine, College of Veterinary Science, Guru Angad Dev Veterinary and Animal Sciences University, Ludhiana, Punjab 141004, India

**Daniel D. Lewis and Matthew D. Winter**
Department of Small Animal Clinical Sciences, College of Veterinary Medicine, University of Florida, Gainesville, FL 32610, USA

**Stephen C. Jones**
Department of Small Animal Clinical Sciences, College of Veterinary Medicine, University of Florida, Gainesville, FL 32610, USA
Department of Veterinary Clinical Sciences, College of Veterinary Medicine, The Ohio State University, 601 Vernon L. Tharp Street, Columbus, OH 43210, USA

**Mario Ricciardi, Antonio De Simone, Pasquale Giannuzzi and Floriana Gernone**
"Pingry" Veterinary Hospital, Via Medaglie d'Oro 5, 70126 Bari, Italy

**Maria Teresa Mandara and Alice Reginato**
Department of Biopathological Science and Hygiene of Food and Animal Productions, Faculty of Veterinary Medicine, University of Perugia, 06126 Perugia, Italy

**C. Bosco, E. Díaz, J. González and R. Gutierrez**
Placenta and Fetal Development Laboratory, Anatomy and Developmental Biology Programme, Institute of Biomedical Sciences, Faculty of Medicine, University of Chile, Independencia 1027, Casilla Postal 70079, 8380453 Santiago, Chile

**Giovanna Bertolini**
San Marco Veterinary Clinic, Diagnostic Imaging Division, Via Sorio 114/c, 35141 Padova, Italy

**Maria C. Fugazzola, Christoph Klaus and Christoph Lischer**
The Department of Veterinary Clinical Sciences, Unit of Equine Medicine and Surgery, University of Teramo (Fugazzola); V.le Crispi-Loc. Cartecchio, 64100 Teramo and Klinik für Pferde, Free University of Berlin (Klaus and Lischer) Oertzenweg 19b, 14163 Berlin, Germany

**Matías Nicolás Tellado**
Facultad de Ciencias Veterinarias, Universidad de Buenos Aires, Avenida Chorroarín 280, C1427CWO Ciudad de Buenos Aires, Argentina

**Sebastián Diego Michinski**
Instituto Tecnológico de Buenos Aires, Avenida Eduardo Madero 399, C1106ACD Ciudad de Buenos Aires, Argentina

Laboratorio de Sistemas Complejos, Facultad de Ciencias Exactas y Naturales, Universidad de Buenos Aires, Intendente Guiraldes 2160, Pabellon I, C1428EGA Ciudad de Buenos Aires, Argentina

**Nahuel Olaiz, Felipe Maglietti and Guillermo Marshall**
Laboratorio de Sistemas Complejos, Facultad de Ciencias Exactas y Naturales, Universidad de Buenos Aires, Intendente Guiraldes 2160, Pabellon I, C1428EGA Ciudad de Buenos Aires, Argentina

**Davoud Kazemi and Gholamreza Assadnassab**
Department of Veterinary Clinical Sciences, Faculty of Veterinary Medicine, Tabriz Branch, Islamic Azad University, Tabriz, Iran

**Yousef Doustar**
Department of Veterinary Pathobiology, Faculty of Veterinary Medicine, Tabriz Branch, Islamic Azad University, Tabriz, Iran

**B. Sudhakara Reddy**
Teaching Veterinary Clinical Complex (Veterinary Medicine), College of Veterinary Science, Sri Venkateswara Veterinary University, Proddatur, Andhra Pradesh 516360, India

**K. Nalini Kumari**
Department of Veterinary Medicine, College of Veterinary Science, Sri Venkateswara Veterinary University, Tirupati, Andhra Pradesh 517502, India

**S. Sivajothi**
Department of Veterinary Parasitology, College of Veterinary Science, Sri Venkateswara Veterinary University, Proddatur, Andhra Pradesh 516360, India

**R. Venkatasivakumar**
Department of Veterinary Medicine, College of Veterinary Science, Sri Venkateswara Veterinary University, Proddatur, Andhra Pradesh 516360, India

**Giovanni Barsotti and Veronica Marchetti**
Department of Veterinary Clinics, Faculty of Veterinary Medicine, University of Pisa, Via Livornese Lato Monte, San Piero a Grado, 56122 Pisa, Italy

**Lorenzo Ressel and Francesca Millanta**
Department of Animal Pathology, Faculty of Veterinary Medicine, University of Pisa, Delle Piagge 2 Avenue, 56100 Pisa, Italy

**Riccardo Finotello**
Small Animal Teaching Hospital, University of Liverpool, Leahurst, Liverpool, Leahurst Campus Chester High Road, Neston, Wirral CH64 7TE, UK

**O. Balland**
Centre Hospitalier Vétérinaire, 95 rue des Mazurots, 54710 Ludres, France

**I. Raymond**
Department of Clinical Sciences, National Veterinary School, 23 chemin des Capelles, BP 87614, 31076 Toulouse Cedex 3, France

**I. Mathieson**
Eyevet Referrals, 41-43 Halton Station Road, SuttonWeaver, CheshireWA7 3DN, UK

**P. F. Isard, Emilie Vidémont-Drevon and T. Dulaurent**
Centre Hospitalier Vétérinaire, 275 route Impériale, 74370 Saint-Martin Bellevue, France

**Brianne E. Phillips, Sarah A. Cannizzo and Craig A. Harms**
Department of Clinical Sciences, College of Veterinary Medicine, North Carolina State University, 1060William Moore Drive, Raleigh, NC 27607, USA
Center for Marine Sciences and Technology, North Carolina State University, 303 College Circle, Morehead City, NC 28557, USA

**Matthew H. Godfrey**
Department of Clinical Sciences, College of Veterinary Medicine, North Carolina State University, 1060William Moore Drive, Raleigh, NC 27607, USA
3North CarolinaWildlife Resources Commission, 1507 Ann Street, Beaufort, NC 28516, USA

**Brian A. Stacy**
National Marine Fisheries Service, National Oceanic and Atmospheric Administration, University of Florida, 2187 Mowry Road, P.O. Box 110885, Gainesville, FL 32611, USA

**F. Faria**
Department of Immuno-Physiology and Farmacology (AR), Department of Veterinary Clinics (TG) and Department of Pathology and Molecular Immunology (FF, IA and FG) of the Institute of Biomedical Sciences Abel Salazar (ICBAS), University of Porto, Campus Agrário de Vairão, Rua Jorge Viterbo Ferreira no. 228, 4050-313 Porto, Portugal

**A. Rocha and T. Guimarães**
Department of Immuno-Physiology and Farmacology (AR), Department of Veterinary Clinics (TG) and Department of Pathology and Molecular Immunology (FF, IA and FG) of the Institute of Biomedical Sciences Abel Salazar (ICBAS), University of Porto, Campus Agrário de Vairão, Rua Jorge Viterbo Ferreira no. 228,

4050-313 Porto, Portugal
Center for the Study of Animal Sciences (CECA), ICETA, University of Porto, Campus Agrário de Vairão, Rua Padre Armando Quintas 7, 4485-661 Vairão, Portugal

**J. C. Duarte and C. Cosinha**
LusoPecus, Rua da Fábrica-Azinhaga do Catalão, Loja 2-A-Porto Alto, 2135-000 Samora Correia, Portugal

**V. T. A. Lopes**
EVP Lda, Rua Luís Derouet 27, Esquerdo 1, 1250-151 Lisbon, Portugal

**I. Amorim and F. Gärtner**
Institute of Molecular Pathology and Immunology of the University of Porto (IPATIMUP), Rua Dr. Roberto Frias s/n, 4200-465 Porto, Portugal

**Aina Adeogun**
Department of Zoology, University of Ibadan, Ibadan 200005, Nigeria

**Olutayo Omobowale**
Department of Veterinary Medicine, University of Ibadan, Ibadan 200005, Nigeria

**Chiaka Owuamanam**
Zoological Garden, University of Ibadan, Ibadan 200005, Nigeria

**Olugbenga Alaka and Victor Taiwo**
Department of Veterinary Pathology, University of Ibadan, Ibadan 200005, Nigeria

**Dick van Soolingen**
Department of Pulmonary Diseases and Department of Clinical Microbiology, Radboud University, Nijmegen Medical Centre, Nijmegen, Netherlands
Diagnostic Laboratory for Bacteriology and Parasitology (BPD), Center for Infectious Disease Research, Diagnostics and Perinatal Screening (IDS), National Institute for Public Health and the Environment (RIVM), P.O. Box 1, 3720 BA Bilthoven, Netherlands

**Simeon Cadmus**
Tuberculosis and Brucellosis Research Laboratories, Department of Veterinary Public Health & Preventive Medicine, University of Ibadan, Ibadan 200005, Nigeria

**Sergio A. Zanzani, Luigi Cozzi, Alessia L. Gazzonis and Maria Teresa Manfredi**
Dipartimento di Medicina Veterinaria, Universit`a degli Studi di Milano, Via Celoria 10, 20133 Milano, Italy

**Emanuela Olivieri**
Dipartimento di Medicina Veterinaria, Universit`a degli Studi di Perugia, Via S. Costanzo 4, 06126 Perugia, Italy

**M. Gallego**
Centro Veterinario Madrid Exóticos, Calle Meléndez Valdés 17, 28015 Madrid, Spain

**L. Avedillo**
Centro Veterinario Salud Animal, Calle de la Iglesia 10, Griñón, 28971 Madrid, Spain

**Sonja K. Heinrich and Bettina Wachter**
Leibniz Institute for Zoo andWildlife Research, Department Evolutionary Ecology, Alfred-Kowalke-Strasse 17, 10315 Berlin, Germany

**Gudrun Wibbelt**
Leibniz Institute for Zoo and Wildlife Research, DepartmentWildlife Diseases, Alfred-Kowalke-Strasse 17, 10315 Berlin, Germany

**Tsumugi Anne Kurosawa**
Royal Veterinary College, Clinical Science and Services, Royal Veterinary College, Hawkshead Ln, Hatfield AL9 7TA, UK

**Tamilselvam Gunasekaran**
BluePearl Veterinary Partners, 4126 Packard Road, Ann Arbor, MI 48187, USA

**Robert Sanders**
Veterinary Medical Center, Small Animal Clinical Sciences, College of Veterinary Medicine, Michigan State University, 736Wilson Road, East Lansing, MI 48187, USA

**Elizabeth Carr**
Veterinary Medical Center, Large Animal Clinical Sciences, College of Veterinary Medicine, Michigan State University, 736Wilson Road, East Lansing, MI, USA

# Index